Current Opinions
on
Shanghan Lun

Dr. Martin Wang
MD. PhD. R.Acupuncturist

Dedicated to those:

who have developed and funded Chinese medicine;
who have practiced and continue to practice Chinese medicine; and
who are going to learn Chinese medicine and serve his or her people using it.

Contents

Preface

Background

Herbal therapy is one of the essential parts of Traditional Chinese Medicine (TCM). There are several major herbal therapy systems. The most important system among them is the Classical herbal formula system (经方). This system is described in the book *Shanghan Zabing Lun* (伤寒杂病论) by Dr. Zhang Zhongjing from the later Han dynasty of China. The book was later separated into two parts, the *Shanghan Lun* (伤寒论) and *Jin Kui Yao Luo* (金匮要略). The former talks about the diagnosis of exogenous diseases, and the latter about that of miscellaneous diseases. In *Shanghan Lun*, Dr. Zhang Zhongjing proposed the Six Disease diagnosis system, which is also called the Six Jing diagnosis, or Six Syndrome diagnosis. In my understanding, if this diagnosis system is used for an exogenous disease, it might be better called Six Stage Diagnosis system, and if it is used for miscellaneous diseases, it is better called Six Disease Diagnosis system.

There are different opinions about how to understand the naming of the diagnosis system. The main idea in *Shanghan Zabing Lun* is believed to be developed from other earlier books such as *Yi Yin Tang Ye* (伊尹汤液, 汤液经法) and *Fu Xing Jue* (辅行诀), not from the book *Huangdi Nei Jing* (黄帝内经), although there are also different opinions about this.

The *Shanghan Lun* system requires the diagnosis of the stages (disease) of the Shanghan disease first. The six stages are Taiyang, Shaoyang, Yangming, Taiyin, Shaoyin, and Jueyin.[1] Then, a secondary diagnosis searches for indications of which herbal formula should be used for treatment. This is called the Indication differentiation diagnosis. Once the diagnosis of the (herbal) formula indication is established up, the herbal formula needed for the treatment of that clinic condition[2] is known. For example, if the clinical condition is diagnosed as Guizhi Tang condition, it means that the disease condition needs to be treated with the herbal formula Guizhi Tang.

After the secondary diagnosis, the doctor will know the name of the herbal formula required. The function of each herb in a formula for treatment is based on the book *Shennong Bencao Jing* (神农本草经). The herbal formulas introduced in *Shanghan Zabing Lun* are called Classical formulas, or "Jing Fang" (经方).[3]

In a survey, most current famous TCM doctors believe that the essential TCM books are *Shanghan Lun* and *Huangdi Nei Jing*, but not many TCM doctors predominantly practice the *Shanghan Lun* style (the Classical herbal formula system). It is commonly agreed that this TCM system is not easy to learn (though it is easy to practice).

The possible reasons for learning difficulties are:

---

[1] In this book, we transliterally translate the Chinese name of the six stages as Taiyang, Yangming, Shaoyang, Taiyin, Shaoyin and Jueyin stages. The reason is that the meanings of the stage names in *Shanghan Lun* are not the same as explained in book *Huangdi Nei Jing*. For example, In *Huangdi Nei Jing*, the same Chinese terminology of "Taiyang" is translated as "Great Yang", meaning that the intensity of the body Yang Qi is the strongest in the Taiyang meridian. However, this may not be the case in the Taiyang stage in *Shanghan Lun*. In the Taiyang stage of the Shanghan disease, the severity of the disease is not the strongest. The strongest intensity of the disease is in the Yangming stage, not in the Taiyang stage. It can be understood that, the meanings of the Taiyang, Yangming, Shaoyang... in *Shanghan Lun* are different from those in *Huangdi Nei Jing*, though the Chinese characters are the same in the two books.

[2] *Clinic condition*: It means clinic situation, clinic status, disease manifestations, or disease appearance, which include symptoms and body signs (information collected from patient's pulse, tongue, skin color, etc.).

[3] The herbal formulas that are not from this book are called Conventional formulas. For the diagnosis, it uses the Organ-meridian theory introduced in *Huangdi Nei Jing*, with the aim of finding out the location, current status and nature of the disease in the body. Such a methodology is also called the Eight Gang diagnosis system (or Eight Principle diagnosis system, TCM-concept oriented syndrome diagnosis system).

The *Shanghan Zabing Lun* mostly introduces the clinical manifestations of disease, the diagnosis, and the treatment. It does not give reasons for the diagnosis and treatment, nor does it tell the function of each herb. The result is that different doctors interpret the book in different ways, such as from the point of view seen in *Huangdi Nei Jing*, or from the Five-element Organ relationship, and so on. Such explanations do not seem so convincing.

The *Shanghan Za Bing Lun* was written in very early times. It was initially handwritten on pieces of bamboo strips, which were linked with thin ropes made of hemp (or some other material). After storage for many years, the rope became corrupted, and the strips lost their order.

In the early years, the book was hand copied by different people again and again; there could have been mistakes made during this course. When later doctors re-edited the book, they could have inserted their own opinions or notes, mixing their words with the original ones.

Due to the reasons above, there are many versions of this book. It is still difficult to tell which version should be regarded as the most "correct" version. If a version varies, the understanding to the contents would, of course, be different among different doctors.

The structure of the most herbal formulas in this book appears very strict. To change one herb ingredient, or change the dosage of one or more herb ingredients, could change the treatment target dramatically. Without close attention to this, the healing effect could be entirely different and elicit conflicting comments.

Due to the reasons above and others, there have been more than one thousand doctors who have tried to study the book and gave their ideas and opinions. Even the chief editors of the TCM textbook about this book have different ideas.[1] My own experience is that, if we follow an expert's lectures or books, we could feel that they sound reasonable and correct. However, if we attend more lectures or read more books from other experts, we could find differences amongst the experts. We might find that we feel more comfortable with one expert's style of explanation about *Shanghan Lun* and that arguments by others feel cloudy.

My book here is a collection and summary of opinions from different doctors and modern experts. I believe that when the modern doctor studies and practices Classical herbal formulas, they are also learning from the experience and ideas of doctors who came before. When we learn from more recent doctors, it means that we, as students, stand upon their shoulders and that they likewise stand on the shoulders of previous doctors.

There are many modern experts[4] in Shanghan study, such as Dr. Hu Xishu (胡希恕)[2], Liu Duzhou (刘渡舟)[3], Hao Wanshan (郝万山)[4], Ni Haixia (倪海厦)[5], Tan Jiezhong (谭杰中)[6], Li Keshao (李克绍)[7], Di Lengxian (翟冷仙)[8], Xu Chenghe (徐成贺)[9], Gui Liang (桂亮)[10], Cai Changfu (蔡长福)[11], Xiao Xiangru (肖相如)[12], Liao Houze (廖厚泽)[13], Lao Zhuang (老庄)[14], and Huang Huang (黄煌)[15]. In the supplementary reading materials of this book, the opinions of more doctors are included.

Experts in modern times can be roughly separated into three groups:

There is the textbook group. Doctors in this group tend to understand *Shanghan Lun* from *Huangdi Nei Jing* (黄帝内经) and *Bencao Gangmu* (本草纲目). Doctors in this group include Dr. Liu Duzhou (刘渡舟), Dr. Hao Wanshan (郝万山) and many more.

Experts in the second group tend to explain *Shanghan Lun* using *Tang Ye Jing Fa* (汤液经法), *Fu Xing Jue* (辅行决) and the book *Shengnong Ben Cao Jing* (神农本草经). Doctors in this group include Dr. Hu Xishu (胡希恕), Dr. Feng Shilun (冯世纶) and others.

The experts in the third group are mostly from Taiwan. They include Dr. Ni Haixia (倪海厦) and Mr. Tang Jiezhong (谭杰中). Both of them also understand the *Shanghan Lun* from the *Huangdi Nei Jing* and *Five-element theory* perspective, but their lectures are particularly interesting, lively and vivid.

---

[4] Dr.Du Yumao: it has been summarized that, since 1986, there are as many as 541 books that explain and discuss the book *Shanghan Lun*.

They explain body physiology and pathology in a very different, but very easily understandable, way. It is enjoyable to listen to their lectures. Many TCM concepts in their minds seem beyond those that we, TCM doctors from mainland China, are familiar.

This book focuses on the discussion of Six-stage (Six-disease) diagnosis and does not deal with the structure and function of each formula. Such contents will be introduced exclusively in another book of us, *Jingfan Today*.

During the editing of this book, I have tried not to include my own opinion, unless I feel that I have to. This is because I feel that I am not in line the experts shown. This book has reorganized some paragraphs of the original *Shanghan Lun*, with the aim of making the separation of the six diseases more explicit. It is hard to tell if such re-organization is correct or not. Such reorganization has been tried by previous doctors too. This way of reorganization only reflects my understanding and works as a reference only.

Translation

The *Shanghan Lun* was written originally in ancient Chinese and without comma or period in between setense. In some versions of the book, there are always periods between the sentences. It is hard to tell the exact place to start or to stop a sentence. Such a way of writing caused some difficulty in understanding the meaning of the words. I have tried to translate the original texts as it is, without vigorous efforts to "guess" the start or the stop of a sentence. This is to prevent any possible "distortion" of the real meaning of the original texts. Different ways of understanding the grammar of the original texts may result in a different understanding of the meaning of the original texts.

There are many different versions of *Shanghan Lun*. Our book here is based on the commonly used Song version and refers to some parts of the Kangping version too.

It is not easy to understand *Shanghan Lun*, and it is further complicated to translate the Chinese version into an English version. Even for a Chinese-speaking TCM doctor, the understanding of the original text of *Shanghan Lun*, and the understanding of the function of an herbal formula and of an herb in that formula could be different each time it is reviewed. Dr. Zhang Butao (张步桃) said that he had read the book more than 3000 times.[16] Each time he reads it, he gains a different understanding. After my book here, the reader needs to read additional books about *Shanghan Lun*. If the understanding of the original text is different, the English words chosen for translation will also be different.

In the translation of TCM literature, sometimes there are no exact words in English to describe the meaning of the Chinese. One of the ways to prevent misunderstanding of Chinese TCM concepts is to use a capital letter for the first letter of a word. For example, "Liver" is a TCM concept. It includes the anatomic organ, the liver, but also includes both the Liver meridian and the emotion. "Kidney" includes the anatomic organ kidney, but also means the urinary system, the reproductive system, the bone, the bone marrow, the memory, the libido, the Kidney meridian, and so on.

The TCM terminology glossaries in the book here are mostly referred from various current sources, such as WHO TCM terminology glossary,[17] Wiki TCM terminology,[18] Nigel Wiseman (2000),[19] as well as English-Chinese, Chinese-English Professional dictionary (专业英汉汉英词典),[20] as long as there are proper terms that can be chosen from these sources.

This book here is a professional TCM book. Readers should have had education in the basic concepts of Chinese herbal therapy before.

It is my wish that this book helps English-speaking TCM doctors understand more about the Shanghan style of herbal therapy and improves their clinical work efficiency and that they can enjoy further success in their clinic work.

Financial consideration

The selling of this book is to cover the cost for edits (English language correction), prints, and publications, not for my own private profit. Because almost all the information in this book can be collected online for free by everyone, it is understood that my work here is pretty much a reprint (转载) of this online information (from Chinese to English), and such reprint should be allowed, as long as the sources of the information has been indicated (see reference list), and there is no indication in the online sources that such reprint is not allowed. I am happy to contribute voluntarily my own time and effort to introduce Chinese herbal therapy to whoever wishes to learn Chinese medicine.

Many times it is difficult to find the name(s) of the original authors or to contact the authors. If readers find that some information is cited and reprinted but the source is not listed, or if the reader is the original author and does not want the information reprinted, please contact me via e-mail (wenqiw57@hotmail.com). I will correct the mistake as soon as possible.

Note to Readers

The information in this book has been collected, cited and compiled from various sources. The contribution of the author is the English translation only. The book is intended to provide helpful and informative materials on the topics addressed in the publication. It is being sold with the understanding that the author is not engaged in rendering medical, health, or any other kind of personal or professional services in the book. The reader should consult his or her doctor or other competent health professionals before adopting any of the suggestions in this book or drawing inferences from it. The author expressly disclaims all responsibility for any liability, loss, or risk, personal or otherwise, that is incurred as a consequence, directly or indirectly, of the use and application of any of the contents of this book.

Declaration

This publication contains the opinions and ideas of the author. It is intended to provide helpful and informative materials on the subjects addressed in the publication. It is sold with the understanding that the author and publisher are not engaged in rendering medical or any other kind of personal, professional service in the book. The reader should consult his or her medical doctor or other competent professional before adopting any of the suggestions in this book or drawing inferences from it. The author and publisher expressly disclaim all responsibility for any liability, loss, or risk (personal or otherwise) that is incurred as a consequence, directly or indirectly, by the use and application of any of this book's contents.

Basic concept

It has been agreed that *Shanghan Lun* (伤寒论)[5] is the first principle, a bible-like book about effective Chinese herbal therapy ever written. It was written by Dr. Zhang Zhongjing more than 2000 years ago. Here the *Shang* means to "be attacked"; *Han* means "Cold". *Lun* means "special talk and focused discussion about something". So *Shanghan Lun* means discussion about the treatment of diseases that are caused by the attack of Cold.

Classification of diseases

In Chinese medicine, fever diseases are separated into two major classes: Shanghan diseases and epidemic febrile disease.[6]

Shanghan disease is a broad concept. It is furthermore separated into Cold-attack diseases, Wind-attack diseases, Dampness-Warm diseases, Fever diseases, and Warm diseases.

Cold-attack diseases (伤寒, Shanghan): a group of diseases that are caused by an attack of Cold;

Wind-attack diseases (中风, Zhongfeng):[7] a group of diseases that are caused by an attack of Wind;

Dampness-Warm diseases (湿温, Shiwen): a group of diseases that are caused by an attack of Dampness and Hotness.

Fever diseases (热病, Re Bing): a group of diseases that are characterized by high fever, which are caused by the attack of Fire.

Warm diseases (温病, Wen Bing): a group of diseases that are caused by the attack of Hotness.

The book *Shanghan Lun* mostly talks about the diagnosis and treatment of the Cold-attack and Wind-attack diseases using Chinese herbs, though the other types of diseases can also be diagnosed and treated with the ways introduced in *Shanghan Lun*.

Terminology

Pathogenic Qi: *Pathogenic Qi* (e.g. 邪气, Evil Qi) [8] means external factors/agents that can attack the body to cause disease. It can be a Cold, Wind, Hotness, Dampness, Dryness, and Fire or more.

Health-maintaining Qi: *Health-maintaining Qi* (正气, Health Qi) [9] in most case refers to the body's defense system, self-healing ability, constructive, and nutritional essence. It is the opposite concept of pathogenic Qi.

A disease condition is the results of the mutual reaction between the strength of the pathogenic Qi and the Health-maintaining Qi. If the Health-maintaining Qi is strong enough, the pathogenic Qi cannot cause disease or can only cause less severe disease conditions.

TCM always considers the status of the Health-maintaining Qi during treatment. When using a therapy to deplete the pathogenic Qi, the doctor always needs to protect the Health-maintaining Qi so that it is not hurt at the same time. Sometimes the Health-maintaining Qi also includes the body's digestive function, because the normal function of the digestive system is the prophase condition for the body to have a substantial strength of defense function. Normal digestion functions supply strength to the defense system. For example, in the treatment of cancer, if the patient can still eat, we say that there is still a chance to save the life of the patient with proper treatment. If a cancer patient

---

[5] In WHO TCM glossary (hereafter refers to WHO), the book "伤寒论" is translated into Shanghanlun. Similarly, the book "伤寒杂病论" is translated into Shanghanzabinglun. According to such translation principle for book names, the 医学衷从中参西录 should be translated into Yixuezhonzhongcanxilu. This is ridiculous. For such a long name, it is hard even for a Chinese to quickly identify what this book is.

[6] The epidemic febrile diseases are a group of diseases that include large-scale epidemical diseases, such as plague, cholera, smallpox, black fever, etc. In this group of diseases, every patient, no matter if the body is healthy or sick before being attacked by pathogenic Qi this time, or if they are children, adult or elderly, the symptoms are pretty much the same. On the contrary, Shanghan diseases (broad concept) can be variable among patients when attacked by pathogenic Qi.

[7] The *Cold-attack*, and the *Wind-attack* here are sometimes translated as "Cold-damage" and "Wind-damage", respectively by others.

[8] The Chinese word 邪气 was translated as the "evil energy" in some books.

[9] The Chiese word 正气 was translated as "Healthy Qi", "Right Qi", "Proper Qi", "Upright Qi", or "Body resistance", in some books.

has no desire to eat and cannot digest food, there will be no chance to save his or her life.

The word *condition* (证) following the name of an herb or an herbal formula means a group of symptoms and body signs (such as pulse, tongue, stomach touch, and so on.), which indicate the use of that herb or herbal formula for treatment. It means that to use that herb or herbal formula will have a high chance of success (方证). For example, Guizhi Tang condition means a body condition that can be treated with Guizhi Tang with high success. Chaihu condition means a body condition that can be treated with herbal formulas containing the herb Chaihu.

The *Formula Indication Differentiation diagnosis* (方证辩证) is to identify the indications (evidence) for the use of a given herbal formula for treatment, from a group of symptoms and signs in the body. A disease condition may manifest many symptoms and body signs, which may indicate the use of one or more herbal formulas. For example, the body condition may indicate the use of Guizhi Tang alone or that of Guizhi Tang and Xiao Chaihu Tang together. In former, the body condition is Guizhi Tang condition, and in the latter, it is the Guizhi Tang condition plus Xiao Chaihu Tang condition. To identify the formula conditions (evidence) from various symptoms and body signs is to perform the Formula Indication Differentiation diagnosis. [10]

The word *disease condition* (疾病现状) means the disease's manifestations or disease's status (symptoms plus body signs).

The word *Fire* (火) or Excessive Fire (实火) refers to a fever condition of the body. High body temperature is caused by the invasion of a virus or bacteria or other pathogenic agents, and the body defense system is strong. It can mostly be seen in acute infectious disease or an acute inflammation condition, such as a fever in acute pneumonia.

The word *Deficient Fire* (虚火) also refers to a fever condition of the body. The patient feels hot, with or without a body temperature increase. The hot feeling is mostly due to a disorder of the metabolism or hormone disorder, such as in hyperthyroidism, or in menopause. It can also occur in later stages of a Fire disease when the body condition is very weak.

The word *Excess condition* (实证) refers to a body condition, in which a patient feels pain, fullness, bloating or hardness in some part of the body. Such body condition is caused by the presence of a solid mass/knob/bind in the body. For example, an Excess condition in the Yangming stage means that the digestive duct is blocked by some concrete thing such as phlegm, garbage water, garbage food, firm stool, a worm, a blood clot, and so on.

The word *deficient condition* (虚证) refers to a body condition in which patient can also feel pain, fullness, bloating or hardness, but there is no concrete or solid mass/knob/bind to cause that feeling. For example, a deficient bloating feeling in the abdomen means that the patient feels bloating in the abdomen region, but there isn't a solid mass inside the abdomen, such as phlegm, retained water, detained food, hardness stool, blood clot, purulent mass or worm to cause the bloating feeling.

Coldness condition (寒证): With the Coldness condition in the body, the patient feels cold, chilly, tired, abdominal pain, cold hands and feet, and can't sweat. The patient has a desire to

---

[10] The word "方证辩证" (Formula Indication differentiation diagnosis) has been recommended (personal communications) into *Formula syndrome diagnosis*. This might not be a proper translation. Syndrome means a group of symptoms and body signs. Traditionally, the symptoms and body signs for a given syndrome is standardized and fixed. However in the indications for the use of one herbal formula could be more than one syndrome. There are many different groups of clinic conditions can indicate the use of Guizhi Tang, or Xiao Chaihu Tang. It is said in *Shanghan Lun* that, with one of the symptoms or body signs, the Xiao Chaihu Tang can be used, such as bitter taste in mouth, dryness in throat, dizziness or blurring in vision, pain under the flank region, alternating hot-cold feeling, annoyance and has profuse nausea. Here means: if such symptoms or body signs is identified from various other symptoms or body signs, the Xiao Chaihu Tang can be used. The word *syndrome* can not well describe such multiple conditions

indicating the use of the Xiao Chaihu Tang. This term has also been recommended to translate as formula presentations diagnosis or formula evidence diagnosis. The latter might be relatively better.

drink warm water. If there is diarrhea, there is undigested food, or even pure water, in the stool. There is no stool retention feeling inside the anus (Tenesmus). The urine is clear as water. Urination takes a long time. The face looks pale. The tongue is pale. The pulse feels weak or slow. With a warm environment or a warm drink, the patient can feel better.

Hotness condition (热证): Patient feels hot, sweaty, anxious, annoyed or vexed, dry mouth or throat, thirsty. Patient has a desire to drink cold water and a large volume of cold water. If there is diarrhea, the stool has a terrible odor, and there is tenesmus. Urine volume is small, and the urine is red. The tongue is red and dry. The pulse feels big and strong.

Dampness (湿): Patient feels heavy, and there could be swelling in the whole body or one part of the body. The tongue coating is thick and greasy. The Dampness condition can co-exist with the Coldness or Hotness condition, to form a Coldness-Dampness or a Hotness-Dampness condition.

Fluid or water-fluid (饮证): *Fluid* means the water in the body that does not participate in normal water metabolism and circulation. It stays in some part of the body to cause bloating, nausea, dizziness, dry mouth and difficulty in urination.[11] It can be regarded as less condensed phlegm in the body. The *Fluid* is easier than Phlegm to follow air rushing upwards in the body to attack and to assault the stomach, diaphragm, chest or brain, to cause nausea, palpitation, pain, dizziness, or even a panicked feeling. Such *fluid* is actually the retained water inside the body, so we choose the word "retained water" or "garbage water" to mean it and to allow a reader to understand the meaning easily.

Phlegm (痰证): *Phlegm* in TCM is a broad concept. The phlegm spit after coughing (sputum) is a narrow concept. The phlegm can move to any part of the body to block blood circulation or Qi circulation, to cause pain, heaviness, swelling or numbness. The *retained water or garbage water* above can be regarded as less condensed phlegm.

Body surface conditions (表证): In this book, whenever the "*body surface condition*" is mentioned, it means the symptoms in the body surface layer. It refers to symptoms or body signs, such as a headache, chilliness, sneezing, running nose, sore throat, coughing, sweating or inability to sweat, fever or no fever. The disease in the body surface involves skin, muscle, head, sensory orifices, joints.

On the other side, the term *body inner condition* (里证) refers to a disease in the inside of the body, which involves inner solid organs or hollow organs. In different disease stages, the organ(s) involved is different. For example, in the Yangming stage, it involves Stomach, Small intestine, and Large intestine, but in the Shaoyin stage, it involves Heart and Kidney.

Traditionally the body surface condition and the inner condition are translated into Exterior and Interior, respectively. It is suitable for Eight-gang diagnosis system, but not so much in the Six-stage diagnosis in *Shanghan Lun*. Each stage has both body surface condition and inner condition; the three Yang stages are body Exterior stages, and the three Yin stages are Interior stages; the Shaoyang stage is Interior to the Taiyang stage, but it belongs to Interior to Yangming and the Jueyin stages. Urine bladder belongs to Interior to the Taiyang body surface condition, but it is the Exterior to the Shaoyin (Kidney) stage. Therefore, the meaning of the Exterior and Interior in the Shanghan Lun system is mostly variable. To prevent such confusion, we choose to use the simple way of indicating the body surface phase or inner phase in each stage.

Uprush feeling (上冲): This is a unique symptom described in TCM.[12] The patient feels something rushing from the bottom of the abdomen up to the stomach, chest, throat or brain. During the up-rushing time, the patient feels as if something moves quickly to pound the stomach and cause nausea, to the diaphragm to cause dizziness, to the throat to cause a choked feeling and difficulty breathing, to the brain to cause dizziness or even loss of consciousness.

---

[11] The Chinese word 饮证 was translated as "*retained fluid*", "Thin Mucus", or "rheum" in some books.

[12] The Chinese word "上冲" here is translated as "Upcast", "Gush Upward", or "upflushing" in some other books.

Bi syndrome (痹证): This is a feeling of long-term discomfort in one part of the body.[13] The feeling can be pain, stiffness, bloating or swelling. It is always there, though the feeling is sometimes stronger and sometimes weaker. It is difficult to make it disappear. It is an intractable and sticky problem in the body. A typical example of Bi syndrome is arthritis. The Bi syndrome is usually caused by entanglement of Wind, Cold, Hot, or Dampness, mostly a combination of them, in one part of the body. If the Bi syndrome occurs in a blood phase, it is called Blood Bi syndrome. The patient feels mostly numbness. If it occurs in the chest, it is called Chest Bi syndrome, which shows as coronary heart disease or pleurisy. If it occurs in the throat, it is called Throat Bi syndrome. The patient with it feels choked, pain, or swelling in the throat for a long time.

Pi syndrome (痞证): This syndrome refers to fullness or a bloating feeling in the upper part of the abdomen (stomach region).[14] The diseased area is soft upon pressing, and there is no concrete mass there to be touched and no pain.

Chest-bind syndrome (结胸): The patient feels hardness and discomfort in the upper abdomen. If there is no pain or pressure pain, this is called Small Chest-bind condition.[15] If the patient feels hardness and pain, and pressure pain in the whole abdomen, it is called Big Chest-bind condition. The small Chest-bind syndrome can be seen in localized infections in the upper part of the abdomen, as in localized gastric ulcer. The Big Chest-bind syndrome can be seen in general peritonitis.

Triple Jiao (三焦): This term means the chest cavity (Upper Jiao), above-naval abdominal region (Middle Jiao) and below-navel region (Lower Jiao) regions.[16] One of the primary functions of the Triple Jiao is to conduct water transportation. Some other TCM doctors believe that there is no concrete physical structure for the "Triple Jiao", and that the Triple Jiao is only a functional concept of some particular structure in the body, such as connective tissue.

Healing crisis (暝眩反应): The healing crisis means a body reaction after usage of therapy, more often seen with herbal therapy than acupuncture. Patients may feel more annoyed, hot, have a nosebleed or a shaking of the body. After such reactions, the disease gets better dramatically. Such a healing crisis can last from seconds to minutes or hours. Mostly it seems to happen more easily when the pathogenic Qi is strong, but the body condition is weak. The herbal therapy strengthens the body defense system to struggle against the pathogenic Qi, to cause such a reaction. Sometimes it might be difficult to identify if there is a substantial body reaction. It depends on the doctor's clinical experience to judge this.

Special disease syndrome

Lily disease (百合病): The patient looks quiet and silent; has a desire to eat, but stops eating after just eating a little bit. The patient has a desire to lie but gets up after lying down for just a while. The patient has a desire to go out, but returns after several minutes. The patient feels that food is delicious for some time, but then has no taste for food at other times. The patient looks cold, but the person says that he or she does not feel cold; the patient looks hot, dresses lightly, but the patient says that he or she does not feel hot. The patient tastes bitterness. Urination is short and yellow. Such conditions can happen after a wrong treatment. It is difficult to treat. The patient could vomit after drinking the herbal tea. There could be no clear indication for a physical disease in the body. The pulse may feel slightly fast. Such diseases

---

[13] The Chinese word "痹证" here was translated as "Bi syndrome", "impediment disease", "painful obstruction syndrome", "rheumatic or rheumatoid arthritis" or "impediment pattern" in some other books.
[14] The Chinese word "痞证" was translated as "Stuffiness", "Focal Distention" or "Flatulence" in some other books.
[15] The Chinese word "结胸" here was translated as "Chest-bind", "Clumping In the chest", "Accumulation of qi in the chest", or "Accumulation of excessive harmful factor in the chest" in some other books.

---

[16] The Chinese word "三焦" was translated as "Sanjiao"," Triple Burner", "Triple energizers", "Triple heater", "Triple warmer" and "Triple energizer". The Burner, Energizer, Warmer, or Heater cannot express out the meaning of water conduction function of the *Sanjiao* in original TCM concept. They are only a word-to-word translation.

need to be distinguished from Shaoyang disease and Xiao Chaihu Tang condition (see later).

Fox–bewilderment disease (狐惑病): The patient could feel hot or chilly, or pain in the body. They may be silent and quiet and desire to sleep, but cannot close their eyes for a nap. It may be challenging to stay lying down or remaining up, being restless. There could be ulcers in the mouth or vagina (or mucus in other parts of the body). If the ulcer is in the throat, there could be a loss of voice. The patient dislikes the smell of food. The face looks reddish but quickly changes to black, or white in flashes of color. Such conditions can be seen in Behcet's syndrome.

Herbal therapies

In *Shanghan Lun*, various treatment principles are introduced. These treatment principles are still the most essential and fundamental principles used in current Chinese herbal therapy.

Sweating therapy (汗法): Herbal formulas are used to expel disease via sweat. The most commonly used herbal formulas are Mahuang Tang and Da Qinglong Tang. Whenever the word Sweating therapy is indicated in *Shanghan Lun* (and also here in this book), it refers to these herbal formulas. Some other herbal formulas can also create sweat, such as Guizhi Tang, but to create sweat is not the aim of these formulas.

Vomiting therapy (吐法): The herbal therapy is used to expel a disease via vomiting. The most commonly used herbal formula is Guadi San.

Purging therapy (下法): The herbal therapy is used to expel disease via stool. Examples are the herbal formulas Tiaowei Chengqi Tang, Xiao Chengqi Tang, Da Chengqi Tang, Taohe Chengqi Tang, Didang Tang, Da Xianxiong Tang, and so on.

Reconciliating therapy (和法): This kind of therapy is used when the Qi and the blood are in disharmony, the water distribution is in disorder, or the distribution of Fire and Cold in the body is in disorder. Herbal formulas used include Xiao Chaihu Tang, Chaihu Guizhi Shengjiang Tang, and Xiexin Tang. They are used to balance, to adjust, to harmonize, to make the movement of the Qi and blood in the body smoothly, or to release the entangled Qi, blood, phlegm or water in the body.

Warming therapy (温法): Used to increase the body metabolism, and to warm up the inside Cold condition. The formulas used include Lizhong Tang, Si Ni Tang, Tongmai Si Ni Tang, Baitong Tang, and so on.

Fire therapy (火疗): Fire therapy means to use a therapy to warm the patient, such as to warm the patient's face, or let the patient sleep on a hotbed, electric hot blanket, using moxibustion on the skin, using Fire acupuncture (the acupuncture needle is warmed with Moxibustion cylinder), and so on. It may be used in the treatment of Cold-attack disease, but it is wrong to use it for Warm diseases or Wind-Warm diseases.

Fire-cleansing therapy (清法): Used to reduce the Fire condition inside the body. Herbal formulas used include Zhizi Chi Tang, Baihu Tang, and Huangqin Tang.

Nourishing therapy (补法): Used to nourish and to strengthen the body Qi or blood, or both. Formulas used include Xiao Jianzhong Tang and Zhigancao Tang.

Dissolving therapy (消法): Used to remove mass (such as phlegm mass, dead blood clots, or even tumors). Formulas used include Didang Wan.

Arresting therapy (涩法): Used to make the bowel movement not abrupt, or to reduce the frequency of bowel movement or urination. Formulas used include Chishizhi Yuyuliang Tang and Taohua Tang.

Translation of herbal formula names

Currently, the name of an herbal formula is translated with various ways. It may be translated with word-for-word translation, such as to translate 麻黄汤 as Ephedra decoction; or with transliteration, such as to translate 甘草干姜汤 into Gancao Ganjiang decoction. I choose complete transliteration, such as translate the 甘草干姜汤 into Gancao Ganjiang Tang. One of the critical principles in the translation is retro-translation. If after English translation, Chinese terminology can be understood by English-speaking people but becomes hard to understand by Chinese-speaking people, the translation is neither perfect. "Ephedra decoction" may be understood by English-speaking people, but it is hard for Chinese.[17] Such a problem would be a ban for communication between English and the Chinese world. We should not make one problem into two problems after a translation. In discussion with English-speaking TCM students, I found that to talk the transliteration of a formula name has no any problem, but if an English speaking student mentions a word-for-word translated formula name, it is hard for our Chinese to understand. Such a situation definitely affects professional communication.

The word *Tang* (汤): The word *Tang* following the name of an herb or an herbal formula means decoction. It means that the herb or the herbal ingredients of the herbal formula are cooked in water for a specific time in a pot. The supernatant (the liquid part) in the pot is collected for drinking (e.g., the herbal tea).

The word *San* (散): The word S*an* following the name of an herb or an herbal formula means the powdered form of the ingredients of the herbal formula.

The word *Wan* (丸): The word *Wan* following the name of an herb or an herbal formula means the pill form of the ingredients of the herbal formula.

The word *herbal formula* (方剂): This is the herbal prescription, which is well recognized by most TCM doctors. A formula includes fixed (standardized) herb names, dosages of the herb ingredients; the way to prepare the herbs (such as to cook in water, to make the ingredients into power or pill form, or other forms), the way to take it (to drink, to smell, or to smear on skin, and so on.), and the frequency to take it. A TCM doctor may use some herbs for the treatment without following any well-recognized formulas. If other doctors do not well recognize the herbs on his prescription, the prescription is called prescription (处方), not an herbal formula. The Indication Differentiation diagnosis (方证辩证) is to identify the evidence to use a formula, not a prescription.

---

[17] Most of Chinese TCM doctors have no proper knowledge of English name or Latin name of herbs.

Brief Introduction of the Six-stage Diagnosis System

There are several diagnosis systems in TCM. The Six-stage diagnosis system is one of them. [18]

Upon being attacked by external pathogenic Qi, our body will launch its defense mechanisms to protect the body's structures and functions. The body activates the defense Qi from the inner digestive system to the body surface to expel the pathogenic Qi out of the body. In total, there are six stages/phases of a disease's development course in the body after being attacked by pathogenic Qi. [19] These include the Taiyang stage, Yangming stage, Shaoyang stage, Taiyin stage, Shaoyin stage, and the Jueyin stage.

Upon being attacked by a pathogenic Qi, a disease can manifest in the Taiyang stage first, then if the pathogenic Qi is too strong, if the body is weak, or if the treatment is insufficient, the pathogenic Qi can invade further deep into Yangming, Shaoyang, Taiyin, Shaoyin, or Jueyin stages. The pathogenic Qi can also cause disease directly in any of these stages without following this typical pass pattern, depending on the part of the body that is weak before becoming sick this time.

The Taiyang, Shaoyang, and the Yangming stages all belong to Yang stages of a disease. [20] It means that the disease is not more profound to affect body solid organs [21] yet. The Taiyin, Shaoyin and the Jueyin stages, all belong to Yin stages of a disease. It means that the disease is deep in the body affecting body solid organs and that the disease is severe and life is in danger. The Yang means that the body's reaction to pathogenic stimulation is active and robust. The Yin means that the body's reaction to pathogenic stimulation is passive and insufficient and that the patient may die relatively quickly.

To set up a diagnosis of a disease, the doctor needs to tell which stage a disease locates in (Six-stage differentiation), and then tell

---

[18] In *Shanghan Lun*, an exogenous disease course is separated into six diseases, such as Taiyang disease, Yangming disease, Shaoyang disease, Taiyin disease, Shaoyin disease and the Jueyin disease. The original word is "病" (it can be translated as "disease" by word). The six diseases are actually six stages (periods, phases, or steps) of the exogenous disease. Therefore I translated the diagnosis system in *Shanghan Lun* as Six-stage differentiation diagnosis.

If a disease is not caused by an external pathogenic Qi invasion, but by some other reasons, such as extreme emotional disorder, trauma, improper diet, and the clinical manifestations are the same as in the six stages, the treatment is the same. In this case, the clinical condition can be diagnosed and termed as "disease", such as Taiyang disease, Yangming disease, Shaoyang disease, Taiyin disease, Shaoyin disease and Jueyin disease. (These diseases may also be due to a Shanghan stage a long time ago, which was not successfully resolved for a long time before becoming sick again this time.) In such case, this diagnosis system can be called Six-disease differentiation system. Other scholars translate this diagnosis system as Six-Jing diagnosis system, for the reason that the original word "病" means meridian (Jing here means meridian). It may have also been translated as Six-gang diagnosis system (meaning Six-principle diagnosis system).

[19]

---

[20] Please note that the meaning of the Yin and Yang in the book here is variable. One of the reasons is that the real meaning of them is not explained clearly in *Shanghan Lun* and that the data here are collected from various sources. For example, the meaning of the Yang pulse and the Yin pulse is different among TCM doctors.

[21] "Solid organs" mean Heart, Liver, Spleen, Kidney, and lungs. The opposite concept is "hollow organs", which include Stomach, Small intestine, Large intestine, Urine bladder, Gallbladder, and pericardium. The *"Solid organ"* refers to the "藏" in Chinese and the *"Hollow organ"* refers to "腑" in Chinese.

which formula should be used for the treatment (Formula indication differentiation).

Every disease stage has two phases: body surface phase and internal phase, and has several syndromes in each phase. Each of the syndromes needs a different formula for treatment. The formula needed can be only one formula or can be two or more formulas together.

1. Taiyang stage:[22]

In the early stages of the disease, the pathogenic Qi locates near the body surface (mostly under the skin). The body defense Qi moves from the inner digestive system to the body surface struggles against the pathogenic Qi and expels the pathogenic Qi out of the body through sweat. If the defense Qi successfully expels the pathogenic Qi from the body, it will return to the digestive system. When the disease locates in the body surface phase, the stage is called Taiyang stage. If the pathogenic Qi invades into a deeper phase of the Taiyang stage, the stage is called Taiyang inner stage. In the latter phase, the pathogenic Qi is mostly in the urine bladder or lungs.[23]

There are two essential sub-types of Taiyang body surface conditions (伤寒表证): Taiyang Wind-attack,[24] and Taiyang Cold-attack.[25]

---

[22] Dr. Hao Wanshan: The meaning of the Taiyang stage, Shaoyang stage, Yangming stage, Taiyin stage, Shaoyin stage, and Jueyin stage, are not the same as the Taiyang meridian, Shaoyang meridian, Yangming meridian, Taiyin meridian, Shaoyin meridian, and the Jueyin meridian, which are concepts in the acupuncture system.

For example, in the acupuncture meridian system, the Taiyang meridian includes the foot Taiyang urine bladder, and the hand Taiyang small intestine. Stimulating these meridians can treat diseases in the urine bladder and small intestine, respectively (as well as diseases along the distribution of these meridians on the body surface). However, the Taiyang stage in the six-stage (disease) system involves the diseases in the body surface, the urine bladder, and the respiratory system, but not the small intestine.

Diseases in the acupuncture Shaoyang meridian system involve diseases in the gallbladder (the foot Shaoyang meridian), and the Triple Jiao (hand Shaoyang meridian), as well as diseases on the body surface along the distribution of the two meridians. However, the Shaoyang stage in the Six-stage diagnosis system involves more diseases, such as in the eyes and throat.

In the acupuncture meridian, the Taiyin meridian includes the foot Taiyin spleen (digestive system) and hand Taiyin lung (respiratory system). However, in the six-stage system, the Taiyin stage only involves the digestive system, nothing in the lung.

Dr. Martin Wang: It is recommended that readers follow the concept of the six-stage system introduced in *Shanghan Lun*, and not link these terms with those in the acupuncture meridian system, or with the terms used in the book *Huangdi Nei Jing*. The Taiyang stage diseases are mostly the common cold or flu, or the early stages of infectious diseases.

[23] Dr. Hao Wanshan: The Taiyang inner stage includes the lung, the respiratory diseases, as well as those in the urine bladder.

Dr. Martin Wang: Not many doctors have pointed out that the diseases in the lungs in Six-stage diagnosis system should belong to the inner phase of the Taiyang state. A possible reason might be that the lung meridian is named Taiyin, which is not the couple meridian to the Taiyang (the couple meridian of Taiyang is the Shaoyin Kidney).

[24] Dr. Hu Xishu: Both Wind-attack and the Cold-attack Shanghan diseases should be understood as the body being affected by Cold pathogenic Qi. However, due to differences in the body constitution, some people have stronger Yang Qi on the body surface, and some do not. For those who have a strong body surface Yang Qi, the Cold is sealed in the body surface, the body feels cold and has no sweat. This kind of Shanghan disease is called Cold-attack Shanghan disease. For those whose body surface Yang Qi is weak, the Yang Qi cannot even seal the body sweat holes completely in normal conditions. Upon being attacked by the Cold pathogenic Qi, the pathogenic Qi can penetrate deep into the muscle phase of the body and can also cause sweating. For this group of people with sweating, the term used is Wind-attack Shanghan disease. Readers need to realize that their body is still attacked by the Cold, not the Wind, though throughout this book, we still separate these two groups of patients by discerning Cold-attack or Wind-attack.

[25] The Warm disease and Wind-warm have also body Taiyang stage, though the Taiyang stage in these diseases are very short. Many times, their Taiyang stage moves very quickly to Yangming stage (the

(1)　　Taiyang Wind-attack (中风): The body's defense system is weak. The patient has an aversion to wind (or dislikes to stay in windy weather or air-conditioned rooms), is slightly sweaty. The disease condition needs Muscle-releasing therapy [26] (Guizhi Tang) for treatment.[27]

(2)　　Taiyang Cold-attack (伤寒): The body defense system is active. The patient feels chilly,[28] has an aversion to cold environments, and has no sweat.[29] Sweating therapy (Mahuang Tang or Gegen Tang[30]) is needed for treatment.

There are also two types of Taiyang inner phases:[31]

(1)　　Urine bladder phase (水液储留)

If the pathogenic Qi is in the urine bladder, urination would be difficult. The difficulty is due to retained water in the urine bladder. Use Wu Ling San for treatment.

(2)　　Lung diseases (外邪侵肺)

If the pathogenic Qi is deeper in the lungs to cause a cough, phlegm, short of breath (such as panting), or chest pain, the herbal formulas used are such as Mahuang Tang, Guizhi Jia Houpu Xingzi Tang, Ma Xing Shi Gan Tang, Xiao Qilong Tang, Da Qilong Tang and so on.

2. *Yangming stage:*

If the body is weak, if the pathogenic Qi is too strong, or if the treatment is not correct, the pathogenic Qi can then penetrate deeper into the Yangming stage. The Yangming stage can also be caused by the invasion of either Cold or Wind. The clinic manifestations are different. The Yangming stage also has a body surface phase and inner organ phase. Among the three Yang stages, the disease in the Yangming stage is the severest.

(1) Yangming Wind- attack

In the Yangming body surface phase, the pathogenic Qi is in the muscle, and the patient feels hot, feverish, thirst, an aversion to warmth, and the pulse is big and strong.

---

treatment for their Yangming stage can be pretty much the same as for the Yangming stage of the Shanghan disease.).

[26] Guizhi Tang can cause mild sweating, but it is not called Sweating therapy in this book. Sometimes it is called Muscle-releasing therapy. Whenever the Sweating therapy is mentioned, it means the use of stronger Sweat-stimulating herbal formulas, such as Mahuang Tang, Da Qinglong Tang or others.

[27] Muscle-releasing therapy is used to expel the invading Cold from the muscle phase of the body through sweating. Sweat created by the Muscle-releasing therapy is different from the sweat caused by the invasion of Wind in muscle.

There is an opinion that for Wind-attack diseases, Guizhi Tang works for the body surface deficient condition and Mahuang Tang, Da Qinglong Tang work for body surface excess condition. Xiao Qinglong Tang should be regarded as the main formula for Cold-attack body surface excessive condition (Dengdai Huakai. Discussion about the co-existing conditions in the *Shanghan Lun.*

http://blog.sina.com.cn/s/blog_5f856c9a0101dbpc.html)

[28] Normally after being attacked by Cold, the body activates the defense system to increase body temperature. The body temperature is higher than the surrounding environment so that the patient feels "cold".

[29] The body surface Yang Qi is sufficient to seal the sweat holes and make the patient unable to sweat. The activated body defense Yang Qi cannot move out through the skin, so it rushes up to the upper part of the body, especially to the head to cause headaches, nausea, and tightness in the neck.

[30] There is an opinion that the Gegen Tang, not the commonly believed Mahuang Tang, should be the main formula used for the Cold-attack Taiyang stage.

(Li Yuming. Gegen Tang belongs to the representative herbal formula of the Shanghan Cold-attack disease. Henan TCM. 2011, 31(6). 569-571)

[31] Strictly speaking, the Taiyang inner phases should belong to "Shanghan interior condition (里证)". The Shanghan body surface phases belong to the classically termed "Shanghan surface stage/condition (表证)".

Use Baihu Tang [32] to clear the Hotness from the muscle layer of the body. [33]

In the inner organ phase, the pathogenic Qi penetrates the digestive system. The nature of the disease is Fire. The Fire exhausts the water/liquid in the digestive system to form a firm stool (Dryness), which then blocks the energy movement inside the digestive system. The patient feels hot/feverish, has no bowel movement for several days, and has bloating and pain in the abdomen. The abdomen feels the hardness and painful upon being pressed by hand. This condition requires various Chengqi Tang for treatment.

The Yangming inner organ phase can be developed from Taiyang, Shaoyang, or by the direct attack by the pathogenic Qi in the Yangming stage. It can also start in the Taiyin or Shaoyin stage, as a reverse development of the disease.

(2) Yangming Cold-attack

For the Cold-attack Yangming stage, [34] the patient feels cold, with intense pain in the digestive system, vomiting, and no bowel movement. The patient prefers warm drinks. Such a condition can happen when a person drinks a lot of ice water or beverages (especially in summer seasons [35]). The herbal

formula needed is Mahuang Fuzi Xixin Tang, Wutou Jian, or Wuzhuyu Tang.

The formulas used in the Yangming Wind-attack inner stage, are used to clear the dry-firm stool out of the body. Such therapy is called Purging therapy. [36] The Formulas used in Yangming Cold-attack inner stage is called Warm purging therapy.

3. *Shaoyang stage:*

If a disease involves the chest cavity, abdominal cavity, the immune system, various glands, [37] lymph system, endocrine system, and the side part of the body, it is called the Shaoyang stage. Patients may feel an alternating hot-cold feeling, annoying bloating feeling in the flank region, no desire to eat, annoyance, tend to have nausea, have a bitter taste in the mouth, dryness in the throat, or blurry vision.

The typical herbal formula used for the treatment of the Shaoyang stage is Xiao Chaihu Tang or various Chaihu-containing formulas. The herbal formulas work to balance the Yin and Yang, to harmonize the body condition. Such therapy is called Reconciliating-therapy.

The pathogenic Qi in the Shaoyang stage can come from the Taiyang stage, Yangming, or from the deeper three Yin stages.

4. *Taiyin stage:*

If the pathogenic Qi penetrates deeper into the digestive system, and if the nature of the disease is weak and cold, this is called the Taiyin stage. The Taiyin stage involves the Spleen in the body. The patient easily has diarrhea and pain from time to time. The patient likes to drink warm liquids and eat

---

[32] The Yangming muscle phase includes fever, dry mouth, but no sweating or only very little sweating. This is different from the concept seen in the Chinese medicine textbook (hereafter refers to "the textbook").

[33] Hereafter, the therapy used to clear Fire is called Fire-clearing therapy.

[34] In the book *Shanghan Lun*, there is no indication of the presence of a body surface stage of the Yangming Cold-attack stage. It only introduces the body inner stage. The Cold-attack Yangming stage seemingly is not caused by an external pathogenic Qi from the Taiyang stage or Shaoyang stage to the Yangming stage. It seems more like a casual, scattered or a miscellaneous disease. Many doctors seem to neglect the meaning of the Cold-attack Yangming stage in the Shanghan disease. They tend not to talk at all, or to talk very briefly, about the meaning of the Cold-attack Yangming stage.

[35] According to Chinese medicine, in the summer, the body surface is hot, but the inner side is cold, similar to the temperature on the surface of Earth. A lot of

cold drinks further reduces the warm energy inside the body. The body has no sufficient Yang Qi inside the body to digest, and to move the food debris down to the colon. The result is the blockage of cold stool in the digestive system.

[36] Any therapy with the aim of expelling disease out of the body from the colon can be called Purging therapy.

[37] Such as saliva glands or sweat glands, for instance.

warm food. There is diarrhea, but the patient tends not to feel thirsty,[38] If we say that the scene of the inner abdomen in the Yangming Wind-attack is Hotness, here in the Taiyin stage, it is Coldness. The herbal formula needed is Lizhong Tang, It is needed to warm up the digestive system, to improve the digestive function.[39]

The pathogenic Qi in this Taiyin stage mostly comes from the Shaoyang stage, or from a later Shaoyin stage. It can also develop from the Yangming inner organ stage due to incorrect treatment.

5. Shaoyin stage:

If the pathogenic Qi in the Taiyin stage lasts for a too long and exhausts the body too much, the disease will affect the Heart and the Kidney system of the body. This stage is called the Shaoyin stage. It is a very hazardous stage. Many deaths happen in this stage. The patient can have frequent diarrhea with strong thirst (the patient has the desire to drink, but cannot drink large volumes of water each time). The hands and feet are cold. The pulse is deep and weak. The main herbal formula used for treatment is Si Ni Tang. It is used mostly to warm up the whole body, to improve the circulation and urinary functions.

The pathogenic Qi in this stage can come from the Taiyin stage, Shaoyang stage, or directly from the Taiyang stage.

6. Jueyin stage:

If a disease further develops, or if it is not treated correctly, the pathogenic Qi attacks the Liver and Pericardium systems. This stage is called the Jueyin stage. This stage is also a very hazardous stage and may cause death, but the disease also has a chance to heal naturally.

There are three primary characteristics of the Jueyin stage:

(1) Mixed Coldness and Hotness in the body. The patient can feel both feverish and hot in some part of the body (or on some days), but cold in other parts of the body (or on other days). Alternatively, the patient has Hotness in the Liver, but cold in Spleen, or has Hotness in the chest cavity but Coldness in the intestine (causing vomiting of roundworm). Use Wumei Tang for treatment.

(2) Jue syndrome (厥证). Patient has a cold feeling in hands and feet, and such cold feeling can reversely develop up to the level of elbow or knee. Such a cold feeling is termed the Jue syndrome.[40] For treatment, use Danggui Si Ni Tang.

(3) Alternating fever and Jue condition.

Patient has the Jue condition (with or without diarrhea) for some days, but hot in some other dasy.

The Jueyin stage can be caused by the further development of the disease in the Shaoyang stage or Shaoyin stage.

A disease progressing from the Yang stage to the Yin stage means that the disease is becoming worse while moving from the Yin stages back to the Yang stages means that it is getting better.

Chinese medicine aims to cure the disease in the first Taiyang stage. The reason is that the early symptoms of many severe diseases appear the same as those for the common cold or flu. To work hard to solve the disease in the Taiyang stage can save much effort in the future.

---

[38] The extent of dehydration is not severe yet.
[39] The therapy using herbs or herbal formula to warm up the inner side of the body is called Middle-warming therapy.

[40] The TCM term"厥证" has been translated as "Reversal cold of the extremities", "Reversal of qi", "Syncope", "Reverse" and "Collapse" in some other books.

Six-stage diagnosis and treatment

1. *Taiyang stage*

太阳之为病, 脉浮, 头项强痛而恶寒。

The Taiyang stage[41] means that the pulse feels floating,[42] the patient has pain and tightness on the head and nape[43] and feels an aversion to cold. [44]

1.1 Taiyang body surface conditions

(1) Taiyang Wind-attack (中风) [45]

太阳中风，阳浮而阴弱，阳浮者热自发，阴弱者汗自出，啬啬恶寒，淅淅恶风，翕翕发热，鼻鸣，干呕者，桂枝汤主之。

In Wind-attack Taiyang stage,[46] Yang is floating, and Yin is weak. The floating Yang results in fever (or hot feeling). The weak Yin results in spontaneous sweat. The patient

---

[41] Only when the floating pulse, pain on the head and the nape, and feeling chilly, are all present, can the diagnosis of Taiyang body surface stage be set up. Any single one of these three alone cannot be used to secure diagnosis. Basically, in this book, the pulse means the pulse that is felt on the inner side of the wrist, close to the Scratching bone (both sides).

Dr. Ni Haixia: For any patients, no matter what the diagnosis by Western medicine, if the patient has a floating pulse, pain and stiffness in the neck, and feels chilly, you can make a TCM diagnosis of Shanghan diseases. Even if a cancer patient has such symptoms and pulse, treat him as a Shanghan disease.

Taiyang stage diseases can be seen in the common cold, flu, in the early stages of many infectious diseases, or in epidemic diseases.

[42] In *Shanghan Lun*, the pulse in most instances is felt on the wrist (both sides). Each side is separated into the Cun, Guan and Chi positions. The Cun position is close to the rasceta, the Chi position is towards the elbow, the Guan position is between the Cun and the Chi position.

Floating pulse: The pulse can be felt upon slight touching. The pulse must feel strong. If the pulse can be felt upon slight touching of the skin but is weak or even difficult to feel upon further pressing down, it is not what we mean the floating pulse here.

Dr. Hao Wanshan: The floating pulse alone indicates that the disease is in the body surface. It can be in the Shanghan Taiyang stage, but can also indicate some other disease, such as urticaria, eczema, psoriasis, or jaundice. It can also be a Shaoyang meridian disease (the patient feels pain on the side of the head or neck, migraines, has reduced hearing ability or red color in the eyes) or a Yangming meridian disease (the patient feels pain on the front of the head, has dry nose and pain in the eyes, has red color of face, etc.).

Be careful that, in slim person, the pulse is easy to feel, but it may not be the floating pulse. In an obese person, the pulse is ordinarily deep, so it is hard to feel the "floating" pulse (it may not be the deep pulse either).

[43] The nape region belongs to Taiyang; the side of the neck belongs to Shaoyang.

Dr. Ni Haixia: The Cold pathogenic Qi slows down blood circulation and reduces nutrition to the nerves so that the nerves sense the pain.

[44] The *aversion to cold* feeling is an obligatory condition for the diagnosis of the Taiyang stage. Without the chilly feeling, the diagnosis of the Taiyang stage (disease) is questionable.

Dr. Du Yumao: The aversion to cold is more seen in the Taiyang stage, but it can also occur in other stages, such as in the Yangming and Shaoyin stages. It can furthermore occur in other conditions after an improper treatment (Yin deficiency after a Sweating therapy) or in other diseases, such as in cholera.

[45] Dr. Hao Wanshan: The clinical manifestation of Wind-attack or Cold-attack is the overall result of the nature of the pathogenic Qi and the status of the body's Heath-maintaining Qi. A patient who is weak in body surface defense system tends to be in the Wind-attack phase of the Taiyang stage. A patient who has a strong body surface defense system tends to be in the Cold-attack phase of the Taiyang stage. It is hard to tell if the pathogenic factor is the Wind or the Cold. (Dr. Hu Xishu has a similar opinion about this comment).

Dr. Liu Duzhou: The Wind causes the Wind-attack Taiyang stage, and the Cold causes the Cold-attack Taiyang.

[46] As mentioned before, here the "Wind-attack" could still be an attack by Cold. The different manifestations from a typical Cold-attack condition are due to the weaker body condition of the patient before becoming sick. However, we still use the term "Wind-attack" throughout this book.

has an aversion to cold, aversion to windy weather or environments, has sweat;[47] has or has no fever,[48] has a stuffy nose[49] and retches.[50] Use Guizhi Tang as the primary treatment.[51]

(The pulse feels floating-soft [52] upon being pressed slightly but feels weak upon being pressed harder. The body may feel generalized pain but the pain is less in intensity, and it mostly occurs in the upper parts of the body.)[53]

太阳病，发热汗出者，此为荣弱卫强，故使汗出，欲救邪风者，宜 桂枝 汤。

In the Taiyang stage, fever and sweating are due to stronger Defensive Qi (卫气) (out of blood vessels) but weaker Nutrient Qi (荣气，营气) (inside the blood vessels). To expel the pathogenic Wind, better to try Guizhi Tang for treatment.[54]

太阳病，外证未解，脉浮弱者，当以汗解，宜 桂枝 汤。

In the Taiyang stage,[55] if the body surface condition remains, and if the pulse feels floating and weak, solve the disease condition with a Sweating therapy. Better to use Guizhi Tang for treatment.[56]

---

[47] This sweating is due to the exhaustion of the Body surface Yang Qi by the invading Cold, so that the body surface Yang Qi becomes weaker and allows further release (escape) of the body's liquids.

Dr. Liu Duzhou: The sweating in the Taiyang Wind-attack stage is usually not with clear water (sweat). It is mostly a wet skin. For this reason, the doctor needs to touch the skin and feel if the skin is wet.

Dr. Hao Wanshan: There are two reasons for sweating in the Wind-attack condition. First, the Wind belongs to Yang-nature pathogenic Qi, which attacks the body surface defense Qi (Wei Qi), reducing the ability of the body defense Qi to seal the sweat. Second, the Wind can evaporate water, such as wind blowing wet clothes dry. It releases the water out of the bloodstream to form sweat.

[48] A patient in the Wind-attack stage has a much higher chance of having a fever and having fever earlier than a patient in the Cold-attack stage.

[49] Here also includes a runny nose and sneezing.

[50] The stuffy nose and retching are not unique for the diagnosis.

[51] In the book Shanghan Lun, whenever a formula is introduced for treatment, it (original texts) means that use this formula as and main and primary choice for the treatment. For short of translation, we only indicate as "Use … for treatment".

Dr. Xu Chenghe: The patient has sweat with the Wind-attack diseases. After the use of the Guizhi Tang, the patient will also have sweat. The two types of sweat are different in meaning. The Former is called disease-sweat and the latter is called healing-sweat. In the disease-sweat, the sweat feels cold, and the patient looks pale on the face. The sweat lasts for a long time, and the disease remains not improved. In the healing-sweat, the sweat feels warm, and the patient's face looks warm in color. The healing-sweat occurs within a short time (after the drink of the herbal tea), and the disease gets better after sweating.

[52] Floating pulse found when pressing slightly is due to the heat inside. A soft pulse when pressing harder is due to the loss of body liquids through sweating. (If there is no sweat, the pulse should feel tight.)

Dr. Xu Chenghe: The pulse is floating-soft, not floating-slow. It is relative to the floating-tight pulse. However, it should be reminded that the floating-soft pulse can also be felt in Cold-attack diseases and the floating-tight pulse can also be felt with Wind-attack diseases. If the body condition is stronger, the pulse feels floating-tight. If the body condition is weak, the pulse feels floating-soft.

[53] The information in the parenthesis following the translation of a Chinese paragraph is the supplementary information, which is collected from various sources for the aim to better understand and to complete the meaning of the original paragraph.

[54] Dr. Liao Houze: Whenever using Guizhi Tang, let the patient drink rice porridge (or hot water) after drinking the herbal tea. Also, whenever the Sweating therapy and Purging therapy are used, let the patient lie down for a while after drinking the herbal tea. Otherwise, the herbal tea does not work properly.

[55] In the Shanghan stage" or "With a Shanghan disease" mean the symptoms in either Wind-attack or Cold-attack condition.

[56] The typical pulse of the Cold-attack Taiyang stage is floating and tight, and that of the Wind-attack Taiyang stage is floating and soft. Floating-soft pulse suggests that the body's liquids are insufficient, so only Guizhi Tang, not Mahuang Tang, can be used.

Dr. Hao Wanshan: If the pulse is not floating, Guizhi Tang should not be used.

太阳病，头痛发热，汗出恶风者，桂枝 汤主之。

In the Taiyang stage,[57] when there is a headache, fever, sweat, and aversion to wind, use Guizhi Tang as the primary treatment. [58]

太阳病, 项背强几几, 反汗出恶风者, 桂枝 加 葛根 汤主之。

In the Taiyang stage, when there is tightness feeling on the nape [59] and back, sweat and aversion to wind (such as when air conditioning blows), use Guizhi Jia Gegen Tang as the primary treatment.[60]

Dr. Liao Houze: If the fever is high, use Guizhi Tang, but also add some detoxifying herbs, such as Jingjie, Fangfeng, Erhua, and Lianqiao.

Dr. Li Keshao: Whenever the Sweating therapy is mentioned in the *Shanghan Lun*, it refers to the use of Mahuang Tang or Guizhi Tang, which can create sweat in the body.

Dr. Martin Wang: There are different opinions about whether Guizhi Tang belongs to the Sweating therapy. It should belong to Muscle-releasing therapy, though there is also sweat being created upon its use.

[57] Whenever we mention the Taiyang stage, it includes the Wind-attack and the Cold-attack stages.

[58] It does not matter if originally the disease is in the Cold-attack or Wind-attack stage. When we have these four symptoms, use Guizhi Tang. For example, a patient might be in the Cold-attack stage: he feels chilly and pain in the whole body and has no sweat. Mahuang Tang should be used. After some treatment, such as the use of Aspirin (or even without any treatment) he starts to have headaches, sweating, fever, and dislikes wind. Now Guizhi Tang should be used.

Dr. Liu Duzhou: Pay attention to the fever, sweat, wind-dislike feeling and floating-weak-soft pulse. With these, use Guizhi Tang, even if the disease is hives, malaria, or dysentery.

Dr. Ni Haixia: Wind belongs to a pathogenic Qi of Yang nature. The Yang tends to go up. The body muscle is folded by the pathogenic Qi, the body temperature cannot be evaporated via skin, the Yang Qi (body warm) goes up to the head to cause headaches.

[59] The side of the neck belongs to Shaoyang.

[60] Dr. Ni Haixia: Because there is dead water accumulated in the muscle, the neck and back feel tight. The herb Gegen works to remove the dead water from the muscle and move it to under the skin,

(2)　Taiyang Cold-attack (伤寒)

太阳病, 或已发热, 或未发热, 必恶寒, 体痛, 呕逆, 脉阴阳俱紧者, 名曰伤寒.

In the Taiyang stage, with or without fever,[61] there is chilly,[62] aversion to cold environments, generalized pain in the body, nausea, and retch, and the pulse feels floating and tight (on the Cun, Guan and Chi

---

and Guizhi Tang works to expel the dead water via sweat. The Gegen also works to bring and lift the water from the digestive system to the throat to solve dry throat.

Gegen works to solve arthritis and muscle numbness, lift puss masses (tumor) and lift water to the face and head. To solve arthritis and numbness, it is used for the treatment of muscle tightness and numbness. To lift the tumor mass, it can push the mass to the body skin surface for easy treatment. Lifting water to the face is used for the treatment of facial paralysis and muscle numbness. To work for facial paralysis, the Gegen used should be a significant amount: double the amount of Guizhi (if the Guizhi usually is three grams, the Gegen should now be six grams).

The sweat-creating capacity of Gegen is strong, so there is no need to drink soup after drinking the herbal tea (Guizhi Tang alone, when used for common cold, requires the drinking of soup after the drinking of the herbal tea).

Dr. Ni Haixia: For treatment with acupuncture, do acupuncture on Shenmai, Houxi, Dazhui points. Alternatively, use a bleeding technique on the points, followed with cupping. This condition is more commonly seen in children. The child has played actively with heavy sweating and then caught a cold. It can also be seen in labor workers who have been working in the winter and sweating, and the disease shows up in spring of the next year. Such cases can also be treated with Gegen Tang.

[61] If there is no fever, it might belong to Shaoyin Cold-attack (see below). In Taiyang Cold-attack, the fever may occur later than the fever in the Taiyang Wind-attack condition. In other words, the fever occurs earlier in the Wind-attack stage than that in the Cold-attack stage.

[62] The chilly feeling cannot be overcome by covering the body with clothes or blankets.

position[63]). In such a case, the disease is in the Cold-attack Taiyang stage.[64]

(The patient will have more or less fever. These symptoms are due to the Cold nature of the pathogenic Qi, which restricts the body Yang Qi's rising and falling down movement. The pulse on the wrist is floating and tight.)

太阳病，头痛发热，身疼，腰痛，骨节疼痛，恶风，无汗而喘者，麻黄汤主之。

In Taiyang stage, when there is a headache, fever (or has no fever yet), pain in the back or the joints,[65] aversion to cold, no sweat but pant (or has shortness of breath or asthma),[66] use Mahuang Tang as the primary treatment.[67]

(There is the opinion that the herbal formula Gegen Tang should be used.[21]) If the patient has body Cold-attack surface condition, and

---

[63] The floating-tight pulse can be felt from the Cun to Chi position of the wrist pulse. If the pulse on the Chi position is slow, Sweating therapy should not be used (such a pulse suggests that the blood is insufficient and that the disease condition might belong to the Cold-attack Shaoyin stage).

Dr. Hao Wanshan: In the Cold-attack Taiyang stage, the patient might also have disorders in the digestive system, having nausea or retching, poor appetite, slight bloating in the stomach and no bowel movement for several days. This is because during the movement of body defense Qi from the digestive system to the body surface, the digestive system is relatively weak, and the up-down movement of the inner Qi is in disorder. There is no need to use herbs for the treatment for the disorder in the digestive system unless such a disorder is very severe and causes body liquid depletion.

TCM doctor needs to remind patients not overeat, but to eat easily-digested food during a common cold. Even if on ordinary days, to overeat will attract body surface defense energy to the inside of the body for digestion and the body surface defense Qi is relatively weak. Such persons tend to have frequent colds, especially children.

[64] The most significant difference between the Cold-attack and the Wind-attack Shanghan disease is that the former has no sweating and pulse feels floating-tight; the latter has sweated, and the pulse feels floating-soft.

[65] The nature of the Cold is to contract (the nature of the Wind is to expand, to release, to loosen). The Cold contracts the muscle to make the muscle spasm and the blood vessels contract (so to retard the blood supply to the tissues) to cause pain. Body pain is the second characteristics of the Cold-attack Taiyang stage.

---

[66] Cold (pathogenic Qi) contracts and seals body Yang Qi to cause various painful feelings. It compresses the Lung Qi to cause shortness of breath, panting, or asthma. The pulse should be floating-tight.

[67] Mahuang Tang creates sweating. The Cold Qi is released out of the body through the sweat. To use Mahuang Tang, the pulse must be floating-tight, or floating-fast on the whole pulse position (from the Cun to the Chi position of the wrist pulse). It should not be used if the pulse on the Chi position is weak or slow (see below).

Dr. Tan Jiezhong: For some patients, their Taiyang disease may get better via more urination, not sweating, after drinking Mahuang Tang. Or, there is no more sweat or urination, but the disease can subside after the use of Sweating therapy. This might be due to the depletion of Cold through breathing. For some patients, the urination may become rough after the use of Mahuang Tang. Use Zhenwu Tang to improve urination.

Dr. Ni Haixia: The master (Dr. Zhang Zhongjing) did not indicate the pulse for this paragraph (case). Generally speaking, in the Cold-attack body surface condition, the pulse is floating and tight. Floating means the disease is in the body surface and tight means the pathogenic Qi is Cold. Therefore the body Surface condition as such needs Mahuang Tang to create sweat, to release the pathogenic Qi out of the body. However, if only when the pulse is floating-tight could Mahuang Tang be used, the master would have written it down, as he did for Guizhi Tang and Gegen Tang. However, he did not. The reason is that, if the disease condition is severe, the patient has nearly no pulse to feel. Mahuang Tang can still be used to bring the life back. For such severe case, some doctors use a hundred grams of the herb Pao Fuzi. It is not necessary. Mahuang Tang is good enough. Mahuang Tang has another nickname: spirit-returning formula. A patient who lives in the north side of the country usually has tight sweat holes in the skin. Mahuang Tang may not create sweat easily for him but induces more urination.

also feels asthma and a fullness feeling in the chest, use Mahuang Tang.[68]

太阳病，脉浮紧，无汗，发热，身疼痛，八九日不解，表证仍在，此当发其汗。服药已，微除，其人发烦目瞑。剧者必衄，衄乃解，所以然者，阳气重故也。麻黄汤主之。

In the Taiyang stage,[69] the pulse feels floating and tight, the patient has no sweat but has fever and pain in the body. After seven to eight days, if the body surface condition remains, Sweating therapy can still be used. (Mahuang Tang is a significant consideration.) After drinking the herbal tea, if the surface condition is improved somehow, and if the patient feels annoyed, the eyes feel challenging to open, and if such symptoms are intense, the patient will also have nosebleeds.[70] The reason is that the body Yang Qi is abundant. (After the nosebleed, the body surface condition will subside.)[71] Use Mahuang Tang as the primary treatment.

伤寒脉浮紧，不发汗，因致衄者，麻黄汤主之。

In Cold-attack Taiyang stage, if the pulse is floating and tight, the patient has no sweat but has nosebleeds,[72] use Mahuang Tang as the primary treatment.

Tang (and some other stronger Sweating therapy) is used, rather than Guizhi Tang (mild Sweating therapy).

Dr. Liu Duzhou: A healing crisis (such as body shaking and nosebleed) occurs more easily when the pathogenic Qi is strong, and the patient has a stronger body constitution. Before the nosebleed, the patient may feel a flash of annoyance (vexation), aversion to light, and feel dizziness. Because this, in the clinic, we can use acupuncture to cause bleeding (especially for patients with high fever): puncture the Quchi (LI11), Shaoshang (LU11) and Taiyang (EX3) points to make several drops of blood appear, to speed up the healing process of the disease.

Dr. Tan Jiezhong: Some people have recurrent nosebleeds. This may be because there is Cold in the blood. Use Mahuang Tang (or even Guizhi Tang) to expel the Cold for the treatment. Nosebleeds are one of the ways by which the pathogenic Qi is expelled out of the body. If there is a nosebleed but the symptoms remain, use Mahuang Tang to help the body. Mahuang works more in the blood phase (Nutrient Qi side). Guizhi Tang works more in the outside of the blood (in the Defensive Qi side). For a similar reason, to stop a bleeding situation as in cerebral hemorrhage, use Mahuang Tang. After depletion of Cold Qi, the body Yang Qi can seal the blood vessels to stop the bleeding. There is no need to worry about the blood pressure increase due to the use of a Mahuang-containing herbal formula.

Dr. Tan Jiezhong: If the nosebleed is due to Cold, the patient usually feels pain in the front of the head before the nosebleed. This is difficult to distinguish from the Yangming body surface condition. However, in the Cold condition, the pulse is floating, and the patient feels chilly (aversion to cold).

---

[68] Dr. Hu Xishu: This condition is not the Taiyang-Yangming co-existing condition (see below).

There is an opinion that this paragraph describes the Wind-attack body surface excessive condition. It is not the cold-attack condition. (Dengdai Huakai. Discussion about the co-existing conditions in the *Shanghan Lun*. http://blog.sina.com.cn/s/blog_5f856c9a0101dbpc.html)

[69] This Taiyang stage should mean Cold-attack Taiyang body surface condition, because the pulse is floating and tight, and there is no sweat.

[70] For some patients, after the nosebleed, the disease will improve. If not, still use Mahuang Tang.

[71] This is a healing crisis. A healing crisis refers to the symptoms that appear as the disease seems to gets worse but is not. It means that the body, with the help of the treatment remedy, has more energy to struggle against the disease, so that the body reaction is stronger than before. In Chinese medicine, blood and sweat are believed to share the same source. Such a nosebleed is also regarded as a kind of sweat. Therefore the pathogenic Qi can be released out of the body through the nosebleed, the same way as through sweat.

Dr. Hu Xishu: Such a healing crisis can happen quite often in clinics. It occurs more often when the disease has lasted for a long time, or if the body condition is weak. It is more common when Mahuang

[72] Dr. Hao Wanshan: Commonly with nosebleeds, the Taiyang disease improves. Now it is not improved. This phenomenon suggests that the nosebleed is not sufficient to release pathogenic Qi. Therefore, use the Mahuang Tang to release it through sweat, instead of waiting for the improvement via nosebleed. Nowadays, such phenomenon is rare to see: once a person gets a common cold or flu with fever, headache, and no sweating, the person will go to a doctor for treatment, rather than stay at home to

(3). Warm disease

太阳病，发热而渴，不恶寒者，为温病。

In the Taiyang stage, if a patient has a fever[73] and feels thirsty,[74] but has no aversion to cold,[75] such a disease belongs to Warm disease.[76]

(Fire-clearing therapy (Baihu Tang or Yuebi Tang) is needed. Sweating therapy should not be used at all. This disease condition is pretty much similar to the Yangming body surface condition.[77]

太阳病，项背强几几，无汗，恶风，葛根汤主之。

In the Taiyang stage, when there is tightness on the nape and back, sweat, aversion to wind, use Gegen Tang as the primary treatment.[78]

(4). Wind-Warm disease

若发汗已，身灼热者，名曰风温。风温为病，脉阴阳俱浮，自汗出，身重，多眠睡，鼻息必鼾，语言难出。若被下者，小便不利，直视，失溲；若被火者，微发黄色，

---

allow the disease to finish its natural development-improvement course.

Dr. Tan Jiezhong: The bleeding, in this case, can be a nosebleed, or bleeding from the mouth or even the brain.

[73] Similar to the Wind-attack Shanghan disease, the fever occurs very quickly in the early stage.

[74] In a Warm disease, the pathogenic Qi strongly exhausts the body's liquids, so that thirst occurs quickly.

[75] Because the patient does not feel chilly, the disease is not a Shanghan disease.

[76] The Shanghan and the Warm diseases are different diseases.

[77] Warm diseases and Wind-Warm diseases (see next paragraph) are both caused by Cold (pathogenic Qi). According to book *Huangdi Nei Jing*, if the Cold attacks the body in colder seasons (such as between October 22-23 and June 21-22) and the disease was not cured properly, the disease will show up later again. If such diseases show up in following spring season, they are called Warm diseases. If the diseases show up again after next June 22-23, they belong to the febrile diseases or Dampness-Hotness diseases.

Dr. Ni Haixia: Warm diseases easily strike when the body has had a heavy sweat due to exercise or labor work, or after running around vigorously as children do. With the heavy sweating, the body loses water from the blood. The warmth of the body is normally in the bloodstream. If the blood is lost, the body feels cold or chilly. If only the water part of the blood is lost, the body feels hot/feverish, but not chilly.

Dr. Liao Houze: The diagnosis and the treatment of the Yangming stage and later Yin stages are also suitable for Warm diseases. If sweating is continuous without stop, dry-fry the herb Sangye (Mulberry leaves) for a while, grind it into powder, then let the

patient drink one to two grams of the powder with warm rice porridge to stop the sweating.

Dr. Du Yumao: Warm diseases (温病) include Wind-Warm diseases (风温), Dampness-Hotness diseases (湿热), Hidden-Qi diseases (伏气), Spring-Warm diseases (春温), and Fushu (heatstroke) diseases (伏暑).

[78] If a patient in the Taiyang stage has tightness in the nape and back and has sweat, use Guizhi Jia Gegen Tang for treatment. If there is no sweat, use Gegen Tang.

Dr. Liu Duzhou: In clinics, many patients with tightness and pain in the nape can be treated with Gegen Tang. After drinking the herbal tea, the patients feel warmth in the back first, then has mild sweating, followed by the release of the tightness and pain.

Some doctors believe that the Gegen Tang condition belongs to Yangming body surface stage (e.g., the Gegen Tang is used in the Yangming body surface stage), similar to another formula called Baihu Tang. In the Gegen Tang condition, the patient has fever, chills, no sweat, has a frontal headache, red face, sore eyes, and dry nose.

Dr. Ni Haixia: Gegen Tang is the formula for the Taiyang stage of Warm diseases. Such common cold happens mostly when a person sweats during labor, physical exercise or hot weather. The herb Gegen works to lift water. Whenever there is a sore throat and dry mouth and throat, use Gegen Tang.

Dr. Di Lengxian: The prerequisite condition for Warm diseases is the loss of body liquid before being attacked by Cold Qi. Thirst and tightness in the neck and back are signs of body liquid loss. If the patient has no sweat, use Gegen Tang. If there is sweat, use Guizhi Jia Gegen Tang for the treatment.

剧则如惊痫，时瘛疭；若火熏之，一逆尚引日，再逆促命期。

After Sweating therapy, a patient feels burning hot/fever. This is a Wind-Warm disease (风温).[79] The Wind-Warm disease means that pulse feels floating,[80] the patient has a very high fever, sweats,[81] feels a generalized heavy feeling,[82] tends to fall asleep[83] with a heavy snore, and has difficulty in speaking.[84]

If Purging therapy were used,[85] the patient would have difficulty in urinating.[86] The eyes would stare forward.[87] The patient would have leaking urination.[88] If the patient were treated by mistake with Fire therapy,[89] the patient would have yellow skin (not jaundice). In severe cases, the patients may have convulsive epilepsy,[90] and muscle spasm from time to time.[91] If the disease is mistreated with a Smoking therapy for once or twice, the patient can still live for several days. If the wrong treatment is repeated more times, the patient will die soon.[92]

---

[79] Dr. Hao Wanshan: The Shanghan, Warm diseases, and Wind-Warm diseases should be regarded as independent and individual diseases. For the Wind-Warm diseases here, even if there is no Sweating therapy being applied, the patient has a high fever and heavy sweat. For any disease, if the body has sweat but the fever remains, the diagnosis of Wind-Warm disease should be considered.

Dr. Ni Haixia: Nowadays, such Wind-Warm disease is caused mostly by medicine used to create sweat, but without supplying sufficient liquid.

[80] The pulse feels floating-fast, strong and slippery here. The pulse in Shanghan disease is floating, not strong and not slippery.

[81] The sweat in the Wind-Warm disease is more profuse than that in the Shanghan Wind-attack Taiyang stage.

[82] Heavy body: There is still much more Dampness in the skin and muscle, which causes the heaviness feeling.

[83] The *fall asleep* here does not mean coma.

[84] The *snore and the difficulty speaking* are due to the Hotness uprush.

Dr. Ni Haixia: The Spleen dominates the muscles in the arms and legs. The body needs water to bring the blood and move on. With insufficient water, the nutrition supply from the blood slows down, so the body feels heavy, slow in action and reaction. The patient becomes lazy to speak and has a snore.

[85] Purging therapy can be used only if there is a firm stool in the bowels (e.g., there is an indication for the use of Da Chengqi Tang, with the addition of some other herbs, such as Shengdi (生地) and Maidong (麦冬), to clear Fire and also to nourish the Yin.).

[86] This is because the Purging therapy can deplete more body liquid. There will be no more liquid to become urine.

[87] With an insufficient volume of blood, the eyes have no sufficient nutrition from the blood. With sufficient supply from blood, the eyes can function normally.

Dr. Ni Haixia: The food in the digestive system is kept continuous digesting to supply nutrition and energy to the body. With the Purging therapy, the source of the nutrition is depleted. Without the sufficient supply of nutrition and energy, the Liver blood is exhausted. The Liver dominates vision so that the visual function of the eyes is damaged.

[88] If there is no firm stool in the bowels, the use of Purging therapy will deplete Qi from the inner side of the body, including the depletion of Kidney Qi. Without sufficient Kidney Qi to control the urine, the urine leaks.

Dr. Liu Duzhou: Both the urine and stool can become out of control, not only the urine.

Dr. Hao Wanshan: It is only the urine that is out of control. The leak of stool is a sign of impending death.

[89] Fire therapy means to use therapy to warm the patient, such as letting a patient face a fire, or letting the patient sleep on hotbed, electric hot blanket, or using moxibustion on the skin, or using Fire acupuncture, and so on. It may be used in the treatment of Cold-attack disease, but it is wrong to use it for Warm disease or Wind-Warm disease.

[90] Convulsive epilepsy is caused by an insufficient supply of blood to the brain.

[91] Muscle spasm from time to time: Insufficient blood supply to the tendon/sinew (the tendon in the body belongs to the Liver system).

[92] Dr. Ni Haixia: The water in the stomach can be evaporated (the Stomach is hot) to the Lungs and distributed to the body surface. The water in the food can move down to the intestine to be absorbed into the blood. Intravenous infusion of liquid can supply water to the bloodstream, but the water will become urine and lost. Only the water absorbed from intestine can remain in the bloodstream to solve the

(In this stage of the Wind-Warm disease, also use Baihu Tang as the primary treatment.[93] If in such case the patient also feels very thirsty, use Baihu Jia Ginseng Tang.)

1.2 Taiyang inner condition

Water-retention in urine bladder

(1)　　太阳病，小便利者，以饮水多，必心下悸。小便少者，必苦里急也。

In the Taiyang stage, if a patient has frequent urination, the frequent urination must be due to too much drink of water. The patient must feel palpitation in the upper abdomen (Use Fuling Gancao Tang for treatment.). If such patient feels reduced urination,[94] the patient must also feel fullness, bloating and even urgent pain in the lower abdomen. (Use formula Wu Ling San for treatment.[95])

(2)　　中风发热，六七日不解而烦，有表里证，渴欲饮水，水入则吐者，名曰水逆。五苓散主之。

In Wind-attack Taiyang stage, there is a fever. After six or seven days without recovery, the patient feels annoyed, and the body surface condition remains. The patient feels very thirsty, has a desire to drink water, but the water is vomited out once it is drunk.[96] Such a situation is termed Water reversing syndrome.[97] Use Wu Ling San as the primary treatment.

Lung Diseases

(1)　　太阳中风，脉浮紧，发热恶寒，身疼痛，不汗出而烦躁者，大青龙汤主之。若脉微弱，汗出恶风者，不可服。服之则厥逆，筋惕肉瞤，此为逆也。

In Wind-attack Taiyang stage,[98] the pulse is floating, and tight,[99] the patient feels feverish, aversion to cold, generalized pain in the body, has no sweat, feels annoyed (vexed)[100] and has irritable emotions. For such a case, use Da Qinglong Tang[101] as the primary

---

insufficient water part of the blood. (This concept sounds strange in current medical theory, but in clinics, it appears as such).
[93] Dr. Hu Xishu: Guizhi Tang should not be used. Even the herbal formula Yinqiao San (银翘散) and Sangju Yin (桑菊饮) should not be used.
[94] The reason is that the stomach can not distribute the water to the body surface and the body has insufficient Yang Qi to take the urine out of the body.
[95] Dr. Liu Duzhou: The water-retention condition can be due to drinking too much water during common cold or flu, or due to the body surface fever sinking in the urine bladder.
[96] The patient does not vomit food.
[97] Dr. Hu Xishu: The Water reverse condition is due to previous accumulation of garbage water in the stomach.

Dr. Liu Duzhou: This condition is due to accumulation of garbage water in the urine bladder.
[98] The original text here is 中风 (Wind-attack). There is an opinion that this paragraph describes the Cold-attack body excessive condition, rather than the Wind-attack deficient condition (Guizhi Tang is used for Wind-attack body deficient condition). (Dengdai Huakai. Discussion about the co-existing conditions in Shanghan Lun. http://blog.sina.com.cn/s/blog_5f856c9a0101dbpc.html)
[99] With Wind-invasion, the pulse is floating and soft. With Cold-invasion, it is floating. A floating and tight pulse suggests the invasion of both Wind and Cold. The formula Da Qinglong Tang is the combination of both Guizhi Tang (for Wind) and Mahuang Tang (for Cold), plus the herb Shigao (to remove more Fire inside) and it is proper to use in this condition.
[100] The annoyed (vexation) feeling indicates inner Fire condition. The patient may also have a dry mouth or dry throat.
[101] The Da Qinglong Tang is the potent herbal formula used to create sweat.
Dr. Ni Haixia: In this formula, there are both Mahuang and Shigao. Shigao can restrict the Mahuang and prevent the Mahuang from creating sweat. Part of the Mhuang works with the Shigao to bring Fire in the lung downwards to be expelled. Another part of the Mahuang works together with Xinren (almond) to improve body surface condition. In the formula Yuebie Tang, there are both herb Mahuang and Shigao too, but no almond; the patient will have frequent urine (to remove swelling and edema). The Yuebi Tang is, therefore, the formula to solve edema. The Guizhi Two Yuebi One Tang is for the early stage of edema.
Dr. Ni Haixia: If the patient feels chilly, itchy in the throat, coughs, has stuffy nose and thirst, and has yellow phlegm, it means that there is Cold in the body

treatment.[102] However, if the pulse is weak and the patient has sweat and has an aversion to wind, the herbal formula should not be used. Otherwise, the patient will have a reversing cold in the hands and feet, irritable body movements, muscle jumping, and spasms – it is the wrong treatment. (Herb Zhenwu Tang should be used to correct the problem.)

(2)   伤寒脉浮缓，身不疼，但重，乍有轻时，无少阴证者，大青龙汤发之。

In Cold-attack Taiyang stage, the pulse is floating and slow,[103] the patient has no pain but a generalized heavy feeling from time to time (not always). If there are no more indications of Shaoyin disease,[104] use Da Qinglong Tang as the primary treatment.[105]

---

[102] The Da Qinglong Tang condition usually happens in patients with stronger body constitution. In clinics, there are many people with anxiety (not meaning they are sometimes happy and sometimes sad), who are in the Taiyang stage (and have no other health disorders), Da Qinglong Tang is an excellent choice (better than Xiao Chaihu Tang – though the latter is commonly recommended in the TCM Textbook). The Mahuang Tang condition and the Da Qinglong Tang condition can occur when a person has a strong sweat (such as in hot summer) and then goes into a very cold room (a very cold environment, such as a deep well, or refrigerated room).

[103] The slow pulse indicates Dampness in the body.

surface and Fire in the lung. Use Da Qinglong Tang for the treatment. The reason for the itchy feeling in the throat is that normally the water in the stomach is evaporated to the lungs, and from the lungs, it is then distributed to the skin to become sweat. Now, due to the Cold in the body surface, the water cannot be expelled via sweat, so it returns to the inner side of the body, but not back to the stomach completely, but to the regions behind and out of the stomach, and the regions around the diaphragm. Therefore, the breath flutters the water to stimulate the throat and causes an itchy feeling in the throat. The Da Qinglong Tang condition is similar to Ma Xin Shi Gan Tang. If the appetite is not affected, use the latter. If the appetite is reduced due to a frequent cough, use Da Qinglong Tang. Poor appetite means that the digestive system has been hurt. In other words, if a patient usually has a reasonable good appetite, when he catches a cough, it is the Ma Xin Shi Gan Tang condition. If a patient usually has a poor appetite, and now has a cough, it might be the Da Qinglong Tang condition.

[104] Shaoyin stage: The patient feels weak and has a desire to lie down for a break; the pulse feels deep and weak. The body is not heavy but weak. The weakness feeling feels constant. Another clinical condition with a heavy body is the Dampness-invasion, in which the heavy feeling is also always there,

 Dr. Liao Houze: If a patient easily gets swelling on the hip, hands, or feet, after drinking water, and the swelling can subside after a while, use formula Xiao Qinglong Tang for the treatment. This is the Floating-swelling condition.

[105] Here is another clinical indication for the use of Da Qinglong Tang: a heavy feeling in the body from time to time. There are other kinds of clinical conditions with the heaviness of body: the Dampness-invasion condition and Dampness-accumulation condition. For the Dampness-invasion condition, the patient feels heavy always and feels it in the whole body. In the Dampness-accumulation condition (the Dampness accumulated in the body due to a disorder of water metabolism, to lack of Yang Qi, and so on.), the patient feels heaviness mostly in the lower back or below (such as in the legs).

There are very hot debates about how to understand this paragraph.

Dr. Hu Xishu: This condition is not a Shanghan disease. It is a garbage-water retention disease. There is water accumulated under the skin. The water can move according to body posture; therefore, the patient sometimes feels heavy and at other times not. Here, use Da Qilong Tang to evaporate the Water (early stage of swelling).

Remember that the condition for the use of the Da Qinglong Tang is that the pulse is floating, with either annoyance (irritable emotion and body) or heaviness in the body.

Dr. Liu Duzhou: That the pulse from typical floating-tight changes into floating-soft in the Cold-attack stage means that the body surface Cold is going to penetrate deeply and change into Fire. Therefore the patient must also have a fever and an annoyed feeling. The heavy feeling is due to the obstruction of body Yang Qi under the skin. The pathogenic Qi is between the body surface and the inner side so that the heavy feeling can become less severe from time to time.

Dr. Hao Wanshan: This is a condition in which Dampness accumulates in the body surface, the Yang inside the body is astricted, and it changes into Fire.

(3)　伤寒表不解，心下有水气，干呕发热而咳，或渴，或利，或噎，或小便不利，少腹满，或喘者，小青龙汤主之。

In Cold-attack Taiyang stage, the body surface condition remains. There is retained water in the stomach;[106] the patient has retch, fever, and cough. The patient can also be thirsty,[107] have diarrhea, burping, difficulty urinating, feel fullness in the lower abdomen, or have panting. For this condition, use Xiao Qinglong Tang as the primary treatment.[108]

The Fire will stimulate the heart to cause annoyed feelings. Due to the annoyed feeling, this condition involves necessarily the Shaoyin aspect, though the annoyed feeling was not clearly written here.

Dr. Ni Haixia: The Shaoyin condition can also have a floating-slow pulse, but patients in the Shaoyin stage feel a desire to lie down for a break. Here, the patient has Dampness in the middle part of the body (Spleen). The Dampness also expands to, and accumulates in, the muscles and joints, so as to cause a heavy feeling. If the Dampness is only in the Spleen, use herb Baizhu and Fuling to deplete the Dampness via urination. If the Dampness accumulates in the muscles and joints, use Da Qinglong Tang to remove the Dampness via sweating.

Dr. Lao Zhuang: There is Hotness inside the body because the pulse feels floating and slow. The Cold transforms into Fire, but the transformation is a slow course. Hotness causes the relaxation (loosen) of the pulse and tendons/sinews. The relaxation of tendons makes turning of the body difficult, so the patient feels heaviness in the body.

[106] The original text said there is water accumulation in "under heart". In TCM, the "under heart" region should be understood as the stomach region.
[107] With garbage water retention in the upper abdomen (in original Chinese, it is "under the heart"), only if there is difficulty in urination will there be thirst. Otherwise, there is no thirst. After the use of the Xiao Qinglong Tang and if the patient starts to feel thirsty, it means that the garbage water has been expelled and the stomach becomes dry.
[108] Xiao Qinglong Tang removes Cold Water inside the body. Da Qinglong Tang is a strong Sweating therapy. Whenever there is body surface condition and also inner garbage water accumulation, the herbal formula must include some additional other herbs that work to remove the garbage water out of the body, such as the use of the formula Guizhi Tang

(If the patient also has an annoyed feeling, add Shigao to the formula.)

(4)　伤寒，心下有水气，咳而微喘，发热不渴。服汤已渴者，此寒去欲解也。小青龙汤主之。

In Cold-attack Taiyang stage, there is retained water in the stomach. The patient has a cough, slight pant (or wheeze), has a fever but no thirst. (Use Xiao Qinglong Tang as the primary treatment.) After the treatment, if the patient starts to feel thirsty, the thirsty suggests that the disease is getting better.[109]

1.3 Special types of the Taiyang stage

Although most of the patients show the above typical conditions for the Taiyang stage, and the disease condition is treated with the formula Guizhi Tang or Mahuang Tang mostly, some patients may have different or variable clinical manifestations, due to some illness that existed before the Shanghan disease this time. Some can be caused by the wrong treatment during the Shanghan disease and require different herbal formulas to correct the mistreatment.

(1)　太阳病，得之八九日，如疟状，发热恶寒，热多寒少，其人不呕，清便欲自可，一日二三度发，脉微缓者，为欲愈也。脉微而恶寒者，此阴阳俱虚，不可更发汗、更下、更吐也。面色反有热色者，未欲解

---

without herb Shaoyao but with herb Fuling and herb Baizhu.

Dr. Liao Houze: For people with Water-fluid inside the body, their pulse is usually deep, big and slow. For asthma in children, use Xiao Qinglong Tang Jia Shigao (but the amount of Shigao should not be large) for treatment.
[109] Dr. Hao Wanshan: The thirsty feeling comes from the use of the herbal formula that contains Warm herbs that consume body liquids.

For the thirsty feeling after drinking Xiao Qinglong Tang, there is no need to use particular herbal therapy. Let the patient drink water a little bit by little bit. Do not let the patient drink too much water at once. Otherwise, there will be garbage water accumulation in the stomach that causes nausea and vomiting.

也，以其不能得小汗出，身必痒，宜 桂枝 麻黄 各半汤。

In the Taiyang stage for eight to nine days, the disease is similar to malaria. The patient feels feverish and an aversion to cold, with more fever than chills,[110] and no nausea. The bowel movement and urination are normal. Such fever-chills can happen twice to three times per day.[111] If the pulse feels slightly slow, the disease is to get better. The faint pulse and the aversion to cold feeling mean that both the Yin and Yang are deficient, neither the Sweating therapy, Purging therapy, or Vomiting therapy should be used again.[112] That the patient has an unexpected pink color of the face means that the disease is not ready to improve yet, because the body cannot sweat slightly. The patient will have a skin itch. It is better to use Guizhi Mahuang Half-half Tang for treatment.[113]

---

[110] Fever represents the body Yang Qi. Chilly represents pathogenic Qi. More fever means that the body Yang Qi is abundant.

[111] Dr. Lao Zhuang: The transformation of the Cold into the Fever is a progressive course so that the patient sometimes feels cold and at other times hot. The Taiyang disease here might mean the Cold-attack disease.

[112] In such cases, herbal formula Si Ni Tang, or Shaoyao Ganco Fuzi Tang can be used.

Because of the alternating fever-chills, this condition should be distinguished from the Shaoyang stage.

[113] Dr. Ni Haixia: This formula only works to deplete the water that is accumulated under the skin, not the body liquid. The herb Mahuang and the almond should be combined. Mahuang works to "open" the bronchus in the lung and the sweat holes on the skin. It increases the function of the heart and promotes blood circulation. Without the almond, the lung could become dry. The almond works to supply more water to the lung to cool the lung. The Guizhi Tang here works to supply more water from the digestive system to the skin.

Dr. Ni Haixia: If the patient has fever and chills of the same length, such as fever for one hour and chilly feeling also for one hour, use Guizhi Mahuang Half-half Tang. If the patient has more fever and progressive chills, use Guizhi Two Mahuang One Tang. The longer length of fever suggests that the body defense energy is stronger.

(2)　　　太阳病，发热恶寒，热多寒少，脉微弱者，此无阳也，不可更汗，宜 桂枝 二越婢一汤。

In the Taiyang stage, if a patient has a fever [114] and an aversion to cold, the fever is more than the aversion to cold, the pulse feels tiny-weak,[115] such a situation suggests that the body is lack of Yang. Sweating therapy should not be used again. Use Guizhi Two Yuebi One Tang for treatment.[116]

(3)　　　伤寒不大便六七日，头痛有热者，与承气汤。其小便清者，知不在里，仍在表也，当须发汗。若头痛者必衄。宜 桂枝 汤。

Dr. Liao Houze: For malaria, the fever and chills occurs once a day, or once every two or three days and the symptoms occurs mostly in the afternoon. The Taiyang alternating fever-chill condition occurs twice or three times a day.

[114] The patient may feel dry mouth or throat.

[115] Dr. Hu Xishu: The tiny-weak pulse indicates that the body liquid is insufficient. Regular Sweating therapy (Mahuang Tang) should not be used. The Guizhi Two Yuebi One Tang is the weakest herbal formula used to create sweat.

Dr. Hao Wanshan: In this case, the patient has alternating fever-chill several times a day, should also have a red face and have itches and an annoyed feeling. This is a Cold-folding-on-body-surface phenomenon with inner hotness condition, though the extent is not as strong as in the Da Qinglong Tang condition. Due to the weak pulse and the annoyed feeling, this condition should be ragared as in the Shaoyin stage.

Dr. Ni Haixia: Normally there is no annoyed feeling in a common cold. The annoyed feeling here is due to Fire in the lung. The weak pulse suggests that the inner side of the body is weak and there is insufficient body liquid (the Yang here), so that Sweating therapy should not be used. A patient with the Fire in the lung has dry tongue. When herb Shigao and Mahuang are used at the same time, the herbal formula will not create sweat.

[116] In this formula, the Shigao works to clear the lung of Fire.

Dr. Li Keshao: This formula is good for treating the early stage of Warm diseases.

In Cold-attack Taiyang stage (body surface condition with fever and headache),[117] when there is no bowel movement for six to seven days,[118] there is a headache and a fever, use Chengqi Tang for treatment. If the urine is clear (not strong yellow), the disease is not inside of the body (not in Yangming stage[119]), Sweating therapy (Mahuang Tang) should be used for treatment.[120] (After sweating,) If a headache remains, the patient would have nosebleeds. In such case, use Guizhi Tang for treatment.[121]

---

[117] Fever and headaches can be seen in both Taiyang and Yangming stages. In the Taiyang, the urine is clear (slightly yellow); in Yangming stage, it is darker yellow (a fire inside). The headache in the Taiyang stage is due to the Qi uprushing. Guizhi Tang works better than the Mahuang Tang to treat the headache, because the herb Guizhi can reduce the uprushing Qi.

Dr. Ni Haixia: If the headache is caused by dry stool in the intestine, the pain locates on the front of the head, between the inner sides of the eyebrows (the Yingtang point of acupuncture). The face of the patient appears to be covered with a thin layer of dust. The headache is due to the uprushing of dirty gas from the intestine. If there are micro-blood vessels apparent at this skin region, it means that the patient has hemorrhoids.

[118] In the Taiyang stage, the patient has more body energy in the body surface and has relatively less energy in the inner side for digestion, so that the patient can have no bowel movement for several days (some patients may have diarrhea), a similar condition as in Yangming inner condition. In this case, check the color of urine to identify.

[119] If the disease is in the Shaoyin stage, the urine can be clear as pure water. If the Taiyang stage is regarded as "Exterior", the Yangming and the Shaoao both can be regarded as "Interior". If it is indeed a shaoyang disease, the formula here is not proper.

[120] Dr. Hao Wanshan: Use Guizhi Tang, not Mahuang Tang at all. Mahuang Tang can cause heavy sweating to deplete body liquid and so change the body condition into the Yangming stage.

[121] Only after the use of Mahuang Tang, and the patient has already sweated, should Guizhi Tang be used. Guizhi Tang should not be used directly in the Taiyang Cold-attack condition.

Dr. Tan Jiezhong: This is an additional disease condition which needs to be distinguished between the Mahuang Tang condition and the Guizhi Tang

(4)　　伤寒脉结代，心动悸，炙甘草汤主之。

In Cold-attack Taiyang stage, when there is throbbing and when the pulse is intermittent and bound, use Zhi Gancao Tang as the primary treatment.[122]

(5)　　伤寒二三日，心中悸而烦者，小建中汤主之。

In Cold-attack Taiyang stage for two to three days, if a patient feels palpitations and annoyance,[123] use Xiao Jianzhong Tang as the primary treatment.[124]

(6)　　服　桂枝　汤，或下之，仍头项强痛，翕翕发热，无汗，心下满，微痛，小便不利者，桂枝　汤去桂，加　茯苓白术　汤主之。

After having drunk Guizhi Tang or having had a Purging therapy, if the patient still has tightness and pain on the nape, headaches, mild fever, no sweat, feels fullness and

---

condition. If the patient has no bowel movement for several days, use Guizhi Tang, not Mahuang Tang, to prevent further depletion of body liquids, even if the body condition appears more as a Mahuang Tang condition.

[122] This situation happens more in a person who is weak in body constitution and has a deficiency in both blood Qi before the Shanghan disease. That makes the heart unable to manage a regular heartbeat. In this case, Zhigancao Tang works to improve the function of the heart, even if the Shanghan disease still exists. This and the previous paragraph introduced that it is important to support the body inner side first, if the inner side is weak during the Shanghan disease, other than to use Sweating therapy to solve the disease directly.

Zhi: processed.

[123] Palpitation and an annoyed feeling suggest weakness inside the body (insufficient blood to nourish the heart), therefore Sweating therapy should not be used.

[124] Palpitation and an annoyed emotion suggest weakness inside of the body. Xiao Jiangzhong Tang works to improve the condition in the middle part of the body, e.g., it improves the Spleen and Stomach systems to help to expel the disease from the body.

If the palpitation occurs with irregular pulse, use Zhigancao Tang. If the palpitation occurs after heavy Sweating therapy, use Guizhi Gancao Tang for the treatment.

mildly ache in the upper abdomen, and has difficulty in urinating, use Guizhi Qui Shaoyao[125] Jia Fuling Baizhu Tang as the primary treatment.[126]

(7)　　伤寒，无大热，口燥渴，心烦，背微恶寒者，白虎加人参汤主之。

In Cold-attack Taiyang stage, when there is no intense heat, but there are a dry mouth and thirsty, annoyance, and a slight aversion to cold on the back, use Baihu Jia Renshen Tang as the primary treatment.[127]

(8)　　伤寒八九日，风湿相搏，身体疼烦，不能自转侧，不呕不渴，脉浮虚而涩者，桂枝附子汤之。若其人大便硬，小便自利者，去桂枝加白术汤主之。

In Cold-attack situation for eight to nine days, there is Wind and Dampness entanglement (in the muscles and joints).[128] The patient

feels annoying generalized pain in the body, which is so much that the patient can hardly turn the body, has no nausea,[129] no thirsty,[130] and the pulse feels floating, weak and rough.[131] In such a situation, use Guizhi Qui Shaoyao Jia Fuzi Tang as the primary treatment.[132] If the patient has firm stool and urination is frequent, use Guizhi Tang Qui Guizhi Jia Baizhu Tang as the primary treatment.[133]

(9)　　风湿相搏，骨节烦疼，掣痛，不得屈伸，近之则痛剧，汗出短气，小便不利，恶风不欲去衣，或身微肿者，甘草附子汤主之。

With the entanglement of Wind and Dampness, the patient feels much annoying pain in the joints, so much so that the joint

---

[125] In the original version, it is Guizhi Qui Guizhi Jia Fuling Baizhu Tang.

[126] Such a condition may happen when the patient has had garbage water accumulation in the upper abdomen area before sick this time. This condition is also similar to Chest-bind syndrome, but the garbage water accumulation syndrome includes difficulty in urination. This herbal formula removes the garbage water through urination. The Formula Wu Ling San also works to remove garbage water accumulation. It works to remove the garbage water through mild sweating.

There is a very hot debate about this paragraph, about whether Guizhi or Shaoyao should be removed from the original Guizhi Tang.

Dr. Hu Xishu: The herb Shaoyao should be removed, not Guizhi. In this case, the difficulty in urination is due to uprushing Qi. The herb Guizhi works to repress the uprushed Qi and improve urination.

Dr. Liu Duzhou (and other doctors): The herb Guizhi should be removed, not Shaoyao.

[127] In this syndrome, there is inner Fire in the stomach, which causes parched mouth and thirst. Because of the thirst, the body lacks liquid, the regular herbal formula for the body surface condition (e.g., Mahuang Tang or Guizhi Tang) should not be used. Instead, use the Baihu Jia Renshen Tang first, to save body liquid.

[128] The patient had Dampness condition in the muscles or joints before becoming sick this time. Upon being attacked by Cold and/or Wind, the Wind

---

and the Dampness, or the Cold and the Dampness entangled to cause joint pain.

[129] No nausea here suggests that there is no garbage water accumulation in the stomach.

[130] No thirsty feeling here suggests that there is no Fire or the disease condition is not in Shaoyang or Yangming stage. It is on the body surface.

[131] The pulse feels weak and is rough: the body is in a weak condition and has insufficient blood.

[132] This is Wind-Dampness condition in the body. Because the patient has pain in the body, no sweat, and the pulse feels floating, it must be the Taiyang stage.

[133] The patient has frequent urination that causes loss of body liquid, so Guizhi Tang cannot be used as it is. The Guizhi is removed but the herb Baizhu is added to resolve the frequent urination. The herb Baizhu can treat both difficulties in urination or frequency in urination. The herb Guizhi improves urination, so it should be deleted. If there is body liquid (some kind of Qi) uprushing condition, the water moves up along with body liquid to cause difficulty in urination. Guizhi can reverse the body liquid movement, to improve urination. Also because the Guizhi can stimulate sweat and cause more loss of body liquid, it should be removed from the original formula.

Dr. Hu Xishu: For this syndrome, I use the original Guizhi Tang plus herb Fuzi, Cangzhu. If the pain is limited to one side of the body, use Dahuang Fuzi Xixin Tang.

Dr. Ni Haixia: If there is body surface condition, use Guizhi Fuzi Tang, if there is no body surface condition, use Guizhi Fuzi Tang but with the removal of Guizhi while adding herb Baizhu.

cannot extend or bend, and the joint feels more pain upon being pressed. The patient has sweats, feels short of breath (pant),[134] has difficulty in urinating,[135] has an aversion to wind and refuses to remove blankets from the body;[136] or has slight swelling on the body. In such a case, use Gancao Fuzi Tang as the primary treatment.[137]

(10)　太阳病不解，热结膀胱，其人如狂，血自下，下者愈。其外不解者，尚未可攻，当先解外。外解已，但少腹急结者，乃可攻之，宜桃核承气汤。

If the Taiyang stage is not improved and there is Heat entangled in urine bladder,[138] the patient behaves as madness. Blood can leak by itself from lower orifices of the body.[139] With the bleeding, the disease can get better without help. If the body surface condition remains not improved, treat the body surface condition first (with Mahuang Tang or Guizhi Tang).[140] After the surface condition subsides, if the patient still feels

tightness, and urgent and hard feelings in the lower abdomen, use Taohe Chengqi Tang,[141] to deplete the dead blood.[142] (Such a therapy belongs to Intensive-purging therapy.)

---

[134] Shortness of breath: There is an accumulation of water in the stomach that presses the diaphragm and affects breathing. The patient can also feel palpitations.

[135] Water accumulated in the stomach and not moving down to form urine.

[136] *Aversion to wind and cold and wants warm*: the body Yang Qi is insufficient.

[137] Dr. Hu Xishu: If the pain is severe, there is uprushing feeling, and the patient has more difficulty in urination. Use Gancao Fuzi Tang.

[138] In the original text, it says that this condition is the entanglement of Fire in the urine bladder.

Dr. Liu Duzhou: This is the entanglement of Fire and blood (dead blood) in the small intestine (the small intestine meridian belongs to the hand Taiyang meridian). The Small intestine and the Heart have a surface-inner meridian relationship. The block in the Small intestine with the dead blood also affects the function of the Heart and causes psychological disorders.

[139] For females, the dead blood may leave the body through menstruation.

Dr. Hao Wanshan: The bleeding can occur via urine, menstruation or stool.

[140] Use Mahuang Tang or Guizhi Tang, or other herbal formulas, depending on clinical manifestations.

[141] Remember, if the disease is in both body surface and the inner organs (the urine bladder, or in the digestive system, e.g., the Yangming stage), first treat the disease in the body surface (e.g., the Taiyang stage), then the one in the inner organ. However, if the disease locates in both body surface (Taiyang stage) and inner solid organs (such as heart and kidney, e.g. the Taiyin stage), improve the functional condition of the heart and kidney first, and treat the body surface condition later.

The formula Taohe Chengqi Tang has a stronger function in reducing the Fire than clearing the dead blood. Use formula Tiaowei Chengqi Tang plus the herbs Taoren and Guizhi. The herbal tea should be drunk on an empty stomach. It is used for the treatment of psychological symptom (such as madness, crying, and so on.). In females, it can work for anxiety, stress, and upset feelings before or during menstruation.

Dr. Hao Wanshan: The Hotness-blood is entangled in the urine bladder (and lower Jiao cavity).

Dr. Xu Chenghe: The location of the Hotness-blood entanglement condition is in the large intestine, not in the urine bladder.

[142] The Heat-blood entanglement here should belong to Shaoyang disease, in consideration of the disease location. It is listed here possibly for the differentiation from the Water retention in urine bladder syndrome. The book here means dead blood that presented in the lower part of the body before sick this time.

Dr. Ni Haixia: This is the entanglement of Fire in the urine bladder. If the blood can go out via urine, the condition will get better. To solve the external condition (not meaning the body surface condition), use Xiao Chaihu Tang. After treatment, if the patient has urgent and tight feelings in the lower abdomen and urination is difficult, use Taohe Chengqi Tang.

Dr. Ni Haixia: To tell if there is stagnated blood in the lower abdomen, there is a pain on the Geshu (UB17) point, Xuehai (SP10) point, and Sanyinjiao (SP6) point, or there is pressure pain on these points. The patient feels dry mouth but has no strong will to drink water. In severe cases, there is blue-purple color on the skin of the abdomen.

Dr. Lao Zhuang: The patient is "mad", or not "mad" yet, suggesting that the Fire is not too high. For

(11)　太阳病六七日，表证仍在，脉微而沉，反不结胸，其人发狂者，以热在下焦，少腹当硬满，小便自利者，下血乃愈，(所以然者，以太阳随经，瘀热在里故也。)抵当汤主之。

In the Taiyang stage for six to seven days without improvement, the pulse feels faint and deep,[143] and there is no Chest-bind syndrome,[144] the patient behaves madness. The reason is that there is Fire in the lower part of the abdomen (the Fire is entangled with the dead blood in the lower part of the abdomen before becoming sick this time.[145]). The lower abdomen should feel painful and hardness when pressed. If urination is normal, the condition can be dissolved by depletion of the dead blood. This condition is caused by the penetration of Heat from body surface into the inner side of the body along the Taiyang meridian. Use Di Dang Tang as the primary treatment. [146]

---

the treatment, using formula Di Dang Tang to remove the entangled dead blood is enough to solve the problem. There is no need to use formula Taohe Chengqi Tang.

[143] If the disease has existed for six to seven days with a deep and faint pulse, if there is no strong emotional disorder, such as madness, the disease condition indicates that the disease is in the Shaoyang stage. Herbal formula Mahuang Fuzi Xixin Tang should be used.

[144] The faint and deep pulse can occur in Chest-bind syndrome, which is due to improper Purging therapy.

[145] Dr. Hu Xishu: The dead blood has been in the lower abdomen before becoming sick this time. It is not due to the Fire from the body surface. The dead blood can be from previous bleeding from the colon, ovary, urine bladder, stomach, or any surgical operations in the abdomen, or any physical trauma. The pulse feels deep and faint, suggesting that the entanglement of dead blood is very deep and that the condition is an obstacle to treatment.

[146] Distinguish between water retention (in urine bladder) and blood entanglement syndrome (in the lower part of the abdomen): in both syndromes, the patient feels fullness and bloating in the lower abdomen and feels hardness and pain in the lower abdomen when pressed. In the former, the urination is abnormal, and the patient can feel annoyed but is

(The normal urine suggests that the bloating and hardness in the lower abdomen are not due to problems inside the urine bladder.)

(12)　太阳病，身黄脉沉结，少腹硬，小便不利者，为无血也；小便自利，其人如狂者，血证谛也，抵当汤主之。

In the Taiyang stage, a patient has yellow color on the skin (jaundice[147]), the pulse is deep and bound, the patient feels hardness and fullness in the lower abdomen, and has difficulty in urinating. Such a situation means that the disease condition is not due to an accumulation of dead blood in the lower abdomen.[148] If the urination is normal and the patient behaves as mad,[149] the situation indicates the retention of dead blood in the lower abdomen (pelvic cavity),[150] Use Di Dang Tang as the primary treatment. [151]

---

not mad-like. In the latter, the patient has normal urination, the stool may be black, and the patient behaves madly (and may have a poor memory).

Dr. Hao Wanshan: If these two syndromes are difficult to distinguish between, treat the disease with both Wu Ling San and Taohe Chengqi Tang.

Dr. Ni Haixia: After using Di Dang Tang, the dead blood is expelled via stool. In Western medicine, after the use of a stomach catheter to supply liquid food, the patient's condition tends to become the Didang Tang condition.

Dr. Lao Zhuang: in this condition, the patient is "mad", suggesting that the inner fire is intense. Here the condition should be treated with Taohe Chengqi Tang, to remove both the Fire and the dead blood.

[147] This is a special type of jaundice. Jaundice cannot be cured without removal of dead blood from the body.

[148] This condition is not due to accumulation of dead blood in the lower abdomen (but due to water retention in urine bladder. Herb formula Wu Ling San, Yinchen Wu Ling San, or Yinchen Tang can be used.

[149] Behaves as mad: the patient is extremely irritated, aggressive, but not as typical insane yet.

[150] There is nothing wrong in the urine bladder.

[151] The dead blood entanglement syndrome and Dampness-Fire condition both can elicit fever, a fullness feeling in the lower abdomen and jaundice. In the former, the patient has normal urination, behaves mad, and has a poor memory. In the latter, the urination can be abnormal or there is no sweat, there is an annoyed feeling but no madness behavior.

(13)　伤寒有热，少腹满，应小便不利，今反利者，为有血也，当下之，不可余药，宜抵挡丸。

In Cold-attack Taiyang stage, when there is a fever and bloating in the lower abdomen. The urination should be difficult, but it is now normal. Such a condition means that there is dead blood entanglement (in the lower abdomen),[152] which should be solved by a Purging therapy. Use Di Dang Wan.[153] The medicinal should be intaken all once.[154]

---

[152] The garbage water retention can happen in either the stomach or in the urine bladder. The garbage water accumulation in the stomach comes from drinking copious amounts of water. The patient will feel palpitation in the stomach area, and the urine is normal. If water accumulates in the urine bladder, the patient will feel bloating and hardness in the lower abdomen and feels an urgent desire to pass urine. The urination is difficult.

Dr. Du Yumao: It is blood entanglement in the urine bladder. In clinics, we see blood coming out of the urine bladder. Urination is relatively more natural in the dead blood entanglement than in the water-entanglement condition. This does not mean that the urination is normal in the former.

[153] If there is retention of either water or dead blood inside the body, the regular treatment with Sweating therapy hardly works. The accumulated water (no matter if it is in the stomach or the urine bladder) or the dead blood must be removed before or along with the regular treatment strategy. In this condition, the patient has only a continuous fever, not the madness or madness-like symptom. The mild herbal formula Di Dang Wan is used.

Dr. Hu Xishu: Di Dang Wan is the only herbal formula to use. After intaking one pill, wait for one day to see if blood comes out of the body (usually through stool). If not, take a second pill on the second day.

Dr. Liu Duzhou: This is mild dead-blood entanglement syndrome, so the patient feels fullness but not hardness in the abdomen and has no madness. Di Dang Wan works less strongly than Di Dang Tang. With the former, the stool may come out on the next day and, in the latter, the stool may come out after several hours. For the treatment of dead blood entanglement, Taohe Chengqi Tang works more for Fever, Di Dang Tang works for more entangled dead blood, and Di Dang Wan works only

(14)　妇人中风，发热恶寒，经水适来，得之七八日，热除而脉迟身凉。胸胁下满，如结胸状，谵语者，此为热入血室也，当刺期门，随其实而泻之。

A female is in the Wind-attack Taiyang stage. The patient has a fever and has an aversion to cold when the menstruation comes.[155] After seven to eight days, the fever stops, the patient is cold in the body, and the pulse feels slow. She feels bloating in the flank region, a situation similar to a Chest-bind syndrome, and has delirious speech.[156] This overall condition is called "Heat invasion in the blood chamber" syndrome.[157] For treatment, use acupuncture on Qimen (LV14) point, to deplete the pathogenic Qi.[158]

---

for fullness in the lower abdomen (the fever and entanglement are not severe).

[154] The meaning of the original text "不可余药" is hard to interpret. There is a different opinion if this means to take all the herbal tea once, or if to use this formula, not any other formula, for the treatment.

[155] During the menstruation, the body Yang Qi is weak in the uterus so that the pathogenic Qi can penetrate and invade the uterus.

[156] Similar to the Heat-blood entanglement in the lower part of the body, here the Blood invasion in blood chamber should also belong to Shaoyang disease, in consideration of disease location (Blood Chamber mostly means uterus). The inclusion of this syndrome in the Taiyang disease is also for the differentiation with Taiyang Water retention syndrome in the Taiyang inner disease. Because the Heat invades the uterus, the body does not feel hot anymore, and the pulse becomes slow. The heat is in the uterus, but the symptoms are under the rib arch. The delirious speech is usually at night. For example, the woman may see a "ghost". During the daytime she is fine. If there are no symptoms for the heart, lung, and stomach, the disease can end by itself. Delirious speech can happen in the Shaoyang Heat invasion in uterus syndrome and the Yangming stage too.

[157] Dr. Ni Haixia: Some doctors believe that Fire can also invade the liver. They think that the blood chamber also includes the liver.

Dr. Du Yumao: Hotness in the blood chamber should mean the Hotness is in the uterus.

[158] This condition means that the Hotness in the blood chamber has affected the function of the Liver.

Dr. Hu Xishu: Xiao Chaihu Tang can be used.

39

(15) 妇人中风，七八日，续得寒热，发作有时，经水适断者，此为热如血室，其血必结，故使如疟状，发作有时，小柴胡汤主之。

A female has been in Wind-attack Taiyang stage for seven to eight days, then started to have alternating cold and hot feelings at a fixed time of the day, and then menstruation stops too, this is also the Heat invasion in blood chamber syndrome. Because the blood is entangled in the body, the body has such alternating hot-cold feeling as in malaria disease. For such as case, use formula Xiao Chaihu Tang as the primary treatment. [159]

(16) 妇人伤寒发热。经水适来。昼日明了。暮则谵语。如见鬼状者。此为热入血室。无犯胃气及上二焦。必自愈。

A Female in Cold-attack Taiyang stage has a fever, and her menstruation occurs. The female behaves normally in the daytime but has insane speech in the evening as she talks with a ghost. Such a situation is Heat in blood chamber syndrome too. If there is no evidence indicating disorders in Stomach function, Yangming inner stage, or Heat in

Pericardium syndrome, the disease can get recovery naturally. [160]

1.4 Turnover of Taiyang stage

For disease in the Taiyang stage, if the patient has proper rest, proper care or treatment, the development of the disease can be stopped, and the patient gets better within seven days.

伤寒一日，太阳受之，脉若静者为不传；颇欲吐，若躁烦，脉数急者，为传也。

With Shanghan disease[161] for one day,[162] the disease is in the Taiyang stage. If the pulse feels stable, the Taiyang stage will not develop further into other stages. If the patient feels nausea,[163] the pulse feels hurried and fast, and the patient feels annoyed and feels restless in the arms and legs,[164] the disease will progress into other stages. If there are no such changes, the Taiyang stage remains without worsening further. [165]

Dr. Hao Wanshan: Xiao Chaihu Tang does not work.

[159] Dr. Hu Xishu: In practice, Xiao Chaihu Tang is not used alone. If the patient has conditions for the use of Purging therapy (there is no bowel movement for several days, and the stool is firm), the Xiao Chaihu Tang is used together with Taohe Chenqi Tang or with Da Chaihu Tang. If the stool is loose (unformed stool), use Xiao Chaihu Tang and Guizhi Fuling Wan together.

Dr. Hao Wanshan: Xiao Chaihu Tang should be used with the addition of other herbs, such as Danpi (丹皮), Chishao (赤芍) and Qiancao (茜草), to remove the entangled dead blood. This condition means that the Heat in the blood chamber affects the Shaoyang Gallbladder.

Dr. Ni Haixia: The use of Sweating therapy in such cases may result in cessation of menstruation, or in reverse menstruation: the blood goes out via nosebleed. In the book *Shanghan Lun*, there are three types of the Fire in the blood chamber syndrome. All refer to a female, because a male has no menstruation.

[160] If the disease condition does not get recovered naturally, use acupuncture (bleeding therapy) on the Qimen (LV14) point for treatment.
[161] The "Shanghan" here includes the Wind-attack and Cold-attack stages.
[162] Dr. Ni Haixia: Here the "one day" should mean six days. There is a rule in nature that the Cold or Fever condition in the body cannot last for more than six days. Upon the seventh day, the condition will change. This is similar to a typhoon; the typhoon cannot last for more than six days. As for cold or hot weather, on the seventh day, the previous cold or hot weather must change. This is a basic rule in nature. Therefore the "one day" in the original text should be understood as "one disease term", which is a six-day term.
[163] The nausea feeling is more significant in the Shaoyang stage.
[164] The annoyed feeling and the restless arms and legs are more often found in the Yangming stage. The fast and hurried pulse indicates that the pathogenic Qi has moved into the Yangming stage and the Cold has changed into Fire.
[165] Dr. Ni Haixia: With a common cold or flu, the patient should keep quiet, take a break from labor or emotional work, have a reasonable diet and sleep, and avoid emotional disturbance as well. A stressful or scary event may hurt the Kidney and change the

伤寒二三日，阳明少阳证不见者，为不传
也。颇欲吐，若烦躁者，为传也。

With a Shanghan disease for two to three
days, if there are no signs of the Yangming or
Shaoyang stage, the Taiyang stage will not
pass into these two stages. If there is a desire
to vomit, or if the patient feels annoyed, the
Taiyang stage will develop into deeper other
stages.[166]

太阳病，头痛至七日已上自愈者，以行其
经尽故也。若欲作再经者，针足阳明，使
经不传则愈。

In the Taiyang stage,[167] the headache
subsides naturally before the seventh day.
This situation means that the disease will not
develop into another stage(s), because the
disease has finished the movement in whole
"Jing".[168] If there is a sign of advancing into

the next stage, perform acupuncture on
acupuncture points on the foot Yangming
meridian[169] to prevent its development.

风家，表解而不了了者，十二日愈。

For a patient who is easy to suffer from a
Wind-attack disease, if the significant
symptoms of the Shanghan disease (Cold-
attack or Wind-attack stage[170]) have
subsided but there are still some minor
symptoms, (such as mild coughing or a runny
nose, there is no need for further treatment),
the remaining symptoms will subside after
twelve days.[171]

Taiyang stage into the Shaoyin stage. An upset
emotion could hurt the Liver to change the Taiyang
stage into the Jueyin stage. If the patient has been
taking synthesized medicine, the tongue has become
map-tongue, which indicates pain to the Heart, and
the Taiyang stage can easily develop into the Shaoyin
stage.

[166] In the original text, it says, "within two or three
days there are no changes". In fact, no matter how
many days have passed, if there is no change in
symptoms and pulse, the Taiyang stage remains
unchanged.

If there is retch, nausea or vomiting, the Taiyang
stage will develop into Shaoyang stage. If there is an
annoyed feeling, it will develop into the Yangming
stage.

Dr. Ni Haixia: This means the period from the
seventh to the fourteenth day, and from the
fourteenth to the twenty-first day of the Taiyang
stage.

[167] Dr. Liu Duzhou: It is a clinical experience that many
diseases have a seven-day cycle.

Dr. Ni Haixia: A common cold usually gets better
within one week.

Dr. Martin Wang: Note that Dr. Ni Haixia explains
the "seven days" as seven days, not seven "disease
terms". Previously he explained one day as one
"disease term", and two days as two "disease terms".

[168] The original text there is Jing (经). It should mean
the stages, not the meridians. In the book Shanghan
Lun, whenever it was written as the Jing (经), it should
mean the disease stages, not the meridian.

[169] "Six to seven days" are usually the time when the
Taiyang stage passes into the Yangming stage.
Therefore, perform acupuncture on Zusanli (ST36)
point to prevent further development of the Taiyang
stage.

Dr. Liu Duzhou: The acupuncture as such can
prevent the disease's development into any other
stages, it can also improve the body's defense ability
in struggling against the disease in the Taiyang stage.

Dr. Hao Wanshan: The natural self-healing period
indeed exists. I always emphasize this in my lectures.
For example, in virus infections in children, if the
fever does not subside after the seventh day, we can
expect that it will subside on the thirteenth or
fourteenth day. If it still does not subside, we have to
expect its subside on the twenty-first day. With
proper treatment, the disease course can be
shortened. If a disease in the Taiyang stage does not
subside, then on the second seven-day course, the
disease may remain in the Taiyang stage, but can also
be in other stages. No matter which stage, it is useful
to do acupuncture on the Zusanli point. The
acupuncture can increase the body's defense ability in
struggling against the disease.

Dr. Martin Wang: For the same reason, the third,
fourth and fifth day is the time when the Taiyang
stage may move into the Shaoyang stage. To prevent
this development, perform acupuncture on the
Shaoyang meridian, such as the Zulinqi (GB41) and/or
the Yanglingquan (GB34) points.

[170] Dr. Hu Xishu: This means Wind-attack disease.

Dr. Liu Duzhou: This means both Wind-attack and
Cold-attack Shanghan disease.

[171] Dr. Hao Wanshan: For those of patients who easily
suffer from Wind-attack disease, the course of the
disease is also seven days, but the body does not
recover completely. The body needs another five days

太阳病，脉浮紧，发热身无汗，自衄者愈。

In the Taiyang stage, if the pulse feels floating and tight, the patient has a fever, but no sweating, and if the patient starts to have nosebleeds, the disease will get better.[172]

凡病若发汗。若吐。若下。若亡血。亡津液。阴阳自和者。必自愈。

For any disease, if it has been treated with Sweating therapy, Vomiting therapy, or a Purging therapy, and the body blood or body liquid has been depleted, but the body Yin and Yang are still in harmony (equally matched), the body will recover naturally

---

to get complete recovery. The reason is that the body energy must go through all five organs (heart, lungs, liver, kidney, and spleen).

Dr. Liu Duzhou and Dr. Hu Xishu: Twelve days is a rough number of days only.

Dr. Ni Haixia: After treatment for the common cold, if the body surface condition has been improved but the patient still feels slightly annoyed or vexation, or feels slightly lazy, the condition can be solved by the body alone after twelve days. If happy, the body can get better sooner.

[172] The nosebleed signals a healing crisis in the Taiyang Cold-attack stage. The Taiyang stage here should mean the Cold-attack stage because the pulse is floating and tight and there is no sweat.

Dr. Hao Wanshan: There are several meanings for nosebleeding in Shanghan disease: (1) Healing crisis. The disease improves after the nosebleeding (the body has the nosebleeding by itself); (2) After treatment with Mahuang Tang, the patient has nosebleeding and the disease gets better (also belongs to healing crisis); (3) There is nosebleeding but the bleeding is not smooth and the symptoms remain unimproved. In this case, use Mahuang Tang to create sweating. Let the pathogenic Qi be depleted through sweat; (4) The patient has nosebleeding and high fever. The nosebleeding is due to the invasion of pathogenic Qi into the blood, pressing the blood out of the blood vessels. In this case, the Mahuang Tang should not be used at all. It should be treated with Xijiao Dihuang Tang (Fire-clearing therapy). There is another alternating way to create nosebleeding and to release the pathogenic Qi from the blood: use a needle to punch the inside of the nose to make bleeding. Such a way is used in the countryside of China.

(There is no need to give additional treatment).[173]

(Some other signs can also tell if the disease is to get better or worse:

If the patient feels hungry at noon, or at midnight, and if the pulse is less floating but calm and smooth, these conditions indicate that the Taiyang stage is over, and the disease is not going to develop further.

If the disease is in the Taiyang stage for eight to nine days, the patient feels hot and chilly (more hot feeling than chilly), but has no nausea;[174] bowel movement and urination are reasonable;[175] the pulse feels slightly slow, then the patient will recover soon, and no treatment is needed.

In the Taiyang stage and after Sweating therapy (with Mahuang Tang), if a patient has heavy sweating, feels annoyed (irritable in emotion and the body);[176] has a desire to drink water, then give the patient water to drink little by little. The disease condition will get better without medical help. If the patient is allowed to drink a large volume of

---

[173] Dr. Tan Jiezhong: There are several ways to explain the meaning of Yin-Yang harmony. If we use pulse, it means that the pulse on the Cun and the Chi position, or the pulse on the right side and the left side of the wrist, or the pulse upon slight pressure or on deep pressure, are equal in intensity and in pulse shape. If so, do not give extra treatment. Let the body recover by itself. Another way to tell if there is Yin-Yang harmony is that the patient's skin is wet (not sweat) and that there is saliva in the mouth.

Dr. Ni Haixia: Yin-Yang harmony is seen when the pulse beats four times per each breath (inhalation and exhalation), there is slight sweating, a hungry feeling, and the tongue coating is slightly white.

[174] *No nausea*: There is no sign of the Shaoyang stage.

[175] *Regular bowel movement and urination*: No sign of the Yangming stage.

[176] The heavy sweat depletes liquid in the stomach.

water;[177] or if the patient has a shower or bath,[178] the patient will have asthma.)

太阳病，十日以去，脉浮细而嗜卧者，外已解也。设胸满胁痛者，与小柴胡汤。脉但浮者，与麻黄汤。

In the Taiyang stage for more than ten days,[179] the pulse feels floating and thin,[180] the patient feels tired and desires to lie down for rest.[181] Such a situation suggests that the disease is to get better. If the patient starts to feel fullness in the chest and a pain in the flank, use Xiao Chaihu Tang for treatment.[182] If the pulse feels floating only, use Mahuang Tang for treatment. (Though the disease has passed for more than ten days).

(If the patient also feels dry mouth or dry throat, and the tongue coating is white, use Xiao Chaihu Tang Jia Shigao for treatment.)

大下之后，复发汗，小便不利者，亡津液故也。勿治之，得小便利，必自愈。

After the use of an intense Purging therapy, followed by a Sweating therapy, a patient may have difficulty in urination. This situation is because of the exhaustion of body liquid via these therapies. Do not treat the difficulty in urinating. (If there is no further body surface or inner conditions,) the body liquid will restore itself, and urination will be improved automatically.[183]

1.5 Conditions in which the Sweating therapy should not be used

The clinical manifestations of the early stages of many diseases, such as the common cold, flu, infectious diseases, hepatitis, even cancer, are very similar: chills, fever, headaches, stuffy nose, runny nose, coughing, nausea, sore muscle, and so on. For most people, with proper rest, proper diet and water, the symptoms can subside within six days. If the symptoms are very severe or if they do not show signs of diminishing after six days, the patient needs medical help.

In this stage, the pathogenic Qi is in the body surface layer. The easiest way to expel it and to get recovery is to let the pathogenic Qi leave the body through the skin via sweat. Chinese medicine has already had rich experience about how to solve this problem at this stage. A good TCM doctor, therefore, is asked to deal with the early stages of a disease, rather than waiting for a disease to develop and to show its typical symptoms later. Once a disease develops into its later stages, either the treatment is difficult, or it requires much more effort to treat it, or the patient may die.[184]

The Sweating therapy is beneficial for the treatment of Taiyang stage diseases, whereas it should not be used in the following conditions:

(1)   咽喉干燥者，不可发汗。

---

[177] The dried stomach has insufficient Yang Qi to evaporate a large volume of water. The water remains in the stomach and prevents movement of the diaphragm to cause shortness of breath (or pant).
[178] Water shower, bath, or using an ice patch on the body, all will restrict the inner Fire and prevent release the Fire. The entangled Fire stays in the lung to cause asthma (pant or wheeze).
[179] Such post-common-cold fever conditions are very prevalent in clinics.
[180] The thin pulse suggests that the body has an insufficient blood and Qi.
[181] Dr. Hu Xishu: *Has a desire to lie down for rest* is one of the indications of the Shaoyang stage (it is not mentioned in the Shaoyang stage).
[182] *Fullness in the chest and pain in the flank of the abdomen* are typical indications of the Shaoyang stage, so that Xiao Chaihu Tang can be used for treatment.

[183] This paragraph reminds us that if a patient has difficulty urinating, the reason for the difficulty should be verified. If it is due to depletion of body liquid, not due to retention of garbage water or other reasons, then Diuretic therapy should not be used. Otherwise, with more depletion of body liquid through urine, the urination difficulty will become worse.
[184] Dr. Hu Xishu: For severe diseases, however, even if with proper Sweating therapy or with the Muscle-releasing therapy, the disease will still develop into Shaoyang or Yangming stage. The early treatment can only suppress its intensity. With proper treatment, a severe disease usually stops in the Shaoyang stage, or in the Yangming body surface stage.

Do not use Sweating therapy, if a patient feels very thirsty in both mouth and throat.[185]

(2)　　淋家不可发汗，发汗必便血。

If a patient has an infectious disease in the urine bladder; or has a kidney stone or urine bladder stones, do not use Sweating therapy.[186]

(3)　　疮家虽身疼痛，不可发汗，发汗则痉。

If a patient has pus and a big ulcer in the body and the patient feels pain,[187] the Sweating therapy may cause spasms.

(4)　　衄家不可发汗，汗出必额上陷，脉急紧，直视不能眴，不得眠。

If a [patient has a chronic history of nose bleeding,[188] the Sweating therapy should not be used. With the Sweating therapy, the skin on the front of the head loses flexibility; the eyes sink deeply, the pulse feels hurried-fast, the patient may feel difficulty in moving their eyeballs and has difficulty in falling asleep.[189]

(5)　　亡血家，不可发汗，发汗则寒栗而振。

If a patient has lost a large volume of blood,[190] the Sweating therapy can cause body shakes and chills.

(6)　　汗家重发汗，必恍惚心乱，小便已阴疼，与 禹余粮 丸。

If a patient has a long history of easily sweating, the Sweating therapy can make the patient feel cloudy of mind, have poor analysis and evaluation abilities [191] and feel pain in the urinary duct at the end of

---

[185] The dry mouth and throat suggest that there is inner Fire, or the body is lacking liquid (Yin deficiency). The Sweating therapy can be used to release body surface Fire, but not inner Fire. The Sweating therapy will further deplete body liquid. In such cases, if the dryness is not very severe, we may use Guizhi Tang plus Jiegen, or Gegen Tang plus Jiegen. The Sweating therapy must not be used for patients with throat pain. The throat pain belongs to the Shaoyin stage.

　　Dr. Ni Haixia: The dry feeling in the throat suggests Yin deficiency. To solve dry throat, use formula Maimengdong Tang. With common cold or flu, if the patient feels pain in the throat, it is a Warm disease. Consider the use of Gegen Tang for treatment. If there is dry throat, but no pain, it is not the Gegen Tang condition. If the patient has a dry throat and is treated with Sweating therapy, the disease can quickly develop into Zhenwu Tang condition.

[186] Patients with these symptoms already have Yin deficiency. Sweating therapy may make the water in the stomach insufficient; so that there is insufficient water from the stomach to the urine system, to cause bleeding in the urine or stool.

　　Dr. Ni Haixia: Sweating therapy can exhaust the water in the blood. Without sufficient water in the blood, the blood becomes hot and causes fever. The fever can break the blood vessels and cause bleeding. Such cases require formula Zhuling Tang for treatment.

[187] Sweating therapy can still be used if the swelling has not developed into pus, or if the pus is small and the skin or mucus has not broken, and there are no open holes yet. If the infectious disease or inflammation is under the skin, and there is no open hole in the skin, Sweating therapy can move the infectious mass to the skin surface. Then use herb Baishu and Fuzi to expel the pus out of the skin.

[188] This means that the patient has a long history of nose bleeding. Such patients already have insufficient blood.

[189] All the symptoms here suggest that the Yin is exhausted and the Deficient-Fire is uprushing to affect the vision and mind.

　　Dr. Ni Haixia: If the Sweating therapy is essential for those patients who have habitual nosebleeding, use Huanglian Ajiao Jizihuang Tang plus herb shallot and herb Douchi (soybean meal), or use formula Xiao Chaihu Tang.

[190] The body has insufficient liquid for Sweating therapy. Further sweating may make the Yang and Yin separate in the body and cause death.

　　Dr. Ni Haixia: For such patients, use Xiao Jianzhong Tang plus shallot and Douchi; or Xiao Chaihu Tang.

[191] Dr. Hao Wanshan: Sweating therapy causes the exhaustion of both Yin and Yang. The Heart is in poor condition and cannot control the mind. At this moment it is hard to explain the reason for the pain in the urinary duct after urination.

urination. Use formula Yuyuliang Wan for the treatment. [192]

(7)　　病人有寒，复发汗，胃中冷，必吐蚘。

If a patient has (inner, stomach) Coldness condition, the Sweating therapy was used again, which makes the inner much colder. (If the body has roundworm before sick this time,) the worm will move up to spit out. [193]

(8)　　脉浮数者，法当汗出而愈。若下之，身重心悸者，不可发汗，当自汗出乃解。所以然者，尺中脉微，此里虚，须表里实，津液自和，便自汗出愈。

The pulse feels floating and fast. The body surface condition should be treated with Sweating therapy. If Purging therapy is used, the patient will feel palpitations[194] and a heavy feeling[195] in the body. In this case, Sweating therapy should not be used. Wait for the body to have sweat by itself to cure. The reason is that the pulse is faint in the Chi

position (of the wrist pulse), suggesting that the inner body is weak. The disease condition can be cured only when both body surface and inner side are stronger, and the body liquid distribution is even in any part of the body. In such case, the body can have sweat by itself to solve the disease condition. (For treatment, use Xiao Jianzhong Tang or use Guizhi Xin Jia Tang.)

(9)　　脉浮紧者。法当身疼痛。宜以汗解之。假令尺中迟者。不可发汗。何以知然。以荣气不足。血少故也。

If the pulse feels floating-tight, the body should feel pain, and the condition should be improved with Sweating therapy. If the pulse feels slow at the Chi position, this therapy should not be used. The reason is that the slow pulse at the Chi position indicates that the body Qi and Blood is in deficiency condition.

1.6 Modification of Guizhi Tang

(1)　　Patient with Dampness in middle part of the body

If a patient has too much Dampness in Spleen, it is called Middle Dampness syndrome. Patients with this syndrome have an enlarged spleen, which prevents movement of stomach for digestion, the tongue coating is white and thick, and the stool is sticky. If Guizhi Tang is given to such patients, the patients may feel stiffness in the nape and headaches, have a fever from time to time, have bloating and slight pain in the upper stomach, and urination will be rough (not smoothly). If the Guizhi Tang is needed, it is necessary to add more herbs[196] to remove the Dampness.

(2)　　Patient with Yin deficiency

Yin deficiency means that the liquid part of the body is in a deficient condition. The patient usually feels dry mouth and wants to drink cold water, but can only drink a little bit; has dry skin; easily feels hot at night; easily sweats at night. For this condition, if Guizhi Tang is used, the body will lose more liquid. The patient will feel dry in the throat

---

[192] There is no data for the ingredients of this herbal formula.

　　Dr. Ni Haixia: It is sufficient to use herb Ginseng, Gancao, Shengjiang, and jujube, to supply liquid to the body.

[193] Sweating therapy is used for body surface Fire. After the release of body surface Fire, the inner warm Qi will move to the body surface and tend to leave the inner body in cold status. The worm likes warmth but dislikes cold environments, so it will feel discomfort in the cold stomach and move to find warm space to stay. The upper part of the body is usually warmer than the lower part of the body, so it tends to move up to spit out. Therefore, spit-worm suggests the inner Coldness condition.

　　Dr. Ni Haixia: If Guizhi Tang is required, Shengjiang (fresh ginger) should be replaced with Ganjian (dried ginger). The fresh ginger makes the stomach colder.

[194] Purging therapy causes depletion of blood liquid and there will be reduced blood volume to support the heart.

[195] There is water accumulation on the body surface.

　　Dr. Hao Wanshan: The heavy feeling can be caused either by the pathogenic Qi being too strong or because the body Yang Qi and blood are too weak. Here the heavy body feeling is due to the weakness in the body: the patient has palpitations, and the pulse feels slow at the Chi position.

[196] The herbs required include Baizhu, Cangzhu, Fuling, Yiyiren, etc.

and annoyed, feel nauseous and vomit, have cold hands and cold feet, have spasms in feet and have insane speech. For treatment of such patients, it is necessary to nourish the Yin first, before using Sweating therapy. It is common to first use Xiao Jiangzhong Tang with increasing amounts of herb Shaoyao in it.[197]

(3) Patient during a menstrual period

During the female menstrual period, the pathogenic Qi can easily invade the uterus to cause Heat invasion in blood chamber syndrome (see above).[198] If there are no any other symptoms, it is not necessary to treat such a syndrome.[199]

For the treatment, use Chaihu-containing herbal formulas, such as Xiao Chaihu Tang.[200] Sweating therapy used in such cases may stop the menstruation for later life, or cause reverse menstrual period (bleeding from nose).

(4) Patient indulging in alcohol

若酒客病，不可与桂枝汤，得之则呕，以酒客不喜甘故也。

If a patient indulges in alcohol,[201] Guizhi Tang should not be used, because it causes retch or nausea. Such a patient does not like sweet flavor. (Guizhi in the herbal formula could stimulate Dampness in the stomach and cause nausea.[202] It can also stimulate nausea and stomach discomfort when the patient has similar to the Taiyang Wind-attack condition, which is easy to confuse with the Guizhi Tang condition.

Second, such patients indeed become afflicted with the Wind-attack Taiyang disease. In this case, Guizhi Tang should not be used directly. There is an opinion that we should delete Gancao and jujube but add Gehua and Zhijizi, or use Gegen Tang. Such alcohol-abuse conditions should be distinguished from Guizhi Tang condition because such persons can also have hot feelings in the body, sweat easily, have headaches, and be slightly chilly with a headache. However the tongue is red, the tongue coating is white-yellow and thick, and the pulse is slippery-fast. The person can have a poor appetite, bloating feeling in the stomach, and the stool is sticky. All such conditions belong to a Hotness-Dampness disease condition.

[197] Dr. Liao Houze: For patients with a background of an inner Fire condition, or alcoholics, with red tongue and yellow tongue coating, use Guizhi Tang but add Huangqin, and five-fold of Guizhi, for treatment. This formula is called Yindan Tang (阴旦汤).

[198] This syndrome should belong to the Shaoyang stage.

[199] That the common cold (or flu) happens around menstruation may or may not be a bad thing. For most females, the invading pathogenic Qi can be depleted out of the body via the menstrual blood (similar to the depletion via nosebleed). Only if there are additional symptoms, such as bloating in the upper abdomen or flank region, or some other symptoms, is treatment needed.

[200] The Chaihu-containing therapy is called conciliating therapy (see below).

[201] Dr. Hao Wanshan: There are two meanings here. First, it means the patient has alcohol-abuse related diseases. The patient has Fire-Dampness in the stomach. The patient has red dots on the nose, is overweight, has black dots on the tongue, has a yellow tongue coating. The patient can have sweat,

[202] Dr. Hu Xishu: The alcohol brings Fire/Hotness and Dampness inside the body. Guizhi Tang is a warm herb. The warmth from the herbal tea makes the inside much warmer. The nature of warmth or fire is to rush up (as the nature of water to flow downwards), to cause nausea. The upward-flowing warmth/fire can damage the lung and cause vomiting of pus and blood (fire burns the blood vessel). The alcohol-abusing person dislikes sweet food because the sweet food can create Dampness in the body, resulting in stomach discomfort.

Dr. Ni Haixia: Long-term drinking of alcohol makes the stomach cold although the body surface is warm. It damages the stomach Yang Qi and reduces the ability of the stomach to evaporate water. The accumulated water becomes Dampness. The jujube in the Guizhi Tang is sticky and sweet, and it can entangle with the Dampness in the stomach to increase the Dampness and create more discomfort in the stomach. In *Huangdi Nei Jing*, it says that to solve alcohol abuse, use Zexie and Cangshu. Actually, adding these herbs to Guizhi Tang cannot solve the discomfort caused by the Guizhi Tang. Therefore, for such alcohol-abuse patients, it is better not to use Guizhi. It is the Guizhi, not the Zhigancao, which causes the discomfort. Patients who vomit after drinking Guizhi Tang must have a disease in the stomach, either gastric ulcer or cancer. For such patients, use Gegen Huanglian Huangqin Tang, if the inner condition is Dampness-Hotness condition.

stomach cancer or gastric ulcer. For such patients in the Taiyang stage, use Gegen Tang as the primary treatment.[203])

(5)　　Patient who usually has asthma

喘家，作 桂枝 汤，加 厚朴 杏子佳。

If a patient has a history of asthma (or pant, wheeze) and becomes afflicted with Shanghan disease, if a Guizhi Tang is needed, add Houpo and almond to the formula.[204]

(6)　　Patient who has an abscess

凡服桂枝汤吐者，其后必吐脓血也。

If a patient has vomit after intake of the Guizhi Tang, the patient would spit pus and blood later.

(The abscess can be in stomach, liver or lung or other parts of the body. The reason is that there is a Fire-Dampness condition in the body.[205] Guizhi Tang is warm in herbal nature. It can make the disease worse.[206])

---

[203] Dr. Liao Houze: For alcoholism, use Guizhi Tang but add herb Shigao and Huangqin.

[204] Dr. Ni Haixia: The patient has the Guizhi Tang condition and also has shortness of breath (or asthma). This must be Dampness and Hotness inside the lungs. The tongue coating is thick and yellow, and the saliva is sticky. For such patients, after drinking Guizhi Tang, the patient could feel shortness of breath or have an asthma attack. In this case, add almond and Houpo to the Guizhi Tang. The almond can clear the Fire and phlegm in the lung (and lubricate the skin). Houpo works to remove Dampness in the Spleen, and remove the source of phlegm (TCM believes that the Spleen (Soil) is the source of phlegm in the Lung (Metal). The Soil nourishes the Metal).

[205] Dr. Hao Wanshan: Such patients can also have fever, sweating, headaches, and appear similar to the Guizhi Tang condition. Therefore, such disease conditions need to distinguish from the Guizhi Tang condition. In such patients, the tongue is red; the tongue coating is yellow, the pulse is fast, the stool is firm, and urine is red-dark.

[206] Dr. Ni Haixia: If a patient is vomiting (and/or has stomach pain) we usually do not use Guizhi Tang. Such patients must have had a gastric ulcer and easily experience acid reflux after eating. Guizhi Tang can stimulate blood circulation and make the ulcer bigger and cause vomiting of blood.

1.7 Disease condition change with even normal level of sweat via Sweating therapy

Though Sweating therapy is useful and it is the leading therapy used to solve body surface conditions, sometime it may cause unexpected symptoms. The most likely reasons for the variations of the clinical situations are that the body has been in an abnormal condition before becoming sick this time. For example, the body has Yang deficiency, has a poor digestive system, there is water accumulation in the upper or lower abdomen, or there is phlegm accumulation above or beneath the diaphragm, and so on.

(1)　　发汗，病不解，反恶寒者，虚故也，芍药 甘草附子 汤主之。

After Sweating therapy, the body surface condition remains unchanged. The patient feels an unexpected aversion to cold.[207] This situation means that the patient body condition is weak. Use Shaoyao Gancao Fuzi Tang as the primary treatment.

(2)　　发汗后，恶寒者，虚故也；不恶寒，但热者，实也。当和胃气，与调胃承气汤。

In the above case, if the patient does not feel any aversion to cold after Sweating therapy, but feels hot or feverish, such a situation indicates that the disease condition is not weak but excessive (a sufficient condition). The herbal formula Tiaowei Chengqi Tang should be used to conciliate stomach Qi.

(3)　　太阳病，初服 桂枝 汤，反烦不解者，先刺 风池 、风府 ，却与 桂枝 汤则愈。

In the Taiyang stage, after Sweating therapy, a patient feels more annoyed, and the clinical condition is not improved.[208] In this case, use

---

[207] In another version of *Shanghan Lun*, it says that the Taiyang stage ends after Sweating therapy, but the patient feels an aversion to cold. This is because the average dose of Guizhi Tang is insufficient to create sweating in this patient.

[208] Dr. Hao Wanshan: The *annoyed* here belongs to irritating effect. It means that the dose of the treatment is insufficient so that the body is over-reacting. Such an irritating effect can be seen in the treatment of tuberculosis. For this reason, the dose of medicine used for the treatment must be large

acupuncture on Fengchi (GB20) and Fengfu (DU16) points. Then use Guizhi Tang again.

(4)　　伤寒发汗，解半日许，复烦，脉浮数者，可更发汗，宜 桂枝 汤主之。

In Cold-attack Taiyang stage, Sweating therapy has solved the body surface condition. However after half a day, the patient feels annoyed again, and the pulse feels floating and fast.[209] In this case, Sweating therapy can be used again. Use Guizhi Tang as the primary treatment.[210]

(5)　　发汗后，不可更行桂枝汤。若汗出而喘，无大热者，可与麻黄杏子甘草石膏汤。

After Sweating therapy, Guizhi Tang should not be used again.[211] If the patient has

sweating and panting but no strong fever,[212] Mahuang Xingren Shigao Gancao Tang can be used.[213]

(6)　　下后，不可更行桂枝汤。若汗出而喘，无大热者，可与麻黄杏仁甘草石膏汤。

After Purging therapy, Guizhi Tang should not be used again. If the patient has sweat and

---

enough in the beginning of the treatment. Another example is for the treatment of roundworm. If the initial dose of medicine is too small; the roundworm may be irritated and move to the stomach, gallbladder and the bowel to cause much more pain and even obstruction in the bowel.

　　Dr. Ni Haixia: Guizhi Tang activates blood circulation, but the heart was weak before becoming sick this time. The activated Yang Qi normally moves to the head, first, and then moves down to the other parts of the body. Now with the weak heart, the Yang Qi is retarded in the chest and causes the annoyed feeling. Acupuncture here opens the channel for the body Yang Qi to go up to the head and then downwards to other parts of the body. If a common cold is in the Taiyang stage, the patient can have the Stomach Qi restored around lunch time (the patient starts to have an appetite). If the common cold is in the Shaoyin stage, the patient may have stomach Qi restored in the middle of the night, and have an appetite return.

[209] The annoyed feeling and the floating-fast pulse both suggest the presence of body surface Fire.

[210] In the original text, it said that Sweating therapy could be used and the formula recommended is the Guizhi Tang. Such a statement causes confuse. Strictly speaking, Guizhi Tang should not belong to Sweating therapy.

[211] The disease has spread into the lung. Guizhi Tang therapy will enhance the Fire in the lung.

　　Dr. Tan Jiezhong: Because there is no sweat or asthma, Guizhi Tang should not be repeated again. Otherwise, if, after the previous use of Guizhi Tang,

the body surface condition remains, Guizhi Tang can still be used.

[212] Because there is Fire inside the lungs now, Guizhi Tang or Guizhi Jia Houpo and Xingzi Tang should not be used. The sweat is due to the entangled Fire in the lungs. The sweat is sticky and has a strong, odd smell.

　　Principally after Mahuang Tang, the remaining conditions should use Guizhi Tang for treatment. Here the asthma is due to the pathogenic Qi invading the lungs. There is Fire inside the Lungs (nearly the Yangming condition). Therefore Guizhi Tang should not be used. The condition here is sweat and asthma, so Mahuang Tang, which is used for asthma but with an absence of sweat, should not be used.

　　Dr. Liu Duzhou: In clinics, even if there is Fire, even high fever, this Mahuang Xingzi Gancao Shigao Tang can be used, as long as the asthma is not due to typical Fire in the bowels (e.g., not in the Yangming inner stage.), but due to the Fire in the lungs.

　　Dr. Hu Xishu: This condition is also seen often in children. This herbal formula can be used even if there is no sweat.

　　Here it is clearly indicated that Mahuang Xingzi Shigao Gancao Tang can be used for the treatment of asthma and sweating, but not strong fever, after Sweating therapy or after Purging therapy. In practice, even if the person has no history of Sweating therapy or Cleansing therapy but has asthma and sweat, this herbal formula can be tried. If one has asthma but no sweat, Xiao Qinglong Tang is commonly used.

[213] After sweating, *no strong fever and no dislike of cold* suggests that the disease is no longer in the Taiyang stage. *Sweat but no dislike of hot feeling* suggests that the disease is not in Yangming stage. Asthma with sweat only suggests that the disease is in the Taiyin (lung) stage.

　　Remember, asthma following a Purging therapy when the disease is in Taiyang stage requires Guizhi Jia Houpo Xingzi Tang. If, in this case, the patient has asthma, sweat, and diarrhea with a fast pulse, Gegen Huanglian Huangqin Tang is required. *Asthma with sweat but no apparent fever* needs Mahuang Xingzi Cancao Shigao Tang. These are pretty commonly used herbs for asthma.

panting (or wheeze) but no strong fever, Mahuang Xingren Shigao Gancao Tang can be used.[214]

(7)　　伤寒汗出，解之后，胃中不和，心下痞硬，干噫，食臭，胁下有水气，腹中雷鸣下利者，生姜 泻心汤主之。

In Cold-attack Taiyang stage,[215] Sweating therapy was used, original body surface condition stops, but the patient starts to feel discomfort and hardness in the upper abdomen, nausea, has a bad odor from the mouth, burps, there is water Qi on the flank, has big noise in the stomach, and has diarrhea.[216] In this case, use Shengjiang Xiexin Tang as the primary treatment.[217]

(8)　　发汗后，身疼痛，脉沉迟者，桂枝 加芍药 生姜 各一两 人参 三两新加汤主之。

After Sweating therapy, the patient feels generalized pain in the body,[218] and the pulse

feels deep and slow.[219] Use Xinjia Tang as the primary treatment (e.g., Guizhi Tang plus herb Shaoyao, Shengjiang and Ginseng).[220]

(9)　　发汗已，脉浮数，烦渴者，五苓散主之。

After Sweating therapy, if the pulse feels floating and fast, the patient feels thirsty. Use Wu Ling San as the primary treatment.[221]

(10)　　伤寒汗出而渴者，五苓散主之。不渴者，茯苓甘草 汤主之。

In Cold-attack Taiyang stage, a patient has sweat (and is slightly hot) and feels thirsty, (has difficulty urinating,[222] and the pulse is

---

[214] Dr. Tan Jiezhong: In the original text, it says that after the Purging therapy, Guizhi Tang should not be used. This statement is wrong. In fact, after Purging therapy, if the patient has an up-rushing feeling, Guizhi Tang can still be used for treatment.

[215] Here it should mean either the Cold-attack or a Wind-attack Shanghan disease.

[216] Before becoming sick this time, the patient has weakness condition in the stomach.

[217] Hu Xishu: This formula has a higher chance of triggering a healing crisis: the patient feels dizziness.

[218] *Pain in the body*: there is a pain in the body before the Sweating therapy. The pain remains after treatment. It means that the body surface condition remains. Theoretically, it now needs the use of Guizhi Tang. However, the inner side of the body now is in Coldness and weakness condition, so that other herbs are needed (Shaoyao, Shengjiang, and Ginseng).

Dr. Ni Haixia: There is a pain in the body before the treatment. Then, after Sweating therapy, the body still feels pain. Such a disease condition means that the sweat is too profuse and it exhausted the liquid in the micro-network of blood circulation to cause new pain. The fresh ginger works to enhance the distribution of water in the stomach to the lung and then to the body surface. The Ginseng works to nourish more liquid, and the Shaoyao works to enhance returning of blood to the vein. All the herbs work to improve blood micro-circulation. If the

patient feels an aversion to cold after the initial use of Guizhi Tang, use Guizhi Jia Fuzi Tang for treatment.

[219] Slow pulse can indicate Coldness but also liquid insufficiency. Here the slow pulse is due to loss of body liquid after the Sweating therapy.

[220] There could also be nausea and a hardness feeling in the upper abdomen because Ginseng is used. Nausea and hardness in the stomach region indicate the use of Ginseng.

[221] *Floating pulse, thirsty with difficulty urinating* suggests that the disease attacks the Taiyang inner organ phase - urine bladder. If the patient feels thirsty, the pulse is big, and urination is easy, such conditions suggest Baihu Tang condition – the disease is in the Yangming stage, not the Wu Ling San syndrome.

Both Wu Ling San and Fuling Gancao Tang work to correct the disorder in the water metabolism and/or distribution. Compared with the Wu Ling San syndrome, the person has a little bit of a disorder in the water metabolism and distribution: difficult in urinating and is not thirsty in the Fuling Gancao Tang condition.

Note: Upon being attacked by Cold, and if there is water accumulation inside the body, conventional Sweating therapy (with Mahuang Tang), or Muscle-releasing therapy (with Guizhi Tang) must be accompanied by Water-depleting herbs (Ureric therapy). Otherwise, the disease cannot be improved. The formulas introduced in the book *Shanghan Lun* are Xiao Qinglong Tang, Guizhi Qui Shaoyao Jia Fuling and Baizhu Tang, Ling Gui Zhu Gan Tang, Ling Gui Zao Gan Tang, Wu Ling San, Fuling Gancao Tang, and Zhenwu Tang.

[222] The Wu Ling San syndrome must include the *difficulty in urination*, otherwise, the hot, thirsty, floating-fast pulse, all may belong to Yangming body

floating and fast), use Wu Ling San as the primary treatment.[223] If the patient (has sweat, the pulse is floating and fast, but) is not thirsty, use Fuling Gancao Tang as the primary treatment.[224]

(11)　太阳病发汗，汗出不解，其人仍发热，心下悸，头眩，身瞤动，振振欲擗地者，真武汤主之。

In the Taiyang stage, after Sweating therapy, a patient sweated, but the body surface condition remains unchanged.[225] The patient still feels fever/hot,[226] palpitations,[227] dizziness[228] and tremor of the body[229] as almost to fall.[230] In this case, use Zhenwu Tang as the primary treatment.[231]

---

surface condition, e.g. the Baihu Jia Renshen Tang condition.

[223] The patient has accumulated water inside the body before becoming sick. The accumulated water has to be solved along with the body surface condition.

Dr. Lao Zhuang: Here it might be the herbal formula Zhuling San, not Wu Ling San. Choose either Zhuling or Zexie; we do not need to use both of them in the same formula.

[224] Fuling Gancao Tang condition is with garbage water in the weakened stomach. It is due to drinking too much water when the stomach is weak and cannot handle a large amount of water. The patient should also feel fullness and palpitation feeling, water-running noise in the stomach, and have cold hands and feet. Urination can be normal or slightly difficult.

Ling Gui Zhu Gan Tang condition is the uprushing of garbage water from the stomach. Ling Gui Zao Gan Tang condition is the uprushing of the garbage water from the urine bladder.

[225] Too much sweat caused depletion of Yang Qi.

[226] Dr. Hao Wanshan: There are two explanations about the fever here: the fever is part of the body surface condition, or it is part of the floating Yang in the Yin overwhelming condition.

[227] *Palpitation* suggests Weakness inside.

Dr. Liu Duzhou: The palpitation can be felt in the front left chest or the upper abdomen.

[228] It indicates Weakness in the head.

[229] It indicates Weakness in the meridians.

[230] Sweat-therapy causes the Stomach Yang Qi to float up to the head without falling down to other parts of the body, to cause a heavy feeling in the head, but a light feeling in the feet. Without enough Yang Qi in

(Such conditions can usually be seen in old persons and weak persons with Kidney deficiency.)

(12)　发汗后，腹胀满者，厚朴生姜甘草半夏人参 汤主之。

After Sweating therapy, a patient sweated (and the body surface condition subsides), but the patient feels bloating in the abdomen.[232] Use Houpo Shengjiang Banxia Gancao Rehshen Tang as the primary treatment.

(13)　汗不解，腹满痛者，急下之，宜大承气汤。腹满不减，减不足言，当下之，宜大承气汤。

After Sweating therapy, the body surface condition remains. The patient also feels bloating, fullness and pain in the abdomen. (This disease condition indicates that the disease has reached the deeper Yangming inner stage.) Urgent Purging therapy with Da

---

the stomach, the water in the stomach causes dizziness and palpitations in the upper abdomen. Muscles shake because of the lack of water. The water is under the skin (it has not returned to the stomach), not in the muscle. The drunk water remains in the stomach and cannot be evaporated to the skin yet.

[231] The patient had inner Yang deficiency before becoming sick.

[232] The disease has moved into the Taiyin stage. The patient usually also has nausea and poor appetite. The abdomen looks big (not only feeling bloated).

Dr. Hao Wanshan: This is a Spleen deficiency plus Phlegm accumulation condition. The bloated feeling can be severe in the evening but less so in the morning. For example, the bloating feeling is strong sometimes not strong in other times. The tongue is thick. The tongue coating is thick.

Dr. Ni Haixia: The bloating here belongs to Deficient-bloating (e.g., not the Excessive bloat, which is caused by the presence of solid stool inside the bowels, or a tumor in the abdomen, or water in the abdomen, and so on.). For the Deficient-bloating feeling, the patient has frequent farting but has no stool coming out. Houpo can remove the Dampness in the Spleen and move the Dampness to lubricate the bowels, to make the stool movement easier. Ginseng and Gancao work to supply water to the digestive system. Many old ladies have such Deficient-bloating condition.

Chengqi Tang is needed. After treatment, if the bloating level reduced only slightly, this herbal formula can be repeated.[233]

伤寒，发汗已，身目为黄，所以然者，以寒湿在里，不解故也。以为不可下也。（于寒湿中求之。）

In Cold-attack Taiyang stage, after Sweating therapy, a patient has jaundice in the eyes and the whole body. The reason is that the patient had Dampness before becoming sick this time. (The Sweating therapy moved body Yang Qi to the body surface layer, leaving the inner body Coldness. The Coldness becomes entangled with the Dampness to cause jaundice.[234]) For such jaundice condition, Purging therapy should not be used.

1.8 Over-sweat due to the Sweating therapy

Sweating therapy requires that the patient only mildly sweats. A profuse sweat during the Sweating therapy[235] should be avoided. It can cause loss of body liquid and cause various problems, depending on the body's original conditions.

(1)　　未持脉时，病人手叉自冒心，师因教试令咳而不咳者，此必两耳聋无闻也，所以然者，以重发汗虚故如此。

Before pulse diagnosis, a patient crosses his hands over the heart. The patient is asked to have a cough, but the patient does not follow. This situation means that the patient has lost the hearing ability. The reason for this is the repeated Sweating therapy used, which made the body condition weak.[236]

(2)　　发汗过多，其人叉手自冒心，心下悸，欲得按者，桂枝甘草 汤主之。

In above condition, after the intensive Sweating therapy, if the patient crosses hands over the heart region, also feels palpitations (and tends to press the upper stomach), use Guizhi Gancao Tang as the primary treatment.[237]

---

[233] Basically, before Sweating therapy, if the disease is in the Taiyang-Yangming co-existing stage, it is necessary to have Sweating therapy to solve the body Surface condition first, then use Purging therapy to solve the Yangming abdomen condition. Then, the Yangming abdomen condition happens after the Sweating therapy, so the Purging therapy is used, even if the body Surface condition is still present.

[234] If it is Hotness-Dampness jaundice, sweating should reduce the chance of jaundice. For Coldness-Dampness jaundice, use formula Yinchen Lizhong Tang or formula Yinchen Zhu Fu Tang for treatment. The Coldness-Dampness jaundice belongs to the Taiyin stage.

Dr. Liu Duzhou: Yinchen Si Ni Tang can also be considered if the patient with Coldness-Dampness jaundice has cold hands and feet and if the pulse is weak.

Dr. Hao Wanshan: For the treatment of Coldness-Dampness jaundice, Yinchen Wu Ling San, Yinchen Lizhong Tang, or Yinchen Si Ni Tang are choices.

If Purging therapy is used on patients with Dampness before becoming sick this time, the treatment may bring body surface Fire deeper in the body. The Fire becomes entangled with the inner Dampness and also causes jaundice. For such Hotness-Dampness type jaundice, use Yinchen Wu Ling San or Yinchenhao Tang for treatment.

[235] In Western medicine, the use of Aspirin can also cause profuse sweating. Other reasons can be staying in a hot environment (such as sauna), doing heavy exercise, drinking alcohol or being near fire, etc.

[236] The over-sweating exhausted the blood. There is insufficient blood to nourish the ear.

[237] In TCM, the sweat and the blood are connected, sharing the same source. Over sweating reduces the volume of blood. Lack of blood then makes the heart weak in function. Therefore the patient feels palpitations and hollowness in the heart area. Besides, the sweat usually occurs more in the upper half of the body. After sweating, the liquid part of the upper body reduced, the liquid in the lower body will rush up to the upper, causing the Qi uprushing. This is another reason for the palpitations. Whenever Guizhi Gancao Tang is used for the treatment of the palpitations (fast heartbeat), the dose of the formula needs to be large.

Dr. Ni Haixia: The use of Mahuang Tang can exhaust the water in the lungs and chest. The water in the lower abdomen will rush up to fill the space in the chest, causing the palpitation. Guizhi works to warm up the water in the stomach (the Guizhi increases the pumping function of the heart), to evaporate the water into vapor and move it to the arms and legs, to solve the palpitation. Guizhi works to suppress up-

(3)　　发汗后，其人脐下悸者，欲作奔豚，茯苓桂枝甘草大枣 汤主之。

After Sweating therapy, a patient has sweated, feels palpitations in the lower abdomen and has a slight Running-piglet (奔豚) feeling.[238] For such case, Fuling Guizhi Gancao Dazao Tang should be used as the primary treatment.[239]

---

rushing air. The Guizhi Gancao Tang condition is similar to the Xiao Qinglong Tang condition, which also has water accumulation in the upper abdomen, but which also has coughing or shortness of breath.
[238] Running-piglet is a kind of feeling, in which one feels as there is a strong air running from the lower abdomen upwards. It is a very strong movement, but does not feel like a usual bowel movement. The Running-piglet syndrome can happen very quickly, and the patient feels panicked. After several minutes, everything returns to normal as if nothing happened.

Here, the disease condition Bentun condition is about to occur, but not yet. Due to heavy sweating that causes loss of liquid in the upper part of the body, the Qi (the Kidney Qi) in the lower part of the body is disturbed, and it rushes up together with the previously accumulated water in the urine bladder. After over sweating to make the heart weak, e.g., the Heart Fire is weak, the Kidney Water rushes up to attack the Heart. This condition happens in patients who have water accumulation in the urine bladder before becoming sick this time. (In Xiao Qinglong Tang condition, the water accumulates in the upper abdomen.). In clinics, it is very important to ask if the patient has difficulty urinating. If yes, the herbal formula Guizhi Qui Shaoyao Jia Fuling and Baizhu Tang should be used (to deplete the accumulated water, together with the release of the body surface condition).
[239] If there is a typical Bentun syndrome, it means there is extensive Kidney Yin. Guizhi Qui Shaoyao Tang should be used.

Dr. Ni Haixia: The left side of navel belongs to Liver, the right side to the Lung, the lower part of the abdomen to the Heart, and the upper part of the navel to the Kidney. If the beat occurs in the upper side of the navel, it means the disease belongs to the Kidney. The herb Fuling improves the urination, removing water and Jujube works to supply liquid to the digestive system. Patients with this condition are usually those who have had water accumulation in the lower part of the body before becoming sick this time.

(4)　　太阳病，发汗，遂漏不止，其人恶风，小便难，四支微急，难以屈伸者，桂枝 加 附子 汤主之。

In the Taiyang stage, Sweating therapy causes continuous sweat,[240] the patient has an aversion to wind, has difficulty in urinating,[241] the arms and legs feel slightly tight and difficult to bend or stretch.[242] For such case, use Guizhi Jia Fuzi Tang as the primary treatment.[243]

---

[240] Too much sweating could deplete the Yang Qi and liquid of the body. The tissue is "dry", so that muscle movement such as bending or stretching becomes difficult.
[241] Dr. Ni Haixia: After depletion of the body liquid via the heavy sweat, there is insufficient body liquid to form urine.
[242] Dr. Tan Jiezhong: Such conditions can be seen in polio.

Dr. Ni Haixia: The muscle needs water for nourishment. The depletion of water via sweat causes shortness of water in the muscles, so the muscles spasm.
[243] Continuous sweating after Sweating therapy suggests that the patient is weak inside and the body cannot tolerate the ordinary extent of Sweating therapy. The involvement of herb Fuzi here is to support the body condition. The disease condition here means an original Guizhi Tang condition was treated with Mahuang Tang by mistake.

Dr. Liu Duzhou: If the heavy sweat is caused by body surface Yang deficiency, the herb Fuzi is the best choice for treatment. Other herbs, such as Dangshen, Fuxiaomai, Longgu or Muli do not work.

Dr. Hao Wanshan: Heavy sweat can deplete body Yang Qi and Yin liquid as well. For some people, the body Yang Qi is more depleted, and in some others, the body liquid is. It depends on the body condition before becoming sick this time. In this paragraph, it describes a Yin and Yang both-depleted condition. However, in the treatment, the herb Fuzi is used without the addition of regular Yin-nourishing herbs. This is to seal the Yin with the Yang.

Dr. Tan Jiezhong: Note that in this Guizhi with Fuzi Tang condition, the sweat is continuous. The patient feels tired after sweating. This is different from Guizhi Tang condition.

Dr. Ni Haixia: The Fuzi here is the processed (Pao) Fuzi. It works to Warm the Kidney and protects the body surface to stop sweating, but it must be added

(5) 　服 桂枝 汤，大汗出后，大烦，渴不解，脉洪大者，白虎加 人参 汤主之。

After drinking Guizhi Tang, a patient has heavy sweating, feels very annoyed, feels very thirsty, which cannot be solved with drinking water, and the pulse feels as big and surging.[244] Use Baihu Jia Renshen Tang as the primary treatment.[245]

(6) 　太阳病，发汗后，大汗出，胃中干，烦躁不得眠，欲得饮水者，少少与饮之，令胃气和则愈。若脉浮，小便不利，微热消渴者，与五苓散主之。发汗后，水药不得入口，为逆，若更发汗，必吐下不止。

In the Taiyang stage, after Sweating therapy, there is heavy sweating. This situation causes dryness in the stomach, and the patient feels annoyed (vexation) and agitated and feels difficulty falling asleep. If the patient wants to drink water, let the patient drink the water little by little (to conciliate the stomach).[246] If

the pulse feels floating and urination is difficult, there is mild fever and intense thirst,[247] use Wu Ling San as the primary treatment.[248] After Sweat therapy, if the patient cannot drink anything (water or herbal tea), the condition is termed "Reverse" syndrome. If Sweating therapy is used again,

---

to the Guizhi Tang. The Guizhi Tang can bring it to the body surface to "seal" the sweat holes.

[244] The Taiyang body surface condition has changed into Yangming body surface condition.

[245] Dr. Ni Haixia: This condition means that the Taiyang stage has moved into the Yangming stage. Such transfers can happen in the following cases: (1) after drinking the first dose of Guizhi Tang, the body surface condition was solved, but the patient drank more herbal tea and overdosed; (2) the amount of Zhigancao, fresh ginger, and jujube in the Guizhi Tang is not enough, so there is an insufficient supply of water for the digestive system; (3) after drinking Guizhi Tang, the disease moves into the Yangming stage. Guizhi Tang uses the liquid from the digestive system to create sweat. Zhigancao, fresh ginger and jujube work to supply more water or liquid to the digestive system, so it is not easy to create the Yangming Hotness condition. However, for Mahuang Tang, if the dose of the Mahuang is too much and if the almond is not enough, the disease would be easy to enter the Yangming stage. If the sweat depletes more water from the blood, it creates the Yangming body surface condition. If it depletes more water in the stomach-intestine, it creates the Yangming inner organ stage.

[246] This is Yangming dryness condition. If the drinking water does not work, consider the use of Baihu Jia Renshen Tang.

Dr. Ni Haixia: If drinking too much water at once, the stomach cannot handle the excess water, and the extra water would become garbage water in the stomach. The disease condition will develop into Ling Gui Zhu Gan Tang condition.

[247] The thirst is due to difficulty in urination, which prevent more water absorption, or, fever.

[248] This paragraph identifies Stomach Dryness condition and Garbage water in urine bladder condition. *San* here means herb powder.

Dr. Ni Haixia: The floating pulse here does not mean the body surface condition. It is due to the accumulation of water under the skin. The water was brought by the Sweating therapy. After sweating, the pathogenic Qi is depleted and the water should return to the digestive system, but it cannot return because the digestive system is weak (it was weak before becoming sick this time). The accumulation of the water under the skin causes the floating pulse. The digestive function is weak, the drunken water cannot be evaporated and cannot move up to the mouth, so the patient feels thirsty. The water cannot be diverted to urine, so urination is less. The previous Sweat-creating herbs brought the water to the skin, so the patient feels hot.

The herb Zexie can deplete water from the whole of the body (skin and the inner side of the body). Guizhi brings the Zexie to the skin to work. The herb Zexie alone can treat fatty liver. The herb Fuling clears water in the middle part of the body; herb Zhuling clears water in the lower part of the body. The cooperation of the herb Fuling and herb Baizhu can clear the Dampness in the Spleen, to restore the digestion function. The functions of Mahuang and Zexie are opposite: Mahuang brings water to the skin, and the Zexie brings water from the skin back to the inner side of the body. Fulling sends the water to the urine bladder; Zhuling depletes the water from the urine bladder. If a lady feels swollen hands and feet in the morning, it is Wu Ling San condition. If a senior feel swelling in the face and hands in the morning and is thirsty, it is also Wu Ling San condition.

the patient will have continuous vomiting and diarrhea. [249]

(7) 发汗后，饮水多，必喘；以水灌之，亦喘。

After Sweating therapy, if drinking too much water, the patient will have pant (shortness of breath). [250] With a water shower, [251] the patient will also have shortness of breath (pant). [252]

(8) 服 桂枝 汤，大汗出，脉洪大者，与 桂枝 汤如前法；若形如疟，日再发者，汗出必解，宜 桂枝 二 麻黄 一汤。

After drinking Guizhi Tang, there is profuse sweat, and the pulse remains big-surge. [253]

---

[249] The patient has difficulty urinating before becoming sick this time. Heavy Sweating therapy stirs the inner accumulated water. If using Sweating therapy again, the patient will have continuous vomiting and diarrhea.

[250] Too much water in the stomach prevents the movement of the diaphragm, causing shortness of breath.

[251] This is true if the patient uses an ice bag while having a fever and sweating. These ways can prevent the release of Fire from the body. The Fire is entangled inside the lung and causes shortness of breath.

[252] Dr. Ni Haixia: Use Wu Ling San for treatment.

Dr. Ke Yunbo (柯韵伯): For asthma without any treatment, use Mahuang Tang. For asthma that occurs after Purging therapy, use Guizhi with Houpo and Xingzi Tang. For asthma with sweat, use Gegen Qin Lian Tang. If asthma occurs after drinking lots of water, use Wu Ling San for treatment.

[253] Dr. Hu Xishu: In the original text the pulse is "big-surge". If the pulse feels big, and if the patient has heavy sweating and feels very thirsty, the disease may have moved into the Yangming stage. Therefore, Guizhi Tang is recommended, so that the pulse should be "floating", not "big-surge".

Dr. Liu Duzhou: After the use of Guizhi Tang, the pulse changed to big-surge, but the symptoms did not change yet. The pulse suggests that the body Yang Qi is still dominant on the body surface, there is a kind of up-rushing feeling so that the Guizhi Tang can be used again. Because of the pulse, the Guizhi Tang condition needs to be distinguished from Baihu Tang condition. In Baihu Tang condition, the pulse is also big-surge.

Dr. Hao Wanshan: The pulse is big-surge, and the patient has heavy sweating, similar to Yangming body surface condition, but the patient has no thirst,

Use Guizhi Tang again as before. [254] If the patient experiences the same symptoms as malaria (sometimes feverish and sometimes cold) again and again during the day at a fixed time, [255] Sweating therapy would solve the disease condition. Use Guizhi Two Mahuang One Tang. [256]

1.9 Wrong treatment of Taiyang stage

The principle way to solve the disease condition in the Taiyang stage is to create sweating. Let the invading pathogenic Qi leave the body through the sweat. The extent of the perspiration has to be controlled at a proper level: not too much or too little. If the sweating is not sufficient, the pathogenic Qi can penetrate deeper into the Yangming stage, but over-sweat can also cause various more troubles.

(1) 桂枝本为解肌，若其人脉浮紧，发热汗不出者，不可与之也，常需识此，勿令误也。

The function of the Guizhi Tang is to release the muscle. (Its aim is not to create sweating, though it will make the skin wet.) If the pulse feels floating-tight, and the patient has a fever and no sweats, (e.g., the symptoms and the pulse indicate Cold-attack Shanghan disease,) the Guizhi Tang should not be used. This is a general principle. Always keep this principle in mind. [257]

---

therefore the disease condition is not the Yangming stage but remains still in the Taiyang stage.

[254] Usually, after sweating, the pulse should be deeper and becomes soft to the touch. Now, the sweat is strong, but the pulse is big, suggesting that the invading disease is not entirely removed from the body yet. The body is activating its defense system to counteract the disease, so the pulse is big. Guizhi Tang will help the body to do the last expelling work.

[255] Dr. Hao Wanshan: The alternating fever-chills cycle occurs twice a day (not several times). This condition should also display a red face and itchy skin, though it is not written here.

[256] This formula means to take two parts Guizhi Tang and one part of Mahuang Tang. Mix them to drink.

[257] There are nourishing and contracting herbs in the Guizhi Tang. It is a Warm herbal formula. Its capacity to create sweat is weak. If it is used in the Cold-attack

(For the same reason, Guizhi Tang should not be used for Warm diseases or Wind-Warm diseases.)

(2)　　本发汗而复下之，此为逆也；若先发汗，治不为逆。本先下之，而反汗之为逆；若先下之，治不为逆。

If a disease condition is supposed to be treated with a Sweating therapy, but a Purging therapy is used, this is wrong. (If there is both Taiyang body surface condition and Yangming body inner condition,) Use Sweating therapy first, then the Purging therapy. If a condition (inner condition alone) is supposed to be treated with a Purging therapy, but a Sweating therapy is used, it is also a mistake. If there is both body surface condition and Yangming inner bowel condition, use the Purging therapy first, then use Sweating therapy to treat the body surface condition.[258]

(3)　　太阳病，外证未解者，不可下也，下之为逆。欲解外者，宜 桂枝 汤主之。

In the Taiyang stage, body surface condition remains (there is also body inner Yangming stage), the Purging therapy should not be used. To solve the body surface condition, use Guizhi Tang.[259]

(4)　　太阳病，下之后，其气上冲者，可与桂枝汤，方如前法，若不上冲者，不得与之。

In the Taiyang stage, Purging therapy is used (by mistake). A patient feels an uprushing feeling inside the body.[260] Use Guizhi Tang for treatment.[261] If there is no uprushing feeling, it should not be used.

(5)　　太阳病，先发汗不解，而复下之，脉浮者不愈。浮为在外，而反下之，故令不愈。今脉浮，故知在外，当须解外则愈，宜 桂枝 汤主之。

In the Taiyang stage, Sweating therapy created sweating but the disease remains. So a Purging therapy follows. The pulse is still floating, suggesting that the disease is not to get better, because a floating pulse indicates that the disease is still on the body surface.

---

stage, sweating becomes more difficult, and the warmth from the Guizhi Tang can increase the Fire in the body, to bring the disease into the deeper Da Qinglong Tang condition.

　Dr. Ni Haixia: Guizhi Tang increases blood circulation in muscles, not in the skin. More blood in the muscle reduces the amount of blood in the chest, so the patient could feel annoyed, feel pressure in the chest and shortness of breath.

[258] Dr. Hu Xishu: In clinics, there is no case with both body surface condition and Yangming body inner condition that requires Purging therapy first and then Sweating therapy. If a reason to use Purging therapy is strong and reasonable, the body Surface condition is no longer present.

[259] In the Taiyang-Yangming concurrent condition, the principle is to treat the body surface condition first. The most important symptom indicating body surface condition is the feeling of aversion to cold. If there is such an aversion feeling, Purging therapy should not be used.

[260] Dr. Hao Wanshan: The uprushing feeling here should be understood as the remaining pathogenic Qi in the body surface, so the pulse should be floating. It means the mechanism, not the symptom. Otherwise, if it is Lung Qi uprushing, the patient should have coughing or panting. If it is Stomach Qi uprushing, the patient should feel nauseous and vomit. But these symptoms are not mentioned here.

[261] Under normal conditions, the body defense Qi is moving up to the body surface. Purging therapy tends to suppress and bring down the defense Qi. If the down-moving force is powerful, it will cause the defense Qi to shrink. Now the down-moving force causes a rebound of the defense Qi, moving up to the body surface so that the patient feels the up-rushing feeling and Guizhi Tang can still be used.

　Dr. Ni Haixia: Purging therapy tends to bring blood downwards to the colon. The stronger the downwards force, the stronger the rebound force of the bloodstream to the heart to make the patient feel the up-rushing feeling. If there is no upwards rebound, it means that the body Qi has been damaged and is too weak.

　In such inner weak condition, Guizhi Tang should not be used. One of the principles in the use of Guizhi Tang (or herbal formulas that work to solve body surface condition) is that it should not be used if the body inner side is weak. However, if there is both body Surface condition and the inner Yangming condition (such as constipation for several days), we can mix the Surface-releasing therapy and Purging therapy into the same formula.

The Purging therapy should not be used, but it is used so that the disease condition is not to get better. Now the pulse remains floating, knowing that the disease is still on the body surface side. For such a case, the treatment now should focus on to solve the body surface condition. Use Guizhi Tang is as the primary treatment.

(6)　　　伤寒医下之，续得下利，清谷不止，身疼痛者，急当救里；后身疼痛，清便自调者，急当救表。救里宜四逆汤；救表宜桂枝 汤。

In Cold-attack Taiyang stage, a Purging therapy was used by mistake. A patient starts to have constant diarrhea with non-digested food in stool and still has generalized pain in the body. The principle of the treatment should be to treat the inner (Shaoyin) condition first. Use Si Ni Tang. After the release of the inner condition (the bowel movement return normal), and if the body pain remains, use Guizhi Tang to solve the body surface condition. [262]

(7)　　　脉浮紧者，法当身疼痛，宜以汗解之。假令尺中迟者，不可发汗。何以知之然？以荣气不足，血少故也。

If the pulse feels floating and tight, the patient should feel generalized pain in the body. Such a condition should be treated with a Sweating therapy. However, if the pulse feels floating and tight but also slow at the Chi position, the Sweating therapy should not be used. The reason is that the slow pulse indicates that the body has inadequate nutrient Qi, which is again due to insufficient blood (e.g., it is an inner weakness condition).

(8)　　　伤寒脉浮，自汗出，小便数，心烦，微恶寒，脚挛急，反与桂枝汤，欲攻其表，此误也。得之便厥，咽中干，烦燥吐逆者，作甘草干姜汤与之，以复其阳；若厥愈、足温者，更作芍药甘草汤与之，其脚即伸；若胃气不和，谵语者，少与调胃承气汤；若重发汗，复加烧针者，四逆汤主之。

In Cold-attack Taiyang stage, the pulse feels floating, the patient sweats and frequently urinates, is annoyed, feels a slight aversion to cold, and the calf spasms. [263] Guizhi Tang was used to solving the body surface condition. This remedy is wrong. [264] With such a treatment, the patient will have cold hands and feet (Jue condition), [265] feel dry in the throat, [266] feel much more annoyed [267] and even have jumping arms or legs (restlessness). For such a situation, use Gancao Ganjiang Tang to restore the body Yang Qi. [268] If the Jue condition is solved and the feet become warm, use Shaoyao Gancao Tang to stop the calf spasms. If Stomach Qi is in disharmony, the patient still has delirious speech, use a little Tiaowei Chengqi Tang to harmonize the Stomach. [269] If the patient was treated with repeated Sweating therapy and Fire acupuncture, the clinical condition should be treated by using Si Ni Tang as the first formula. [270]

(9)　　　伤寒，若吐，若下后，七八日不解，(热结在里)，表里俱热，时时恶风，大渴，舌上干燥而烦，欲饮水数升者，白虎加人参汤主之，

---

[262] Dr. Ni Haixia: The misuse of Purging therapy in the Taiyang stage may cause Hotness-diarrhea or Coldness-diarrhea. For the former, use Gegen Qin Lian Tang. For the latter, use Si Ni Tang for treatment. If a person usually has a poor digestive function, it could be Coldness-diarrhea. If the digestive function is strong, it could be Hotness-diarrhea.

[263] Dr. Ni Haixia: The annoyed feeling and chills are signs indicating that the body liquid is insufficient. The use of Guizhi Tang can cause further depletion of body liquid. For such a chilly feeling, the patient feels cold from the inner side of the body. It is different from the chilly feeling on the body surface in the Cold-attack stage.

[264] Dr. Ni Haixia: In this case, use Guizhi with Fuzi Tang.

[265] Cold hands and feet: There is insufficient liquid and Yang Qi to be transported to the feet and hands.

[266] *Dry in the throat*: Due to insufficient inner liquid.

[267] Inner Yang Qi is floating up due to insufficient liquid to hold it.

[268] Dr. Ni Haixia: Dried ginger and Zhigancao work to improve Spleen Yang Qi, so the body becomes warm.

[269] Dr. Ni Haixia: When body liquid is insufficient, food becomes attached to mucus in the stomach. Bad odor air will move up to the brain, affecting brain function and causing delirious speech.

[270] Dr. Ni Haixia: This paragraph says that if a patient has had a liquid deficiency, be careful not to use Guizhi Tang for the treatment. Such a weakness condition can be identified in many ways, such as the tongue is thick. The thicker the tongue is, the weaker the body liquid is.

In Cold-attack Taiyang stage, after Vomiting therapy or Purging therapy, the body condition was not improved for seven to eight days, (this is Hot entangled inside the body). The patient still feels fever in both inside and outside of the body, an aversion to wind from time to time,[271] is very thirsty, has a dry mouth, feels annoyed and willing to drink liters of water.[272] In this case, use Baihu Jia Renshen Tang as the primary treatment.[273]

───────────────

[271] Dr. Hao Wanshan: Fire exhausted the Qi, and there is insufficient Qi to seal (to protect) the body surface. Also, because of the heavy sweating, the sweat holes are open. The body cannot tolerate wind. This is the same reason that the body feels chilly on the back in the Baihu Pus Renshen Tang condition.

[272] Dr. Hao Wanshan: Fire exhausts the body Qi. Without sufficient Qi, the water cannot be evaporated into micro-water to be transported (by the spleen) to the body tissue and to the tongue, so the thirsty feeling remains unimproved even with heavy drinking.

[273] Da Qinglong Tang is also for Hotness in both body surface and inside during Taiyang stage. However, there is more Hotness in the surface and less on the inside, so the person does not feel very thirsty. Baihu Tang is used for heat/fever in the body surface and inside condition during the Yangming stage, and because there is more Hotness inside, the person feels thirsty. Here, the patient feels hot, thirsty, sweaty, and aversion to wind, all suggesting that the disease is in both Taiyang (e.g. aversion to wind) and Yangming stages, so Baihu Jia Genshen Tang is used. The addition of Ginseng (Renshen) is to improve the defense system and to nourish the Stomach Qi to supply more body liquid.

This syndrome can be regarded as a Taiyang-Yangming concurrent condition. Due to the heavy loss of body liquid, saving body liquid is urgent, so use Baihu Jia Genshen Tang to save it first. A similar condition is Taiyang-Taiyin concurrent condition, or Taiyang-Shaoyin concurrent condition, in which the diarrhea is so severe so that it is needed to solve Taiyin or Shaoyin first, then the body surface condition.

Dr. Ni Haixia: If there is gourmet powder in food, people could feel thirsty and want to drink lots of water. This is also the case for the Baihu Tang condition. The herb Ginseng works to nourish the body with liquid.

(10)　发汗吐下后，虚烦不得眠，若剧者，必反复颠倒，心中懊侬，栀子豉汤主之；若少气者，栀子甘草豉汤主之。若呕者，栀子生姜豉汤主之。

After Sweating therapy, Vomiting therapy or Purging therapy, a patient feels annoyed and feels difficult to fall asleep. In a severe case, the patient feels very agitated and difficult to have a rest physically and emotionally.[274] Use formula Zhizi Chi Tang as primary treatment.[275] If the patient also feels shortness of breath,[276] use Zhizi Gancao Chi Tang.[277] If

───────────────

[274] The annoyed feeling and the agitated feeling are because of the entangled inner Fire in the chest. All of these symptoms are due to the sinking of body surface Fire in the body, due to the previous Sweating therapy, Vomiting therapy or Purging therapy.

[275] The earlier doctor said that this herbal formula might cause vomiting.

Dr. Hu Xishu: I have used this herbal formula my whole life to many patients. I have never seen a case of vomiting after drinking this herbal tea.

Dr. Liu Duzhou: This formula sometimes causes vomiting and sometimes not. If vomiting occurs, it can be regarded as a healing crisis, because after nausea and/or diarrhea, the disease may subside.

Dr. Ni Haixia: The herb Zhizi clears deficient Fire, and the Fire is mostly in the chest. The herb Shigao clears excessive Fire. In the deficient Fire condition, the tongue coating is slightly yellow, and the pulse feels weak upon applying hard pressure. In the excessive Fire condition, the tongue coating is yellow and dry and the pulse feels strong and big. Zhizi Chi Tang is used in the later stage of Warm diseases after Sweating therapy, Vomiting therapy or Purging therapy. The Warm disease easily exhausts body liquid and leaves a small bit of pathogenic Qi (virus) in the body. The patient feels hot in the afternoon or at night on the hands and feet, has a poor sleep and feels annoyed. Zhizi Chi Tang can also occur in Cold-attack diseases after Sweating therapy and if the patient eats meat.

[276] Dr. Ni Haixia: The original text should be understood as weakness in the arms and legs. If the poor sleep is due to Blood deficiency, use moxibustion on the Sanmao point (on the back of big toe).

[277] Dr. Ni Haixia: Zhizi Gancao Chi Tang can treat gastric diseases arising because the patient ate old food, dirty food, or corrupt food. The patient feels

the patient is nauseous, use Zhizi Shenjiang Chi Tang as the primary treatment.

(11)　　　发汗、若下之而烦热，胸中窒者，栀子豉汤主之。

After Sweating therapy or Purging therapy, a patient feels annoyingly hot and feels discomfort in the esophagus (middle part of the torso). Use Zhizi Chi Tang as the primary treatment.

(12)　　　伤寒下后，心烦、腹满、卧起不安者，栀子厚朴汤主之。

In Cold-attack Taiyang stage, after Purging therapy, a patient feels annoyed, fullness in the abdomen, irritated, so much so that it is difficult to sleep. In such a case, use Zhizi Houpo Tang as the primary treatment.[278]

(13)　　　伤寒，医以丸药大下之，身热不去，微烦者，栀子干姜汤主之。

In Cold-attack Taiyang stage, after Purging therapy (with herb pills), a patient feels continuously hot, mildly annoyed, (and has diarrhea,). In such a case, use Zhizi Ganjiang Tang as the primary treatment.[279]

(14)　　　伤寒，五六日，大下之后，身热不去，心中结痛者，未欲解也，栀子豉汤主之。

In Cold-attack Taiyang stage for five to six days and after an intensive Purging therapy, a patient feels continuously hot, feels knot-pain in the front left chest (the region of the heart).[280] Such a disease condition indicates that the disease is not going to recover. Use Zhizi Chi Tang as the primary treatment.[281]

(15)　　　凡用栀子汤，病人旧微溏者，不可与服之。

In the use of Zhizi-containing herbal formulas, if a patient has a history of mild diarrhea (or loose stool), these formulas should not be given.[282]

---

discomfort in the stomach and vomits. If there is both vomiting and diarrhea, use Gegen Qin Lian Tang.

[278] After Purging therapy, and if the patient feels fullness in the stomach but is not annoyed, if the reason is accumulation of a Hotness in the stomach, Da Chengqi Tang is required. If it is caused by an attack of Cold in the stomach, Hou Jiang Xia Cao Renshen Tang is required. If the patient feels annoyed but no such fullness in the stomach, if it is due to Hotness in the chest, Zhuye Shigao Tang is the best choice. If there is nausea, the herb formula Zhizi Chi Tang is the best choice. If the patient feels both fullness and annoyance, Zhizi Houpo Tang is the best choice.

Dr. Ni Haixia: Houpo can move Dampness out of the Spleen, lubricate the stool, and remove farts from the body. Zhishi can peel off stool that is tightly adhered to the walls of the bowel. It can also work similarly on the chest, the blood vessels, and gallbladder, to remove inner substances. It can open the blood vessel between the heart and the small intestine, to improve bowel movement.

[279] In one book version, it is Zhizi Ganjiang Tang. The use of dried ginger (Ganjiang) suggests that there is

Coldness condition inside. This is a Hotness-Coldness co-existing condition.

Dr. Ni Haixia: Dried ginger can warm up the digestive system and restore the warm temperature of the stomach and intestine. The tongue must be thin and white, the pulse weak. Fresh ginger works to remove Coldness, but cannot warm up the digestive system. To warm up the chest and upper abdomen, use dried ginger; to warm up the lower abdomen, use Fuzi.

[280] Dr. Martin Wang: I suspect that the location of the pain should be in the stomach region, not the left chest.

[281] In another version of the book, the herb formula for this condition is Zhizi Chi Tang.

[282] There are many ways to create the vomiting effect to remove the disease from the stomach and chest area, not only Zhizi Chi Tang. In clinics, it is necessary to identify the reasons for the fullness feeling in the stomach and chest: Coldness, Hotness, Food, Water, Phlegm, or stagnated Qi. If the reason is Coldness, dried ginger and Guipi should be used. If it is due to Hotness, use Zhizi Ku Cha (栀子苦茶). If it is due to accumulation of Food, formula Pingwei San is the choice. If it is due to a retained Water, Wu Ling San and fresh ginger are used. If it is due to Phlegm, orange peel is the choice. And if it is due to stagnated Qi, Zhishi and Houpo are the most widely used herbs. For patients with weak body condition, other herbs that work to support the middle Qi are added. If the body is strong, Guadi and Lilou are added too.

Dr. Liu Duzhou: If Zhizi Chi Tang is really needed for patients with a history of diarrhea, the herbal formula can be used with a low dosage, or with the addition of dried ginger in the formula.

(16)　　太阳病，外证未除，而数下之，遂协热而利，利下不止，心下痞鞕，表里不解者，桂枝人参汤主之。

In the Taiyang stage, the body surface condition remains, but a Purging therapy has been used repeatedly several times. The pathogenic Qi penetrates with the heat downwards to cause diarrhea. The patient has frequent diarrhea and feels fullness and hardness in the upper abdomen. If the body surface condition remains, use Guizhi Renshen Tang as the primary treatment. [283]

(17)　　太阳病，桂枝 证，医反下之，利遂不止，脉促者，表未解也。喘而汗出者，葛根黄连黄芩 汤主之。

In the Taiyang stage with Guizhi Tang condition, a Purging therapy was used, however. It caused constant diarrhea. The pulse feels rapid-irregular,[284] indicating that the body surface condition remains.[285] If the patient feels panting and sweats, use Gegen Huangqin Huanglian Tang as the primary treatment.

(18)　　太阳病，下之后，脉促胸满者，桂枝 去芍药汤主之。若微恶寒者，去芍药方中，加 附子 汤主之。

In the Taiyang stage, after Purging therapy, the pulse feels floating at the Cun position but deep at the Chi position,[286] and the patient feels fullness in the chest. Use Guizhi Qui Shaoyao Tang as the primary treatment.[287] If the patient feels an aversion to

---

Dr. Ni Haixia: If Zhizi Chi Tang is required, but the stool is loose, add herb Baizhu, Fuling and dried ginger to warm up the middle part of the body and to remove the Dampness from the digestive system.

[283] If in this situation, the pulse is not weak, Gancao Xiexin Tang can be considered.

Dr. Hao Wanshan: This is Spleen deficiency diarrhea (coldness-weakness diarrhea). It is not hotness diarrhea.

Dr. Ni Haixia: Guizhi Renshen Tang works for Coldness-weakness diarrhea. Here the condition should not be Guizhi Renshen Tang condition. Baizhu can remove Dampness from the spleen, to lubricate the bowels to solve constipation and to adjust the bowel movement.

[284] The *rapid-irregular pulse* here might be better understood as floating at the Cun position but deep at the Chi position (see below).

[285] Dr. Hao Wanshan: We usually do not regard the rapid-irregular pulse as the indication for body surface condition. The rapid pulse here should be fast and strong, not fast and weak.

Dr. Ni Haixia: Purging therapy makes the blood move down to the intestine rigorously. This makes the pulse feel fast with short breaks from time to time. Here Purging therapy brings the pathogenic Qi deeper into the digestive system. Gegen Tang alone is not suitable for treatment.

Dr. Martin Wang: This disease condition should be regarded as Taiyang-Yangming successive

condition, with less Taiyang but more Yangming condition. It is Fire-Dampness condition in the Yangming. For the treatment, both the Taiyang and the Yangming stages need to be taken into consideration. Note that if diarrhea occurs without treatment, then the Hotness diarrhea is treated with Gegen Tang. If it is due to the use of Purging therapy, the Hotness diarrhea is treated with Gegen Huangqin Huanglian Tang.

[286] Dr. Hu Xishu: The original Chinese text for the pulse here is "rapid-irregular pulse". However the pulse should be understood as the pulse being close to the Cun position (since the Qi is rushing up into the chest), and that it feels deep in the Chi position (since the Purging therapy depletes the inner Yang Qi and makes the abdomen area weak). Therefore the pulse matches the clinical condition: the chest is excessive, but the abdomen is deficient (weak). Shaoyao is usually used with bloating in the abdomen in excessive condition, but not in deficient condition.

Dr. Liu Duzhou: The pulse here should be understood as a fast pulse.

[287] The herb Shaoyao is sour and contracting. It will further suppress the Heart Yang Qi to cause more bloating feeling in the chest. Whenever there is chest bloating, Shaoyao should be omitted. It is, however, used more with abdomen bloating, if the bloating is caused by Spleen Yin deficiency.

Dr. Liu Duzhou: This formula can be used for patients with bloating and pain in the chest (may or may not be coronary heart disease), if the disease condition belongs to chest Yang Qi deficiency.

Dr. Ni Haixia: Purging therapy can bring the blood downwards and increase the return of more blood to the heart via veins so that the patient feels fullness in the chest. Shaoyao can increase the blood returning via the veins to make things worse, so it is omitted from Guizhi Tang.

cold slightly,[288] add herb Fuzi in this formula.[289]

(19)　太阳病，下之微喘者，表未解故也。桂枝 加 厚朴 杏仁汤主之。

In the Taiyang stage, after Purging therapy, a patient has slight panting. This situation means that the body surface condition remains. Use Guizhi Jia Houpo Xingzi Tang as the primary treatment.[290]

(This formula is also useful for patients who usually have asthma.[291])

(20)　伤寒若吐若下后，心下逆满，气上冲胸，起则头眩，脉沉紧，发汗则动经，身为振振摇者，茯苓桂枝白术甘草 汤主之。

In Cold-attack Taiyang stage, after Vomiting therapy,[292] or Purging therapy, a patient feels up-reverse floating in the upper abdomen, an uprushing feeling to the chest, and feels dizziness when the body gets up, and the pulse feels deep and tight. In such a case, the use of Sweating therapy would disturb the Qi movement in meridians, and the body will shake, and the muscles will tremor.[293] For such a situation, use Fuling Guizhi Baishu Gancao Tang as the primary treatment.

(21)　问曰：病有结胸，有藏结，其状何如？答曰：按之痛，寸脉浮，关脉沉，名曰结胸也。何谓藏结？答曰：如结胸状，饮食如故，时时下利，寸脉浮，关脉小细沉紧，名曰藏结。舌上白胎滑者，难治。

Ask: Disease can have Chest-bind and Organ-bind syndromes. What is their difference?

Answer: Feels pain when pressed, pulse feels floating on the Cun position but deep on Guan position. This condition is called Chest-bind syndrome.[294] For the Organ-bind

---

[288] Dr. Hu Xishu: The body feels slightly cold, similar to Guizhi with Fuzi Tang. However, it is not the "cold-dislike" feeling.

Dr. Hao Wanshan: The pulse is tiny, and the body feels chilly. Adding Fuzi means that the body has Kidney deficiency, so the pulse must be tiny and weak. The cold-dislike feeling means that the body Yang Qi is weak. These two formulas are commonly used in the treatment of coronary heart disease that onset during the night or in cold weather.

[289] Improper use of Purging therapy in this Taiyang stage will deplete the body Yang Qi, so the patient feels bloating in the chest with a faster pulse. The dislike-cold feeling suggests the depletion is too much, so Fuzi should be added.

[290] For panting or asthma in the Cold-attack Taiyang stage, this formula works well. If the patient has asthma and diarrhea, Gegen Huangqin Huanglian Tang is considered.

[291] Persons with a long history of asthma are called Asthma persons.

[292] Dr. Ni Haixia: Vomiting therapy can also be used in the treatment of stroke. The patient has lots of phlegm that blocks breathing. For acupuncture, use needle on the Tiantu (CV22) point (on the upper edge of the sternum). With the herbal therapy, let the patient drink herbal tea. The patient could have frequent vomiting, spitting up the phlegm and the herbal tea. Repeat the drink, until no more phlegm and herbal tea is being vomited.

Dr. Martin: If the patient is in an unconscious, use the gastric pipe (catheter).

[293] This is a condition with garbage water in the upper abdomen. The Vomiting therapy and the Purging therapy cause the water up-rush. In a severe case, use formula Zhenwu Tang.

Dr. Ni Haixia: Patients who suffer from this condition are those who have had water accumulation in the diaphragm before becoming sick this time or those who usually drink water very fast, and it results in accumulation of water in the diaphragm. The water in the diaphragm prevents the diaphragm from moving up and down and causes shortness of breath. The water shakes and waves along with the movement of the body, causing dizziness. (If the dizziness occurs when the patient lies down quietly on the bed, it might be the Zhenwu Tang condition). Baizhu removes the Dampness (water) from the diaphragm. Fuling removes the water from the body via urine. If the dizziness is severe, add herb Banxia to this formula. The muscles, blood vessels, and nerves need water for nourishment. The Sweating therapy depleted the water and caused spasms in the muscles. This formula can also be used for patients who usually have muscle spasms for seconds or jumping eyelids.

[294] Chest-bind syndrome: This is caused by the wrong use of Purging therapy which brought the pathogenic Qi (Fire) deep into the body, and the pathogenic Qi entangled with phlegm (and water) up and down the diaphragm. The patient feels the hardness in the upper abdomen and feels pain upon being pressed

syndrome, the symptoms are similar to the Chest-bind, but the patient has a regular diet, has diarrhea from time to time. Pulse is floating on the Cun position, but small, thin, deep and tight on the Chi position. Such condition is called Organ-bind syndrome. For

this syndrome, if the tongue coating is white-slippery, the syndrome is difficult to treat.

(22)　藏结无阳证，不往来寒热，一云寒而不热，其人反静，舌上胎滑者，不可攻也。

In Organ-bind syndrome, there is no Yang condition (e.g., without body surface condition), or alternating fever-cold.[295] If the patient is however quiet,[296] the tongue coating is slippery. Purging therapy should not be used.[297]

(23)　病胁下素有痞，连在脐旁，痛引少腹入筋者，此名藏结，死。

A Patient often has a bloated feeling on the flank region,[298] the bloating feeling expands to the side of the navel, the pain expands to the lower abdomen and then to the sexual organs, and the pain causes the sexual organs to shrink into the abdomen (Organ-contracting syndrome).[299] Such conditions

---

there. The pulse feels floating in the Cun position but deep in the Chi position on the wrist. The patient cannot eat. This syndrome should be understood as the pathogenic Qi shrinking into the Shaoyang stage because the place up and down the diaphragm belongs to Shaoyang.

Dr. Du Yumao: The entanglement condition occurs with diseases involving the upper abdomen, the gallbladder, stomach, and intestine, and is not at all inside the chest, or not at all above the diaphragm. According to the location of Chest-bind syndrome, the diseases should belong to the Yangming stage. If the disease locates above the diaphragm, it is Shi Zao Tang condition.

If a patient has a long history of fullness and bloated feeling in the flank region, and the bloating feeling spreads to the navel, the pain spreads to the lower abdomen and into the genitals, it is also a kind of Organ-bind condition (syndrome). The patient may die. This kind of Organ-bind syndrome refers to cancer or a benign tumor in the abdomen (for example in the liver or spleen). Therefore, the Chest-bind syndrome, the Pi condition (syndrome) and the Organ-bind syndrome need to be identified carefully.

Dr. Hu Xishu: Organ-bind syndrome occurs when Purging therapy is used by mistake in the Yin stages, such as in the Taiyin, Shaoyin, and Jueyin stages, while the Chest-bind syndrome occurs when the Purging therapy is used too early in the three Yang stages, such as in the Taiyang, Shaoyang and Yangming stages.

Dr. Liu Duzhou: Organ-bind syndrome also occurs due to wrong treatment in the Taiyang stage with Purging therapy, which brings the Cold deeper inside the body and the Cold is entangled (or folded) with the inner organs.

Chest-bind syndrome can be seen in acute peritonitis.

Dr. Hao Wanshan: Chest-bind syndrome can be seen in patients with acute peritoneal irritation symptoms. This syndrome is different from Da Chaihu Tang condition (most of the time the latter is acute cholecystitis, localized gastric perforation) and Yangming inner condition (the most time various intestinal obstructions cause the Yangming disease condition).

---

[295] *No alternating fever-cold:* This means that the condition does not belong to the Shaoyang stage. Also, there is *diarrhea from time to time:* This suggests that the condition does not belong to the Yangming stage either (in the Yangming stage, there should be constipation). Therefore, the Organ-bind syndrome belongs to the Yin stages (Taiyin, Shaoyin, and Jueyin stages).

In one version of the Shanghan Lun, it said: "there is cold but not hot".

[296] *The patient is quiet:* this means that the condition does not belong to Zhizi Chi Tang condition.

[297] Dr. Liu Duzhou: For the treatment of Organ-bind syndrome, some doctors suggest using Lizhong Tang with Zhishi.

[298] Dr. Hao Wanshan: The bloated feeling is due to either enlarged spleen or enlarged liver.

[299] Dr. Hao Wanshan: Orgain-contracting syndrome can happen without Organ-bind. It can be caused by swimming in cold water or by sexual activity, for example. For organ-contracting syndrome that is not due to the Organ-bind, use moxibustion on Huiyin (CV1), Guanyuan (CV4) and Qihai (CV6) points.

Dr. Ni Haixia: This Contracting condition is a hernia. If the patient has a history of a hernia and then catches a common cold, it is a dangerous situation because blood circulation during the common cold becomes even worse and results in death. However, with proper acupuncture, it is not so

are called Organ-bind syndrome. The patient will die.

(24)　病发于阳而反下之，热入，因作结胸；病发于阴而反下之，一作汗出，因作痞。所以成结胸者，以下之太早故也。

A disease started from the Yang, but a Purging therapy is used, the Heat so invades deeper to cause the Chest-bind syndrome. A disease started from the Yin, but a Purging therapy is used,[300] so to create the Pi syndrome. The reason for the Chest-bind syndrome is due to the Purging remedy is applied too early.[301]

(25)　结胸者，项亦强，如柔痉状。下之则和，宜大陷胸丸方。

Chest-bind syndrome means that the patient also feels tightness in the nape,[302] similar to Soft-tetany (柔痉) syndrome. Use Purging

therapy for conciliation. Use Da Xianxiong Wan.[303]

(26)　结胸证，其脉浮大者，不可下，下之则死。结胸证悉具，烦躁者，亦死。

In Chest-bind syndrome, if the pulse feels big and floating, Purging therapy should not be used. Otherwise, the patient will die.[304] If the patient has clear evidence for the Chest-bind syndrome and the patient also feels annoyed and restless in the arms and legs,[305] the patient will die too.

---

dangerous. Do acupuncture on Dadun (LV1) point (Liver meridian) and use formula Danggui Si Ni Tang.

Dr. Ni Haixia: Organ-bind syndrome means that Cold and Dampness entangle the networks that contact the inner solid organs (epiploon). The hollow organs are normal, but nutrition cannot be distributed to the solid organs. The solid organs become withered and finally lose function (such as liver failure or kidney failure). The tongue coating is thick and white and slippery, the face seems to have a thin layer of yellow-dark dust, the patient looks inactive and quiet, and the pulse is deep-tight. For treatment, use Chaihu (15g), Baizhu (15g), Fuling (15g), Pao Fuzi (9g) and Fuzi (30g).

[300] In one version of Shanghhan Lun, it said: "Disease started from the Yin, but Sweating therapy was used".

[301] Dr. Ni Haixia: If there is body surface condition, and if Purging therapy is used in a strong person, there will be the Chest-bind syndrome. If it is used on a weak person (the digestive system is weak), there will be Pi syndrome.

Dr. Liao Houze: Whenever the abdomen becomes hard during treatment, quickly change to warm herbal therapy to correct the Pi syndrome. Use Guizhi Tang, Guizhi with Dahuang Tang, or Mahuang Fuzi Xixin Tang.

[302] Be careful. The stiff nape in Taiyang stage needs to be distinguished from Chest-bind condition.

[303] Note: Da Xianxiong Tang and Da Xianxiong Wan are different formulas. Both belong to Purging therapy (similar to Da Chaihu Tang and various Chengqi Tang).

Dr. Ni Haixia: If there is fever, use Da Xianxiong Tang, if there is no fever, use Da Xianxiong Wan. For Da Xianxiong Tang condition, the hardness and pain in the upper stomach go from the upper abdomen down to the lower abdomen, while in the Da Xianxiong Wan syndrome, the hardness and pain go from the upper abdomen up to the chest. Da Xianxiong Wan can also be used to treat obstacle pain in the back and shoulder.

[304] Floating pulse suggests that there is still body Surface condition (the pathogenic Qi is still in the body surface). The use of Xianxiong Wan will further bring the pathogenic Qi in and make the entanglement condition worse. This formula must be used when the pulse feels deep and tight (no body surface condition). It is very crucial to control the proper time to use this herbal formula. (Similar caution as in the use of Da Chengqi Tang).

Dr. Hao Wanshan: The floating-big pulse here does not indicate the presence of body surface condition. It is a sign of body Yang Qi floating, a very severe condition that results in death. For floating-big pulse, it should feel hollow-like and weak when pressing harder.

Dr. Ni Haixia: For Chest-bind syndrome, the pulse should be deep-tight. The floating pulse suggests that the body Yang Qi is floating. It is a dangerous condition. Da Xianxiong Tang can still be used, but it is necessary to explain to the patient and their family members about the risk.

Dr. Liao Houze: In this case, use Chaihu Guizhi Tang for treatment.

[305] Dr. Hao Wanshan: The annoyed feeling and the restless condition are no longer due to Fire in the Chest-bind syndrome, but because the body Yang Qi

(27)　　太阳病，脉浮而动数，浮则为风，数则为热，动则为痛，数则为虚，头痛发热，微盗汗出而反恶寒者，表未解也。医反下之，动数变迟，膈内拒痛一云：头痛即眩，胃中空虚，客气动膈，短气躁烦，心中懊憹，阳气内陷，心下因硬，则为结胸，大陷胸汤主之。若不结胸，但头汗出，余处无汗，剂颈而还，小便不利，身必发黄也。

In the Taiyang stage, the pulse feels floating, agitated (jumping feeling) and fast. The floating means Wind; the fast means Heat; the agitated pulse means pain and the fast also means deficiency. The patient has a headache and fever, slightly sweats at night, and feels an aversion to cold. Such a situation indicates that the body surface condition remains.[306] In this case, Purging therapy should not be used, but it is however used. The agitated-fast pulse turns slow,[307] the patient feels pain upon press the upper abdomen. (In one version, it said that the patient feels dizziness once has a headache.) The Purging therapy caused a deficiency in the stomach, the pathogenic Qi so invaded to disturb diaphragm, resulting in shortness of breath, agitated feeling, restless, vexation. Due to the shrink of Yang Qi inside, the upper abdomen becomes hardness to cause Chest-bind syndrome. Use Da Xianxiong

Tang for the treatment).[308] If the Chest-bind syndrome does not occur, and the patient sweats only on the head (not in any other part of the body below the neck),[309] and has difficulty urinating, there will be Jaundice.[310]

(28)　　伤寒六七日，结胸热实，脉沉而紧，心下痛，按之石硬者，大陷胸汤主之。

In Cold-attack Taiyang stage for about six to seven days, a patient has Chest-bind syndrome (Hotness, Excess), the pulse feels deep and tight, the patient feels pain in the upper abdomen. The upper abdomen feels stone-hard upon being pressed. Use Da Xianxiong Tang as the primary treatment.[311]

(29)　　伤寒十余日，热结在里，复往来寒热者，与大柴胡汤。但结胸无大热者，此为水结在胸胁也，但头微汗出者，大陷胸汤主之。

In Cold-attack Taiyang stage for more than ten days, Fire entangles inside the body (there is no bowel movement, and there is a pain in the upper-side of the abdomen), and there are alternating fever and chills.[312] Use Da Chaihu

---

has to make every effort to struggle against the pathogenic Qi, and cannot counteract it. This is the before-death restless condition.

Dr. Ni Haixia: This is the last stage for many cancer patients. The patient can only sit, feel annoyed, feel difficulty closing the eyes sleep, and has asthma. The annoyed feeling can be treated with Fuling Si Ni Tang.

Dr. You Zaijing: There is another kind of Chest-bind syndrome: The patient had been beaten on the stomach a long time ago. There was bleeding in the abdomen. The blood was entangled with lymph nodes in the abdomen to form a mass of hardness. The upper stomach feels hard, and the patient feels pain upon being pressed. The stomach was compressed to a very small size, but there is no sign of cancer. For treatment, use Da Xianxiong Tang.

[306] Dr. Liu Duzhou: Taiyang-Shaoyang co-existing condition can be treated with Chaihu Guizhi Tang.

[307] The pulse changed from floating-fast to slow and deep, indicating that Chest-bind syndrome has begun.

[308] Dr. Ni Haixia: Da Xianxiong Tang condition can also be seen in acute lung dilation, or acute paralytic ileus, child epilepsy, polio, gastric cancer, lymphoma, pancreatic head cancer, and so on.

[309] Sweat only on the head is a sign of the presence of Fire-Dampness in the body.

[310] Chest-bind syndrome is the entanglement of Fire with water in the body. Jaundice is the entanglement of Fire and Dampness in the body (in the blood phase). The Dampness is entangled by the Fire so that the sweat can only occur on the head (above the neck) and urination is difficult (if the urination is normal, there will be no jaundice).

[311] This paragraph says that Chest-bind syndrome can happen without the misuse of Purging therapy too. Note that the pulse turns deep and tight now, and is no longer floating.

Dr. Ni Haixia: The patient had Fire in the lungs before becoming sick this time. When Cold attacked, the Fire could not leave the body through the skin, and it pushes the sweat to the skin, but the sweat cannot go out through the skin, so the sweat water returns to the Shaoyang spaces (the chest cavity and abdominal cavity) and entangles with the Fire, water and phlegm, to form Chest-bind syndrome.

[312] The *entangled Fire* here suggests that the disease is in the Yangming stage. *Alternating hot and cold*

Tang for treatment. Chest-bind syndrome without strong fever (no alternating fever-cold, or steam-fever) means that such situation is due to the entanglement of water in the chest region. In this case, if there is slight sweating only on the head, use Da Xianxiong Tang as the primary treatment.[313]

(30)　太阳病，重发汗，而复下之，不大便五六日，舌上燥而渴，日晡所小有潮热，一云：日晡所发心胸大烦，从心下至少腹，硬满而痛，不可近者，大陷胸汤主之。

In the Taiyang stage, Sweating therapy was used again, followed by a Purging therapy. The patient has had no bowel movement for five to six days, has dry tongue and feels thirsty, has slight tidal hot feeling in the later afternoon (around 3 pm),[314] feels a hardness, bloated and pain in the whole abdomen. Use Da Xianxiong Tang as the primary treatment.[315]

(31)　太阳病二三日，不能卧，但欲起，心下必结，脉微弱者，此本有寒分也。反下之，若利止，必作结胸；未止者，四日复下之，此作协热利也。

In the Taiyang stage for two to three days, a patient cannot lie down and has a desire to sit up.[316] There should be (garbage water) entanglement in the upper abdomen (before becoming sick this time), and the pulse feels faint and weak. Such a situation indicates that the body has Cold (body surface condition?). If a Purging therapy is used, however, if diarrhea so resulted from stops, there will be a Chest-bind syndrome. If diarrhea continues, (there will not be the Chest-bind syndrome, but) the patient will have Hotness-diarrhea after use of a Purging therapy on the fourth day.[317]

---

indicates the Shaoyang stage. This is the Shaoyang and Yangming successive condition.

[313] Dr. Hu Xishu and Dr. Liu Duzhou: This is not water Chest-bind syndrome. It is still Fire-water Chest-bind syndrome. It is Da Chaihu Tang. For Da Chaihu Tang condition, the patient feels bloated mostly in the flank region, does not feel a hardness in the middle part of the abdomen. *Has alternating hot and cold feeling*: if there is sweat, the sweat is on the whole body, not just on the head. The patient feels pain even without pressure. For Chest-bind syndrome, the patient feels bloated, tightness in the upper abdomen or in the whole abdomen, and may or may not have a fever, but there is no alternating hot and cold. The abdomen feels hard as stone and feels pain when pressed.

[314] In one version of *Shanghan Lun*, it said that there is strong vexation in the heart in the later afternoon.

[315] Due to having no bowel movement, having dry mouth and thirst, fever in the later afternoon and pain in the abdomen, this Chest-bind syndrome is similar to the Yangming inner stage. In the Yangming inner stage, there should be tide-like fever, the fever is strong, the abdomen is not as hard as a stone, and the abdomen pain is near the navel only, not in the whole abdomen.

Dr. Ni Haixia: Usually, if Sweating therapy is used first, then Purging follows, Da Xianxiong Tang condition is not created. However, if Purging therapy is used, then the Sweating therapy follows, it can be created. For Da XIanxiong Tang condition, the pain is in the middle part of the abdomen. In Da Chengqi Tang condition, the pain is on the sides of the abdomen. In Da Xianxiong Tang condition, the patient may also have no bowel movement for several days.

[316] There could be two primary reasons why a patient is unable to lie down: (1) there is something (such as water or phlegm) in the abdomen that affects breath; (2) in the Yangming stage there is accumulated firm stool in the bowel that presses on the diaphragm to affect the breath. In either case, the shortness of breath is worse in the lying position and better in the sitting up position.

Dr. Ni Haixia: If there is water accumulation in the chest, then, after lying down, the water stimulates the lung to cause coughing and vomiting. If the water is in the diaphragm, it causes bloating feeling in the upper abdomen and dizziness (Ling Gui Zhu Gan Tang condition). In water condition, the patient does not feel thirsty, the tongue coating is wet, and the pulse feels strong (a similar pulse as in the Shaoyang stage).

[317] *Hotness-diarrhea*: The patient has diarrhea, an urgent feeling to have a bowel movement, hot in the anus area, or spasming pain in the stomach before and during the bowel movement. The patient may have a fever, and the stool may have blood in it. Because the water and Fire are depleted through diarrhea, the entanglement condition cannot form.

Dr. Liu Duzhou: This paragraph emphasizes that with previous garbage water in the upper abdomen, Purging therapy will cause either Chest-bind syndrome or Hotness-diarrhea.

(32) 小结胸病，正在心下，按之则痛，脉浮滑者，小陷胸汤主之。

Small Chest-bind syndrome means that the disease location is just in the upper abdomen. The patient feels pain upon pressed. The pulse feels floating-slippery.[318] Use Xiao Xianxiong Tang as the primary treatment.[319]

(33) 太阳病下之，其脉促，不结胸者，此为欲解也。脉浮者，必结胸也；脉紧者，必咽痛；脉弦者，必两胁拘急；脉细数者，头痛未止；脉沉紧者，必欲呕；脉沉滑者，协热利；脉浮滑者，必下血。

Dr. Ni Haixia: If diarrhea continues, it brings the pathogenic Qi from body surface deep into the intestine to cause hotness-diarrhea. In such cases, use Gegen Tang, Wu Ling San, or Gegen Qin Lian Tang for treatment.

Dr. Martin Wang: it is hard to understand why Purging therapy would be used when there is diarrhea.

[318] Dr. Hao Wanshan: The floating pulse here is an indication of inner Fire. It can be felt upon slight pressing on the pulse which still feels solid with resistance upon deeper pressing. However, the floating pulse in the Taiyang stage is slightly weak, with less resistance upon deeper pressure.

[319] For Xiao Xianxiong Tang condition, the patient feels fullness and hardness in the upper stomach. The patient feels pain when touched, but no pain if not touched. This condition is less severe than Da Xianxiong Tang condition. In clinics, the two syndromes need to be distinguished. Note that, for Pi syndrome, the person also feels fullness and hardness, but there is no pain even if touched.

Dr. Hu Xishu: The herb Gualu in Xiao Xianxiong Tang should be the whole Gualu, not the kernel.

Dr. Ni Haixia: Xiao Xianxiong Tang is used to deplete phlegm that entangles in the chest. The patient vomits phlegm without coughing. This can be easily seen in persons who smoke. In clinics, if a patient has discomfort in the upper abdomen, if the tongue coating is thick and yellow, and if the condition can be confirmed as Fire-Dampness, Xiao Xianxiong Tang can be used for treatment.

Dr. Liao Houze: Xiao Xianxiong Tang condition is the inflammation of the outside of the stomach. If the patient has discomfort in the stomach and is constipated, add whole Gualou in the formula. If the stool looks like big balls, use Xiao Xianxiong Tang with herb Shengdi.

In the Taiyang stage, a Purging therapy is used. The pulse is still floating on the Cun position[320] and there is no Chest-bind syndrome in the upper abdomen. Such a situation suggests that the Taiyang stage will get better. If the pulse is floating,[321] there will be the Chest-bind syndrome. If the pulse is tight, there will be a sore throat. If the pulse is stringy, there will be spasms in the flank region in both sides. If the pulse is thin-fast, there will be continuous headaches. If the pulse is deep and tight, there will be vomit. If the pulse feels deep and slippery, there will be hot-diarrhea. And if the pulse is floating-slippery, there will be blood in the stool.[322]

(34) 病在阳，应以汗解之，反以冷水潠之，若灌之，其热被劫不得去，弥更益烦，肉上粟起，意欲饮水，反不渴者，服文蛤散。若不差者，与五苓散。

Whenever a disease is in the Yang side, the disease should be treated with a Sweating therapy. If a patient is given cold water, however, to wash or shower, the fever will remain, and the patient will feel more annoyed. There will be lots of millet-like dots on the skin (similar to chicken skin). If the patient has a desire to drink water but does not feel thirsty,[323] use Wenhe Tang[324] as the

---

[320] The original Chinese word for the pulse here is "脉促", the literal translation is "fast-irregular pulse". The floating pulse in the Cun position indicates Chest-bind syndrome. If Chest-bind syndrome does not occur, this suggests the recovery of the Shanghan disease.

[321] Here the "floating" should mean the floating feeling on both Cun and Chi positions.

[322] Dr. Hu Xishu: The text (in the original book) is not trustworthy. Omit it. It is not reliable to use the pulse alone for diagnosis. The diagnosis must consider the pulse, symptoms and body signs together.

[323] The heat is sealed under the skin, not in the stomach, so the patient does not feel thirsty. This is a disease condition in which Fire and water are entangled under the skin (Chest-bind syndrome is Fire and water entangled in the upper and lower diaphragm).

[324] Dr. Hu Xishu: This should be herbal formula Wenhe Tang, not the Wenhe San. They are different formulas. Wenhe Tang works similarly to Guizhi Tang to release body surface condition, while Wenhe San works for patients who feel very thirsty and drink lots of water.

primary treatment. If this herbal formula does not work, try Wu Ling San for treatment.[325]

(35)　　寒实结胸，无热证者，与三物 (小陷胸汤)，白散亦可服。

For Coldness Chest-bind syndrome (which is the entanglement of Coldness and water up and down the diaphragm. The patient can also have fullness and pain in the upper abdomen and have no bowel movement), if there is no fever, use San Wu Bai San (三物白散) for treatment.[326]

It works to release massive thirst. Patients here feel willing to drink water but do not feel thirsty. Besides Wenhe Tang, this condition can also be treated with Mahuang Tang with Shigao (because the patient feels annoyed).

　　Dr. Liu Duzhou: This should be Wenhe San (with Wenhe as the only ingredient). The disease condition here is mild, so use Wenhe San. If the condition is severe, use Wu Ling San.

[325] If the Wenhe Tang does not work, there may be some disease conditions inside the body that prevent the release of the body surface condition, such as accumulated water, phlegm, or dead blood. Wu Ling San here is only one of the possible choices for the treatment.

[326] The entanglement condition has both Hotness and Coldness syndromes. In the Hotness-entanglement syndrome, the patient has a fever and feels thirsty. Here it talks about Coldness entanglement, in which the patient does not feel thirsty or fever. The stomach situation is pretty much the same: fullness. In the original text, it says to use Xiao Xianxiong Tang for the treatment. This is wrong. Xiao Xianxiong Tang works for Hotness Chest-bind syndrome not for Coldness Chest-bind syndrome. Coldness Chest-bind syndrome can be treated with San Wu Bai San. If it does not work, Zhishi Lizhong Tang can be tried.

　　Dr. Liu Duzhou: With Coldness Chest-bind syndrome, the pulse also feels deep-tight, similar to the pulse in Chest-bind syndrome.

　　Dr. Ni Haixia: With Coldness Chest-bind syndrome, the tongue coating is white-slippery, and the pulse should be deep or deep-slow. This condition can be seen in lung abscess, cancer or tumors in the mediastinum, or stomach. If the disease is above the diaphragm, the use of this formula can result in vomiting or spitting lots of phlegm. If it is under the diaphragm, it can result in diarrhea of phlegm.

(36)　　心下痞，按之濡，其脉关上浮者，大黄黄连 泻心汤主之。

If a patient feels fullness or bloating in the upper abdomen, the abdomen feels soft when pressed, and the pulse feels floating at the Guan position on the wrist, use Dahuang Huanglian Xiexin Tang as the primary treatment.[327]

(37)　　伤寒大下后，复发汗心下痞，恶寒者表未解也，不可攻痞，当先解表，表解乃可攻痞，解表宜桂枝汤，攻痞宜大黄黄连泻心汤。

In Cold-attack Taiyang stage, after an intensive Purging therapy, a Sweating therapy was followed. The patient feels fullness in the upper abdomen (Pi syndrome) and feels an aversion to cold. This situation indicates that the disease is still in the body surface level. The treatment should focus on the release of the surface condition first, not on the dissolve of the Pi syndrome. To solve the body surface condition, use Guizhi Tang. To release the Pi syndrome, use Dahuang Huanglian Xiexin Tang for treatment.

(38)　　心下痞而复（不是"后"）恶寒，汗出者，附子泻心汤主之。

---

[327] Dr. Ni Haixia: In the book *Shanghan Lun*, two herbal formulas are mentioned for treating bleeding: Gancao Ganjiang Tang and Dahuang Huanglian Xiexin Tang. Gancao Ganjiang Tang is used for bleeding from the stomach, which is Coldness-Weakness bleeding. Dahuang Huanlian Xixin Tang is used for Fire bleeding. The bleeding occurs from the nose, mouth, gum, eyes, ears, or urine. It is also used for trauma damage, in which the patient may lose consciousness and have continuous bleeding. For a sharp cut wound (such as by a knife), smear the powder of Dahuang Huanglian Xiexin Tang into the wound. To prevent pus formation, add Baizhu to the powder. For chronic ulcer, add herb Ruxiang, Moyao and Sanqi to the formula to expel the pus and to heal the skin wound.

　　Dr. Hu Xishu: Dahuang Huanglian Xiexin Tang is also useful for the treatment of nosebleeds, especially in children.

In Pi syndrome, a patient feels an aversion to cold again[328] and sweats.[329] Use Fuzi Xiexin Tang as the primary treatment.[330]

(39) 表以下之，故心下痞，与泻心汤。痞不解，其人口中渴，而烦躁，小便不利者，五苓散主之。

Body surface condition is treated however with a Purging therapy, so resulting in Pi syndrome. Use Xiexin Tang for treatment. If the Pi syndrome remains and the patient feels thirsty, annoyed, and has difficulty urinating, use Wu Ling San as the primary treatment.[331]

(40) 伤寒，汗出，解之后，胃中不和，心下痞鞕，干噫食臭，胁下有水气，腹中雷鸣，下利者，生姜泻心汤主之。

In Cold-attack Taiyang stage, after sweating, the body surface condition improved. A patient, however, feels discomfort and hardness in the upper abdomen, belches, has a bad odor from the mouth, a bloated feeling in the flank region of the abdomen, big and thunder noises in the abdomen, and the patient has diarrhea. In such case, use Shengjiang Xixin Tang as the primary treatment.[332]

(41) 伤寒中风，医反下之，其人下利，日数十行，谷不化，腹中雷鸣，心下痞硬而满，干呕，心烦不得安。医见心下痞，谓病不尽，复下之，其痞益甚，此非结热，但以胃中虚，客气上逆，故使硬也，甘草泻心汤主之。

In Wind-attack Taiyang stage, a Purging therapy was, however, given. A patient has diarrhea several times a day, with undigested food in the stool,[333] has big noise in the abdomen (abdominal movement), feels hardness and fullness in the stomach, feels belch and nauseous but does not vomit, and feels annoyed (vexation). For such case, the doctor regards the fullness syndrome as Yangming stage, and so uses Purging therapy again. This remedy makes the Pi syndrome worse. This condition is not due to Fire entanglement, but due to weakness in the stomach. In such case, pathogenic Qi uprises to cause the hardness and fullness feeling. Use Gancao Xiexin Tang as the primary treatment.[334]

---

[328] The aversion to cold feeling here is not the body surface condition, but an inner Yang deficiency condition.

[329] The sweating here is body surface Yang deficiency.

[330] Dr. Ni Haixia: the herb Pao Fuzi in the formula works to treat the chills and sweat. It can nourish the body Yang Qi, and solve the chills and sweat, including night sweat. It can also work to reduce frequent urination and to stop slippery sperm (together with Longgu and Muli).

[331] Dr. Ni Haixia: For Pi syndrome, the Fullness did not improve. This means that there is Water accumulation in the stomach region. Use Wu Ling San for treatment. With primitive Water accumulation in the body, both Sweating therapy and Xiexin Tang therapy cannot work correctly.

[332] Dr. Ni Haixia: Normally such Pi syndrome would not happen. It occurs only when the patient has had a disease in the stomach before becoming sick this time. After sweating, the body water should return from body surface back to the stomach. Now it cannot come into the stomach because there is garbage food inside the stomach. It, therefore, goes down to the small intestine. The small intestine is a Fire organ. The

---

water cools down the Fire and goes further down to the large intestine, causing thunder noise in the abdomen and diarrhea. For Shengjiang Xiexin Tang condition, the patient tends to have big noises during diarrhea. For Banxia Xiexin Tang condition, the patient tends to have nausea and acid reflux. For Xiao Chaihu Tang condition, the patient tends to have a bitter taste in mouth in the morning.

[333] Dr. Hao Wanshan: Another disease condition in which there could be non-digested food in the stool is the Shaoyin stage. In the Shaoyin stage, the bowel movement could be just one time a day. Here with Gancao Xiexin Tang condition, the bowel moves fast and the bowel movement can be several times a day and with the undigested food in the stool. Among the three Xiexin Tang, Gancao Xiexin Tang has the weakest Stomach Qi.

[334] Dr. Ni Haixia: This disease condition occurs mostly in acute gastroenteritis. Repeated Purging therapy damaged the stomach and the intestines, and it gives the digestive system Coldness and Weakness condition so that diarrhea has undigested food. Gancao can calm the intestines, slow down the bowel movement, and can also break down the food for digestion to supply nutrition to the body. The Gancao Xiexin Tang condition can also include nausea but with no bad breath. Shengjiang Xiexin Tang condition

(42)　　伤寒服汤药，下利不止，心下痞硬。服泻心汤已，复以他药下之，利不止，医以理中与之，利益甚。(理中者，理中焦，此利在下焦)，赤石脂禹余粮汤主之。(复利不止者，当利其小便。)

After a Purging treatment, a patient had constant diarrhea and hardness in the upper stomach (Pi syndrome). This condition was treated with Xiexin Tang first, then a Purging therapy. Diarrhea continues. The doctor uses Lizhong Tang to treat diarrhea and diarrhea becomes worse.[335] In such case, use Chishizhi Yuyuliang Tang.[336] (If diarrhea continues, use Diuretic therapy.)

(43)　　伤寒吐下后。发汗。虚烦。脉甚微。八九日心下痞鞕。胁下痛，气上冲咽喉。眩冒。经脉动惕者。久而成痿。

In Cold-attack Taiyang stage, after the use of Vomiting therapy or Purging therapy, Sweating therapy was used again. The patient feels annoyed [337] and the pulse feels very faint. On the eighth or ninth day, the patient

feels hardness on the upper abdomen[338] and pain in the flank region, feels gas-rushing feeling up to the throat and dizziness or cloudy mind.[339] If the patient also feels spasms and muscles twisting, the muscle will become withered. (In this case, Fuling Guizhi Baishu Gancao Tang should be used for treatment.) [340]

(44)　　太阳病，先下之而不愈，因复发汗，以此表里俱虚，其人因致冒，冒家汗出自愈。所以然者，汗出表和故也。里未和，然后复下之。

In the Taiyang stage, a Purging therapy was however used. The body surface condition did not improve. A Sweating therapy was then used. Such treatment caused the body inside and outside both to have a deficient state. The patient feels cloudy of mind (and may even lose consciousness) due to loss of blood volume. If the patient sweats (but not from the Sweating therapy), the disease will get better, because the sweat suggests that the inside and the outside of the body become harmonious.[341] If the inner condition remains, treat the inner condition by using Purging therapy.

(45)　　太阳病未解，脉阴阳俱停，必先振慄，汗出而解。但阳脉微者，先汗出而解；但阴脉微者，下之而解。若欲下之，宜调胃承气汤主之

---

includes both bad breath and diarrhea. With Banxia Xiexin Tang, there is vomit or diarrhea.

[335] The chest and the abdomen are regarded as a whole Jiao cavity (the triple Jiao system). The Heart and Lung are in the Upper Jiao cavity, the Spleen and Stomach are in the Middle Jiao cavity, and the Liver and Kidney are in the Lower Jiao cavity. (In a very recent textbook, the Liver is included in the middle Jiao.)

The reason for the failure of Lizhong Tang is that this herbal formula works only in the middle Jiao (middle part of the body).

[336] This formula works to contract the intestine, to reduce its movement, to increase water absorption, and thereby stop diarrhea. If it still does not work, use Diuretic therapy (to increase the urine flow to reduce diarrhea). A familiar concept in TCM is that if the water goes to the colon to cause diarrhea, the person tends to have difficulty in urinating. If a patient has too much urine, there tends to be constipation. Only in very severe conditions does the patient have both too much urine and diarrhea (loss of control in urination and bowel movement).

[337] Dr. Ni Haixia: The vomiting results in an empty in the stomach, so there is no continuous supply of nutrition to the blood. The heart is associated with the blood, so the heart is nervous, shown in the annoyed feeling.

[338] Vomiting and bowel movement depleted liquid in the stomach. The liquid in the lower part of the body rushes up to the stomach to cause the fullness feeling.

[339] Dr. Ni Haixia: Normally the Stomach Qi goes down to the intestine. The Vomiting therapy reversed it upwards to the chest, the throat and the head. This condition can be seen in infantile paralysis.

[340] If the disease is still in the Taiyang stage after Sweating or other therapy, this herb formula is needed. If the disease is or has come into the Shaoyin stage, Zhenwu Tang should be used to treat the body shaking.

[341] Be careful as this paragraph talks about the Cloudy-mind person's body reaction after Purging and Sweating therapy, saying that the patient will quickly lose consciousness. Some people may recover after a bowel movement. A Cloudy-mind person is a person who easily felt cloudy of mind, or dizzy, before becoming sick this time. For such persons, usually, there is water accumulation inside the body.

The Taiyang stage remains not improved. The Yin pulse and Yang pulse both feel very faint and difficult to feel.[342] The patient will shake (as if chilly) then sweat,[343] and then the disease will get better. If only the Yang pulse feels faint (the Yin pulse not faint), the body condition would be improved after the sweat.[344] If only the Yin pulse feels faint, the disease condition can be dissolved with Purging therapy. Use Tiaowei Chengqi Tang as the primary treatment.[345]

(46) 伤寒, 发汗, 若吐, 若下, 解后心下痞 鞕, 噫气不除者, 旋覆代赭石汤主之。

In Cold-attack Taiyang stage, after Sweating therapy, Vomiting therapy or Purging therapy was followed. The body surface condition is no longer present, but the patient has Pi syndrome and has continuous burping.[346] In this case, use Xuanfu Daizheshi Tang as the primary treatment.[347]

---

[342] Here *Yang pulse*: the pulse is felt with a slight press; *Yin pulse*: the pulse is felt with a harder press.

[343] The body shaking and sweat can be regarded as a healing crisis. It is called shaking-sweat.

   Dr. Liu Duzhou: If there is body shaking but no sweat, it means that the body has insufficient body liquid to create sweat. Let the patient eat something, or drink water, wine, or warm soup, or give some herbal therapy, such as Guizhi Tang. The patient should also stay in a warm room (but not too hot or too cold environment). Infectious diseases tend to have such shaking-sweat healing crisis.

[344] The patient should also have a body surface condition.

[345] The patient should also have some other symptoms indicating inner Dryness, such as dry mouth and constipation.

   Dr. Ni Haixia: The Yang pulse here should mean the pulse on the Cun position, and the Yin pulse means the Chi position. Here it means that the pulse changes from original floating-fast to softer. It does not mean the Weakness condition of the body. The softer pulse on the Chi position suggests that there is garbage food accumulated in the stomach.

[346] *Continuous burping* is due to stomach Qi reversing and pushing up.

[347] Pi syndrome is caused after Purging therapy, Sweating therapy or Vomiting therapy. The standard herbal formulas for this condition are various Xiexin Tang. Here, the burping is an additional problem to Pi

---

(47) 下之后，复发汗，必振寒，脉微细。 所以然者，以内外俱虚故也。

After Purging therapy and then Sweating therapy, the patient will feel shaking-chilly, and the pulse will feel faint and thin. Such condition means that the body is in both Yin deficiency and Yang deficiency.[348]

(48) 下之后，复发汗，昼日烦躁，不得 眠，夜而安静，不呕不渴，无表证，脉沉 微，身无大热者，干姜附子 汤主之。

After Purging therapy and then Sweating therapy, a patient feels annoyed and agitated [349] during the daytime but normal at night. [350] There is no nausea,[351] or thirsty.[352]

---

syndrome. So, add Xuanfuhua and Daizhishi to Shenjiang Xiexin Tang to bear the reversed stomach Qi downwards.

[348] Dr. Ni Haixia: Purging therapy can deplete body liquid (the Yin), and Sweating therapy can deplete body Yang Qi (warm energy). In this condition, use Si Ni Tang for treatment. For severe cases, use Si Ni Tang Jia Ginseng.

[349] All six stages can include an annoyed and agitated feeling.

[350] The annoyed feeling only happens during the daytime, but not at night, suggesting that it not be a Zhizi Chi Tang condition.

   Dr. Hao Wanshan: This is the Kidney Yang deficiency condition. During the daytime, with the help of Yang Qi in nature, the Kidney Yang can utilize more energy to struggle against the Yin, and the patient feels annoyed. At night, the Yin in nature is dominated, and body Kidney Yang Qi has no energy to struggle with, so the patient is quiet. The quietness means that the disease condition is worse, not better.

   Dr. Tan Jiezhong: The pathogenic Qi is in the Defensive phase (out of the blood vessels). The body Nutrient Qi (inside the blood vessels) struggles against the pathogenic Qi, so the patient feels annoyed. At night, the Nutrient Qi returns to the blood and stops struggling against the pathogenic Qi, so that the patient feels quiet. This condition is opposite to the Heat invasion in blood chamber syndrome. In the latter, the pathogenic Qi is in the blood phase, the Defensive Qi moves into the blood at night and struggles against the pathogenic Qi, so that the patient feels annoyed and speaks as with ghosts, but is normal during the daytime.

   Dr. Ni Haixia: This is Yang deficiency condition. The Yang Qi is insufficient, so deficient-Fire rushes up

There is no body surface condition.[353] The pulse feels deep and faint.[354] There is no strong fever or hot.[355] In such case, use Ganjiang Fuzi Tang as the primary treatment.[356]

(49) 发汗若下之，病仍不解，烦躁者，茯苓 四逆汤主之。

With Sweating therapy or Purging therapy, the disease remains not improved. The patient feels annoyed and agitated. Use Fuling Sini Tang as the primary treatment.[357]

(50) 伤寒五、六日，已发汗而复下之，胸胁满微结，小便不利，渴而不呕，但头汗出，往来寒热，心烦者，此为未解也，柴胡桂枝干姜汤主之。

On the fifth or sixth day of the Cold-attack Taiyang stage, a Sweating therapy has been used but a Purging therapy was used too. The patient feels bloated and a slight hardness in the chest and flank region, has difficulty urinating and feels thirsty but not nauseous. The patient sweats only on the head.[358] The

to the head, causing difficulty in sleeping, and to the chest to cause an annoyed feeling. In this herbal formula, the dried ginger nourishes the Spleen Yang and Fuzi nourishes the Kidney Yang. If a disease shows up during the daytime but not at night, it means that Yang is insufficient. If it shows up at night but there's no discomfort during the daytime, it means that the Yin is insufficient.

[351] *No nausea*: The condition here does not belong to the Shaoyang stage.

[352] *No thirst*: The condition here does not belong to Yangming stage.

[353] *No body surface condition*: The condition here does not belong to Taiyang stage. It is not Da Qinglong Tang condition.

[354] The deep-tiny pulse: The condition is in the Shaoyin stage.

[355] *No strong heat or fever*: The condition, in this case, does not belong to Yang-repelling or Yang-upcasting condition (due to excessive Yin).

[356] The Purging and Sweating therapy have caused depletion of Yin of the body, taking the condition deep into the Shaoyin stage. Without enough Yin, the Yang is floating. During the daytime, Yang Qi is stronger whereas Yin is weaker, so the patient feels more annoyed. At night, there is relatively more Yin from nature (the night belongs to Yin), so it balances the shortage of Yin in the body and makes Yang combine with Yin (during rest), so the patient is quiet. However, some doctors believe that the annoyance here is due to the depletion of the body Yang Qi, not the Yin Qi.

Note that in the Taiyang stage, the patient feels worse at night, but better during the day. Here it says that the condition seems worse during the daytime – a different picture. Is this condition easily seen in most people with anxiety? They feel annoyed, and their pulse is deep and weak (only a doctor knows this) but there aren't any other problems to complain?

Dr. Tan Jiezhong: Even if we use Ganjiang Fuzi Tang, the body Yang Qi has to wait for 12 hours to recover (the body feels warm).

[357] The previous treatment caused a massive loss of body liquid. The body condition now turns into the inner Yin condition (Coldness and Weakness Shaoyin stage). The patient should also feel palpitations. The herb Fuling also works for palpitations and annoyance.

Note: Fuling Si Ni Tang is used when the Taiyang condition remains, and the annoyance occurs during both day and night. It belongs to a weak annoyance, but not like in Da Qinglong Tang condition, in which there is a real annoyance (the body condition is not weak).

Dr. Liu Duzhou: The agitated feeling, or the restless arms and legs condition, is less strong in Fulin Si Ni Tang syndrome, compared to Ganjiang Fuzi Tang syndrome.

Dr. Hao Wanshan: This disease condition belongs to Kidney Yang deficiency and Heart Yin deficiency.

Dr. Ni Haixia: The wrong treatment of the Taiyang disease can cause either Yang deficiency or Yin deficiency, or both. If it is only Yin deficiency, allow the body to get more liquids via diet, without needing to treat it. If it is Yang deficiency, use Ganjiang Fuzi Tang. If it is both Yin and Yang deficiency, use Fuling Si Ni Tang here. The annoyed feeling and agitation happen because the body is in a weak condition: the chest is hot, and there's no water, so the water in the lower part of the body rushes up to fill in the chest. Using Fuling here depletes the water via urine. Ginseng here nourishes the body Yin (liquid part). If there is no annoyed feeling or agitation, use formula Renshen Si Ni Tang.

[358] Dr. Hao Wanshan: The sweat is only on the head because Fire is entangled in the Shaoyang. The Fire cannot be released through sweat from other parts of the body. The thirsty feeling means the loss of body liquid. *No nausea*: the gallbladder Fire does not bother the Stomach yet. The Chaihu Guizhi Ganjiang Tang condition is the Shaoyang-Taiyin successive

patient has alternating hot-cold feeling and is irritated. This condition means that the body surface condition remains not improved. Use Chaihu Guizhi Ganjiang Tang as the primary treatment.[359]

(51) 本太阳病，医反下之，因而腹满时痛者，属太阴也，桂枝 芍药汤主之。大实痛者，桂枝 加 大黄 汤主之

The Taiyang stage is however treated with a Purging therapy. A patient feels bloating in the abdomen and has abdominal pain from time to time. This situation means that the disease has moved into the Yangming stage.[360] Use Guizhi Jia Shaoyao Tang as the primary treatment. If the pain is constant and severe and the abdomen feels hard, use

---

condition, while the Da Chaihu Tang can work for Shaoyang-Yangming concurrent condition.

[359] In this case, the alternating hot-cold feeling, irritation, bloating and hardness in the chest and flank region suggest that the disease condition is in the Shaoyang stage. Due to sweating and bowel movement, body liquid is lost. The difficulty in urinating can be due to (a) loss of body liquid or (b) gas rushing up. That there is Fire in the stomach means thirst. There is no water accumulation in the stomach, so there is no nausea. There is Fire inside the body, so the patient feels annoyed. The *sweat is only on the head*: air rushes up and does not fall. All of these symptoms suggest the Shaoyang stage.

Dr. Hu Xishu believed that this is a Taiyang-Shaoyang successive condition because the herbal formula, contains the formula Guizhi Gancao Tang and works to solve body Surface condition (e.g., the Taiyang stage).
[360] In the original text, it says "into the Taiyin stage". This condition should be Taiyang-Yangming successive condition, so Guizhi Tang is used with the addition of Shaoyao.

Dr. Hu Xishu: The herb Shaoyao is used to relax muscle spasms and to deplete Fire. Dahuang is also used for Fire-type of diarrhea. For this reason, it is better to understand that the Purging therapy has brought the pathogenic Qi into the Yangming stage, not the Taiyin stage. Shaoyang and Dahuang are definitely not used in the Taiyin stage (the Weakness and Coldness condition).

Guizhi Jia Dahuang Tang as the primary treatment.

(52) 发汗後，水药不得入口为逆，若更发汗，必吐 (下) 不止。

After Sweating therapy, a patient can no longer drink any water or herbal tea. This situation means the disease has been treated in a wrong way. If the Sweating therapy is used again, the patient would have constant vomiting (and diarrhea).

(53) 太阳病，二日反躁，凡熨其背，而大汗出，大热入胃，胃中水竭，躁烦必发谵语，十余日振栗而自下利者，此为欲解也，故其汗从腰以下不得汗，欲小便不得，反呕，欲失溲，足下恶风，大便硬，小便当数而反不数，及不多，大便已，头卓然而痛，其人足心必热，谷气下流故也。

In the Taiyang stage for two days, a patient feels annoyingly restless in the body. The doctor used Fire-toast therapy to treat the disease,[361] which makes the patient have profuse sweating. The strong Fire also invades into the stomach to exhaust liquid in the stomach and makes the stomach very dry.[362] The dryness in stomach results in annoyed, restless and has delirious speech.[363] After ten or more days, if the patient has a shaking feeling in the body and has diarrhea, the disease is going to get better.[364] Due to dryness in the stomach, there is only sweat in

---

[361] On the second day, the patient starts to feel annoyed and restless: the disease has penetrated the Yangming stage. Fire therapy presses the body surface Fire deep into the stomach to make the stomach dry.
[362] Such a disease condition easily happens in patients who often had inner Stomach Fire condition before becoming sick this time. During common cold or flu, treatment with Fire is wrong. Fire therapy includes, but not limits to, touching hot brick, toasting in front of a fire, lying on a hotbed, using a sauna, moxibustion, or Fire needle acupuncture.
[363] *Annoyed, restless and delirious speech*: disease condition is in the Yangming stage.
[364] Here, the shaking body and diarrhea is a kind of healing crisis (similar to shaking-sweat). Here it is shaking-diarrhea. If the disease is in the Taiyang or Shaoyang stage, the healing crisis might be shaking-sweat and if in the Yangming stage, shaking-bowel movement.

the upper part of the body (insufficient stomach liquid to make sweat in the lower part of the body). There is a desire to have urination, but the urine is difficult to come out. The patient feels nauseous, has a tendency to have urine leakage, has an aversion to wind in the soles, has a firm stool. The urination is supposed to be frequent but neither frequent or in large volume. After a bowel movement, the patient feels a sudden headache. There must be hot feeling on soles because dietary Qi bears downwards.

(54)　　太阳病中风，以火劫发汗。邪风被火热，血气流溢，失其常度。两阳相熏灼，其身发黄。阳盛则欲衄，阴虚小便难。阴阳俱虚竭，身体则枯燥，但头汗出，剂颈而还，腹满，微喘，口干咽烂，或不大便。久则谵语，甚者至哕，手足躁扰，捻衣摸床，小便利者，其人可治。

The Wind-attack Taiyang stage was treated with a Fire therapy with the aim to force sweat.[365] The Fire entangles with pathogenic Wind, disturbs blood and Qi running in an abnormal manner. The Fire and the Wind both are Yang in nature, their combination cause jaundice[366] in the body. The excessive Yang causes a nosebleed. The Yin deficiency results in difficulty urinating. After the Yin and Yang both become exhausted, the body becomes wilted. There is sweat, but it is only on the head (not below the neck).[367] The patient feels bloated and fullness in the abdomen,[368] slight panting,[369] has ulcers in the throat and dry mouth[370] or has no bowel

movement. After a long time, the patient may have delirious speech, restless in arms and legs, and a hand touching their bed (picking at bed-clothes) unconsciously.[371] If the patient can still have automatic urination, there is still hope to save the life with treatment.[372]

(55)　　伤寒，脉浮，医以火迫劫之，亡阳，必惊狂，卧起不安者，桂枝 去芍药加蜀漆 牡蛎龙骨 救逆汤主之。

In Cold-attack Taiyang stage, the pulse feels floating. The Doctor used Fire therapy however to force sweat, which causes Yang-exhaust condition (substantial loss of body liquid). (The sweat is usually more present in the upper part of the body. The liquid in the lower part of the body will rush up.) The patient feels scared, frighted[373] and mad,[374] and feels difficulty remaining either sitting up or lying down. Use Guizhi Qui Shaoyao, but With Shuxi, Longgu and Muli Tang.[375]

(56)　　形作伤寒，其脉不弦紧而弱，弱者必渴，被火必谵语，弱者发热，脉浮。

---

[365] Taiyang Wind-attack disease has already put Fire in the body surface. Fire therapy creates more Fire in the body. The double Fire makes the body lose liquid in and out of blood vessels and causes inner body dryness too.

[366] Dr. Hao Wanshan and Dr. Hu Xishu: The yellow skin is not jaundice.

　　Dr. Liu Duzhou: The yellow skin is dynamic jaundice.

[367] No enough body liquid to create whole body sweating.

[368] This is a Yangming stage condition: a firm stool in the bowels.

[369] The Fire rushes up to press the diaphragm.

[370] The ulcer and sore in the throat are due to the Fire, which causing mucus to break. The *dry mouth and no bowel movent* indicate Yangming stage.

---

[371] The *restless arm and leg*, and *hand touching bed unconsciously* are both signs of a hazardous condition leading to death.

[372] The disease conditions described here are the results of using Fire therapy for Shanghan disease. It would be the same result as using Sweating therapy for Warm diseases. Both results are due to the exhaustion of both Yin and Yang in the body.

　　Dr. Ni Haixia: This paragraph and the above one are neglected by some doctors in their studies or teaching because they feel it is difficult to understand and to explain.

[373] Due to the insufficient blood supply to the heart, the patient feels palpitation and feels scared and frighted.

[374] Fire rushes up to affect the emotions and mind. The uprushing Fire also brings water up to attack the heart to cause palpitations and attack the brain to cause emotional disorders.

[375] Because the body Surface condition remained unimproved, use Guizhi Tang as the basic herbal formula for treatment. Mahuang Tang cannot be used at all.

　　Dr. Hu Xishu: Fire therapy causes fear and madness in the Cold-attack condition, but not so in the Wind-attack condition.

A disease situation looks like Cold-attack Taiyang stage. The pulse is not tight-string but faint. Such a patient must have thirst.[376] If a Fire therapy is used, the patient will have delirious speech.[377] Patient with the faint pulse will have a fever and have a floating pulse.[378]

(57)　太阳病，以火熏之，不得汗，其人必燥。到经不解，必清血，名为火邪。

Whenever a Taiyang stage is treated however with a Fire therapy, but no sweat created,[379] such a treatment will result in a dryness condition in the body. If the disease does not get better after seven days, the entangled Fire will hurt blood vessels to cause bleeding in the stool. Such bleeding due to a Fire therapy is called Fire-Xie disease.[380]

(58)　脉浮，熱甚，而反灸之，此为实。实以虚治，因火而动，必咽燥，吐血。

A pulse feels floating, and the fever in the body is very high. Such a disease situation is treated however with a moxibustion therapy. This treatment is wrong. Such a disease condition belongs to excess, but it was treated as a deficient condition. Due to the

disturbance by the Fire, there will be dry mouth and throat, and blood spitting.[381]

(59)　微数之脉，慎不可灸，因火为邪，则为烦逆，追虚逐实，血散脉中，火气虽微，内攻有力，焦骨伤筋，血难复也。脉浮，宜以汗解，用火灸之，邪无从出，因火而盛，病重腰以下必重而痹，火逆也。欲自解者，必当先烦，烦乃有汗而解。(何以知？脉浮，故知汗出解。)

If the pulse is faint and fast, Moxibustion should not be used. The Fire is pathogenic Qi. It causes annoying annoyance. To treat excess disease condition with supplying (nourishing) therapy (such as moxibustion) is wrong. The blood will disperse into the meridians.[382] Though the Fire is mild (from the moxibustion), it can still burn bone and hurt sinews. The blood that was dispersed by the Fire is hard to return back to blood vessels. Disease condition with a floating pulse should be released with sweat, not the Fire therapy. Otherwise, the pathogenic Qi has no outlet to exit. The pathogenic Qi would become overwhelming due to the Fire (from the moxibustion). The body feels heaviness downwards from the lower back and has Bi syndrome. Such a situation is also a Fire-reverse condition. If the disease can be released naturally, the patient would feel annoyance first,[383] because the annoyance indicates the come of sweat,[384] which brings

---

[376] The Floating-weak pulse suggests that body liquid is lacking, so the patient should feel thirsty. This disease condition can be an early stage of a Warm disease, in which the patient can also have a fever, headache, even slight chills too. Therefore it is similar to Shanghan disease. The nature of the Warm disease is Hotness inside the body. With Fire therapy, the inner Fire will be more overwhelming and affect the Heart, causing delirious speech.

[377] The use of Fire therapy on the patient with insufficient body liquid will cause more exhaustion of body liquid via sweat (making the stomach even drier).

[378] Dr. Martin Wagn: This paragraph might be translated as Disease condition looks like Cold-attack Taiyang disease. Pulse is not tight-string, but faint. If the patient is weak in body condition, the patient will feel thirst.[378] If a Fire therapy is used, such a weak patient will have delirious speech. The patient with weak body condition has a fever and a floating pulse.

[379] The patient cannot sweat because the body was often in a blood deficiency condition before becoming sick this time.

[380] The Fire-Xie condition needs to be distinguished from the bleeding due to other reasons.

[381] Moxibustion is also a kind of Fire therapy. It enhances the body Fire. The Fire rushes up to cause dry mouth and throat and burns the mucus to cause bleeding in the throat.

[382] The original text is "血散脉中". It is hard to translate. Does this mean that Fire disperses into the bloodstream?

[383] The *sweat before the disease gets better* indicates a healing crisis.

[384] This paragraph introduces the third condition, which is caused by the misuse of Fire therapy. The Fire does not cause bleeding in the nose or large intestine but does burn the blood inside the bloodstream (causing withering of the tendons and bones). Moxibustion causes sweat by damaging the body much more strongly than other kinds of Fire therapies, such as by toasting the patient on a hotbed.

Dr. Hu Xishu: If the body cannot heal by itself, treatment is needed. To solve the body surface

the pathogenic Qi out of the body. (How to know that the disease will get better? The pulse is floating, so the sweat is coming.)

(60)　　火逆下，因烧针烦躁者，桂枝甘草龙骨牡蛎汤主之。

In Fire-reverse condition, if a patient has an annoying restless due to the use of Fire-needle acupuncture, use Guizhi Gancao Longgu Muli Tang as the primary treatment.[385]

(61)　　烧针令其汗，针处被寒，核起而赤者，必发奔豚，气从少腹上冲心者，灸其核上各一壮，与桂枝加桂汤，更加桂枝二两也。

Fire-needle acupuncture is used with the aim to create sweat. The skin spot where the needle is inserted may become infected, swell and become red. The patient may also feel Running-piglet syndrome[386] or feels like a kind of air rushing up from the lower abdomen to the heart. For treatment, use moxibustion on the infected spot and give Guizhi Jia Gui Tang.[387]

---

condition, use Guizhi Tang. To treat the heavy feeling in the lower back, use Ling Jiang Zhu Gan Tang.

Dr. Liu Duzhou: This is another Yang sink condition. The Fire has sunk into the upper part of the body, and the lower part of the body cannot get warm from the upper Yang Qi. The Yang and the Yin in the body cannot connect. Use Longdan Xie Gan Tang and Da Chaihu Tang to solve such Fire-sink condition. In a clinical setting, remember to identify if an impotence or leg weakness disease condition is due to Fire-sink condition, and is not due to a Yang deficiency condition.

[385] Dr. Ni Haixia: *There is sweat on the head but not on the body,* because the Yang Qi floats on the head, but water remains in the middle part of the body. This condition is more often seen in patients with hyperthyroidism.

[386] Fire needle acupuncture causes heavy sweating and makes the upper part of the body weak so that the energy in the lower part of the body (lower abdomen) rushes up to fill the upper, weakened part of the body. The fear due to the Fire needle can also trigger the Running-piglet syndrome.

[387] Dr. Hu Xishu: The extra Guizhi added should be Guizhi, not Rougui. (In *Shanghan Lun*, the author did not indicate clearly if Guizhi or Rougui should be used.)

---

(62)　　太阳病，当恶寒发热，今自汗出，反不恶寒发热，关上脉细数者，以医吐之过也。一二日吐之者，腹中饥、口不能食；三四日吐之者，不喜糜粥、欲食冷食、朝食暮吐，以医吐之所致也，此为小逆。

In the Taiyang stage, patients should have a fever and an aversion to cold. Now, a patient has sweat but has no more fever and no aversion to cold.[388] The pulse is thin and fast on the Guan position.[389] This body condition is due to a Vomiting therapy previously used by mistake. Vomiting occurred on the first and second day, and the patient feels hungry but cannot eat.[390] (Eating causes nausea.) If the patient has vomit on the third and fourth day, the patient will feel no desire to eat porridge-like warm food, has a desire to eat cold food, and will vomit food consumed in the previous meal.[391] Such a situation is due

---

[388] *No more fever or aversion to cold*: The body Surface condition has been solved after sweating without help.

[389] This is due to Vomiting therapy that damaged Stomach Qi (disturbed the stomach environment). *Heat/fever, sweat, and no chills*, all do not mean that the Vomiting therapy brought the condition into the Yangming stage. In the Yangming stage, the pulse should be big and strong, here the pulse is thin and fast. The thin pulse suggests inner Weakness condition and the fast pulse suggests Fire. The Guan position of the pulse suggests that the Weakness and Fire are in the stomach.

[390] Due to Deficient-Fire in the stomach, the patient can feel hungry, but due to the Weakness, the patient cannot eat (cannot digest food).

[391] Dr. Liu Duzhou: This is Coldness-Weakness condition in the stomach. The thin-fast pulse can also be an indication of Weakness and Coldness. If vomiting occurs right after eating, it is an indication of Fire.

Dr. Ni Haixia: For stomach Coldness condition, the patient has an appetite but cannot eat. Use Da Banxia Tang for treatment. Wuzhuyu Tang is stronger and works for Spleen. If a child eats too much and feels discomfort in the stomach, use Da Banxia Tang for treatment. If the patient vomits food that was eaten in previous meals (gastroptosis), use Wuzhuyu Tang. If the patient has hiccups, use Xuanfuhua Daizheshi Tang. For gastroptosis, the pulse in the left Cun position is weak, and it is big in the right Guan position.

to last wrong Vomiting therapy, though it is not a big mistake yet.[392]

(63)　太阳病，吐之，但太阳病当恶寒，今反不恶寒，不欲近衣，此为吐之内烦也。

In the Taiyang stage, a Vomiting therapy was used, however. The patient should have an aversion to cold but no more now, and the patient dislikes being covered with blankets, (Such a condition suggests that the Vomiting therapy brought body surface Fire deep into the Yangming stage.) [393] This condition is the result of annoyance caused by the improper use of Vomiting therapy.

(64)　病人脉数，数为热，当消谷引食，而反吐者，此以发汗，令阳气微，膈气虚，脉乃数也。数为客热，不能消谷，以胃中虚冷，故吐也。

Pulse is fast. The fast pulse means Hotness. The patient should feel strong hungry (high appetite), but now the patient vomits.[394] The reason is that the body has had a sweat before. The sweat exhausted the liquid in the body surface, diaphragm and stomach. The invading pathogenic Qi (Fire) penetrates the diaphragm due to weakness condition there. The weakness condition there is the reason for the fast pulse. Fast pulse indicates the pathogenic Fire in the body. Such Fire cannot improve the appetite. The vomit is due to Weakness-Coldness in the stomach.

---

[392] Dr. Hu Xishu: For treatment, Tiaowei Chengqi Tang can be used.

[393] Dr. Liu Duzhou: This is a Deficient-Fire condition in the stomach after Vomiting therapy. Use Tiaowei Chengqi Tang for treatment.

　Dr. Ni Haixia: After vomiting, the stomach may or may not be dry yet. If it has not been dried, and the patient feels annoyed, use Da Banxia Tang. If the stomach has been dried, and the patient feels annoyed and dry in the mouth, use Ginseng Baihu Tang. If the patient feels hot but not thirsty, use Guizhi Baihu Tang.

[394] If the fast pulse is due to the Yangming stage, the patient should feel hungry. Fire should enable the body to digest food. Here the patient cannot eat, because the stomach is in a Coldness and Weakness condition. The pathogenic Qi invaded and entangled in the diaphragm but not in the stomach.

(65)　太阳病三日，已发汗，若吐，若下，若温针，仍不解者，此为坏病，桂枝 不中与之也。观其脉证，知犯何逆，随证治之。

In the Taiyang stage for three days, after Sweating therapy, the patient was also given Vomiting therapy, or Purging therapy, or Fire-needle acupuncture. The body surface condition remains not improved. The patient has more unexpected symptoms, meaning the disease situation becomes complicated. Guizhi Tang will no longer work. The following treatment has to be based on the current exact disease condition.

1.10　Differentiating the Taiyang stage from other conditions

The body surface condition in the Taiyang stage might be confused with some other clinical states. It is essential to identify these states before beginning any treatment correctly.

(1)　病常自汗出者，此为荣气和。荣气和者，外不谐，以卫气不共荣气和谐故尔。以荣行脉中，卫行脉外，复发其汗，荣卫和则愈，宜 桂枝 汤。

A patient often sweats from time to time. [395]...Nutrient Qi goes inside blood vessels, and Defensive Qi travels outside of the blood vessels. Use Sweat therapy to bring the Nutrient Qi and the Defensive Qi in harmony to stop the spontaneous sweat. (If no other symptoms indicating any other diseases,[396]) use Guizhi Tang for treatment.[397]

---

[395] The original text is "此为荣气和。荣气和者，外不谐". It is difficult to understand and to translate.

[396] The spontaneous sweating symptom is due to insufficient Defensive Qi in the outside of the blood vessels. The Defensive Qi outside of the blood vessels is called "Defensive Qi". The Qi inside the blood vessels is called "Nutrient Qi". These two kinds of Qi normally are in balance. This is called "Nutrient-Defensive Qi (Ying-Wei) harmony". One of the functions of this Defensive Qi is to seal the body surface and to protect the blood vessels. Insufficient Defensive Qi fails to seal them, causing leaking of blood to form sweat. Guizhi Tang works to regulate

(2)　　　病人藏无他病，时发热，自汗出，而不愈者，此卫气不和也。先其时发汗则愈，宜 桂枝 汤主之。

A patient has no symptoms indicating any other diseases,[398] except feels hot and sweats at a fixed time of the day. This condition is the disharmony between the Defensive Qi and the Nutrient Qi. For the treatment, drink herbal tea to create sweat before the onset of the fever and sweat.[399] Use Guizhi Tang for treatment.[400]

(3)　　　证如桂枝证，头不痛，项不强，寸脉微浮，胸中痞硬，气上冲咽，不得息者，此为胸有寒也，当吐之，宜瓜蒂散。

A patient has a disease condition suggesting the use of Guizhi Tang, but the patient has no headache and no stiffness in the nape. The pulse on the Cun position is slight floating. The patient feels fullness and hardness in the chest, and feels reverse uprushing gas even up to the throat and feels difficulty breathing. All of these suggest the presence of retained

water[401] in the chest. Vomiting therapy should be used. Use Guadi San.[402]

(4)　　　伤寒，无大热，口燥渴，心烦，背微恶寒者，白虎加 人参 汤主之。

In Cold-attack Taiyang stage, a patient has no intensive fever, feels very annoyed, feels very thirsty, but drinking water does not help and has a slight aversion to cold on the back. For such case, use Baihu Jia Renshen Tang as the primary treatment.

(This condition belongs to Yangming muscle stage. The aversion to cold on the back of the body can mislead to a wrong diagnosis of the Taiyang stage. In severe cases, the patient may feel very cold, have cold hands and feet[403] but does not want any blanket to cover the body, and wants to drink more water (especially more cold water). This situation is false Coldness in the body surface but true Hotness inside.[404] It is called the Hotness Jue syndrome (see below in Yangming stage). Use Baihu Tang as the primary treatment.)

(5)　　　病有发热恶寒者，发于阳也；无热恶寒者，发于阴也。发于阳，七日愈，发于阴，六日愈。以阳数七、阴数六故也。

If there is a fever and an aversion to cold, a disease started from Yang. If there is no fever but has an aversion to cold, the disease started from Yin. For a disease condition that begins from the Yang, the patient will get better after seven days. If it starts from the Yin, the patient will recover after six days,

---

the Nutrient-Defensive Qi in harmonized status so to solve the unexpected sweat.

[397] Dr. Tan Jiezhong: Guizhi Tang can also be used to treat half body sweat. This happens when there is sweat only on one side of the body.

[398] Dr. Tan Jiezhong: It is necessary to exclude Qi deficiency and Blood deficiency condition. Both conditions can also cause fever and sweating from time to time.

[399] Dr. Liu Duzhou: The natural sweating condition can be seen in menopause. If regular treatment does not work, try to use Guizhi Tang.

Dr. Hao Wanshan: If there is a fixed time pattern to the fever and sweating, drink the herbal tea before its onset. If there is no fixed pattern, drink the tea after the onset, but do not drink it when sweating. Guizhi Tang is one of the best choices for treatment.

Because of the fever and sweating, this condition needs to be distinguished from Taiyang Wind-attack condition, though the treatment is the same herbal formula.

[400] Here again, the Guizhi Tang is used to create sweat like a "Sweating therapy", though the sweat created by the Guizhi Tang is explained as a "Healing sweat". Due to the spontaneous sweat and fever, this Nutrient-Defensive Qi disharmony syndrome needs to be differentiated with the Wind-attack Taiyang disease.

---

[401] The original text is *cold*.

　　Dr. Hao Wanshan: Cold should be understood as *phlegm*.

[402] This is Cold Chest-bind syndrome. It needs to be also distinguished from (Hotness-Phlegm) Chest-bind conditions.

[403] The aversion to cold feeling and the cold hands and feet are easily wrongly diagnosed as the Taiyang stage.

[404] If the patient feels hot and warm in the body but wants more blankets to cover the body and wants to drink hot water, the disease condition is false Hotness on body surface but true Coldness inside of the body. It requires Warm-up therapy. Use Si Ni Tang. This disease condition can be seen in the Shaoyin stage. Deep pulse also indicates water. The herb Xixin in Mahuang Xixin Tang also works to remove water.

because seven is a Yang figure and six is a Yin figure.[405]

[405] Dr. Hao Wanshan: There are three ways to understand Yin and Yang here. First, some doctors believe that Yang means the three Yang stages (Taiyang, Shaoyang, and Yangming) and that Yin means the three Yin stages (Taiyin, Shaoyin, and Jueyin). Secondly, Yang means the Taiyang stage and Yin means the Shaoyin stage. Third, Yang means Taiyang Wind-attack and Yin means Taiyang Cold-attack. Take into the consideration that the patient can recover after seven days or six days whether it starts from Yang or Yin, respectively. The third explanation is more trustworthy. Many diseases have a time cycle for recovery. This means that after seven or six days, the patient gets better without any special treatment. According to Chinese medicine, the recovery cycle is determined by the cycle of the Moon. However, as a TCM doctor, we need to prevent the disease from worsening or further unexpected conditions.

Dr. Liu Duzhou: Yang means the three Yang stages. Yin means the three Yin stages. The *seven* and the *six* here have no useful meaning. The Yang stage is treated with Guizhi Tang. The Yin stage is treated with Si Ni Tang. The intensity of body Yang Qi has a seven-day cycle. It means that the body surface becomes strongest again after seven days so that the patient can get recover after seven days.

Dr. Hu Xishu: Yang means the Taiyang stage and Yin means Shaoyin stage. The *seven* or *six* is a rough estimate; they have no true meaning. I never emphasize this concept. (A doctor still has to do what it is necessary to help patients get better soon.) The number has nothing to do with the Five Elements.

Dr. Martin Wang: The cycle of a disease can be disturbed after intervention by Western medicine, wrong treatment, careless diet, short sleep, improper physical exercise, heavy labor work, or even due to sexual stimulation, and so on.

Dr. Ni Haixia: If the disease is obtained during the daytime, it means that it is obtained in the Yang. If it is obtained at night, it means that it is obtained in the Yin. If it is obtained in the Yang, the length of the disease cycle starts to count on the next day, so there will be an additional six days (totaling seven days) before recovery. Whether the disease starts during the daytime or at night, after six days, the patient will recover (it's the natural course of a disease).

Dr. Li Keshao: Yang here means Yang overwhelming body constitution. Yin means Yang

(6) 病发热，头痛，脉反沉，若不差，身体疼痛，当救其里，宜四逆汤。

A Patient feels hot or feverish and has a headache. The pulse feels however deep (rather than floating).[406] (Use Mahuang Fuzi Xixin Tang for treatment.) After the treatment, if the body still feels generalized pain, the following procedure should focus to save the inner side of the body. For this aim, use Si Ni Tang for treatment.[407]

(7) 伤寒，脉缓，发热，无汗，其表不解，当发汗，不可与白虎汤，渴欲饮水，无表证者，白虎加人参汤主之。

In Cold-attack Taiyang stage, a patient has a fever, does not sweat and the pulse feels soft. This condition means the body surface condition remains not improved yet. Use Sweating therapy for treatment. The herbal formula Baihu Tang should not be used. If the patient feels thirsty and has a strong desire to drink water, and there is no body surface condition, use Baihu Jia Renshen Tang as the primary treatment.

deficient body constitution. The number of days can only be used as a general reference.

Dr. Gui Liang: There is a mistake in the time. It should read like this: If the disease starts from the Yang, the patient will get better after six days, and if it starts from the Yin, the patient will get better after seven days. Here, Yang should mean Yang body constitution. The body is usually in warm and active status. Yin means that the body constitution is in a Yang deficient condition (Yin condition). It is the body constitution that determines the disease's development course. My opinion matches the idea in the book *Huangdi Nei Jing* and the clinical reality and is also the same as the opinion of Dr. Ke Yunbo.

[406] Seniors easily suffer from Taiyang-Shaoyin body surface condition. It is the Shaoyin stage because the pulse is deep. The older patient may not feel hot, but their body temperature is high.

[407] Mahuang Fuzi Xixin Tang works to improve both body surface Coldness and inner Shaoyin Coldness. After treatment, if the body still feels pain, e.g., if the body surface disease condition remains, then it means that the inner Coldness is too heavy. It is, therefore, necessary to focus on treating the inner Coldness with the use of Si Ni Tang.

(8)　　病人身大热，反欲得近衣者，热在皮肤，寒在骨髓也；身大寒，反不欲近衣者，寒在皮肤，热在骨髓也。

A patient has a high fever but wants to cover the body more. This situation means that the heat is false (on the skin), and Coldness (in the bone marrow) is the actual disease status.[408] On the other hand, if a patient feels cold, but refuses to have additional cover for the body, the situation means that the cold is false (on the skin) and that the heat (in the bone marrow) is the actual disease condition.[409]

2. *Yangming stage*

In the Yangming stage (disease), there can be Wind-attack and Cold-attack conditions. The Yangming stage mostly involves muscles and the digestive system.[410]

阳明之为病，胃家实是也。

The nature of Yangming diseases is Stomach Excess condition.(either Hotness Excess or Coldness Excess syndrome.)

2.1 Yangming Wind-attack stage

(1)　　Yangming body surface stage

In Yangming body surface stage, if a patient feels fever, chills, doesn't sweat, has pain in the front of the head, and has dryness in the nose. Gegen Tang is usually used for treatment.[411]

脉浮发热，口乾鼻燥，能食者，则衄.

If the pulse feels floating, the patient has fever, dry nose and mouth, and there is no

problem eating, the patient will have nosebleeds.[412]

伤寒转系阳明者，其人濈然微汗出也。

That a Shanghan disease has moved into the Yangming stage means there is tidal, continuous, and mild sweat.[413]

伤寒发热，无汗，呕不能食，而反汗出濈濈然者，是转属阳明也。

With a Shanghan disease, if a patient has a fever, no sweat, is nauseous and cannot eat, and if the patient starts to have constant sweating, such situation means that the disease has turned into the Yangming stage.[414]

伤寒三日，阳明脉大者。

With a Shanghan disease for three days, if the pulse becomes big,[415] the Taiyang stage has moved into the Yangming stage.

热在上焦，心中懊憹，舌上胎者，用 栀子 鼓汤治疗。

When Fire is mostly in the upper part of the body (Upper Jiao), the patient feels annoyed,

---

[408] This is a condition in which Yin is overwhelming, so it rejects Yang. Use Tongmai Si Ni Tang for treatment.

[409] This is a condition in which Yang is overwhelming, so it rejects Yin. Use Baihu Tang for treatment.

[410] Basically, Warm disease and Wind-Warm disease have a short period in the Taiyang stage and the disease usually a very quickly moves into the Yangming stage.

[411] Some doctors call this stage the Yangming meridian stage.

[412] Here, the *floating pulse and fever, dry nose and mouth* all suggest that Fire is in the Yangming meridian, not in the inner organ level. The patient has a normal appetite because the Fire is in the meridian, not in the organ level. Note that there is no sweat, in this case, so the Fire has to find an outlet via bleeding from the nose. (Yangming meridian goes to the nose). If the fever in the Taiyang stage cannot be depleted through sweating (e.g., the patient has no sweat), the disease can be released via nosebleeds. Here, for the same reason, if the Fire in the Yangming body surface stage cannot be released via sweat, nosebleeding is also one of the ways to release the Fire. For the treatment of such body surface condition, use Gegen Tang.

[413] Dr. Liu Duzhou believed that this paragraph meant the Wind-attack Yangming stage.

　　Dr. Ni Haixia: If the sweat is only on the hands and feet, it is Weakness condition in the stomach.

[414] Dr. Liu Duzhou believed that this paragraph also meant the Wind-attack Yangming stage.

[415] Dr. Ni Haixia: The pulse is big, but it feels hollow inside the pulse.

and there is a thick tongue coat, use Zhizi Chi Tang for treatment.[416]

If the patient has a fever,[417] mildly sweats,[418] is thirsty,[419] is of cloudy mind, has an aversion to heat but not to cold, and the pulse feels big,[420] the disease is already in the Yangming Qi stage. In this stage, the patient feels feverish (Fire and Hotness), not cold or chilly at all.

伤寒脉浮滑，(此表有热、里有寒)，白虎汤主之。

With a Shanghan disease, if the pulse is floating and slippery,[421] (There is heat in the body surface but cold inside),[422] use Baihu Tang as the primary treatment.[423]

伤寒脉滑而厥者，里有热也，白虎汤主之。

With a Shanghan disease, if the pulse feels slippery and the patient has Jue syndrome (This is Hot Jue syndrome), use Baihu Tang as the primary treatment.

若渴欲饮水，口干舌燥者，白虎加 人参汤主之。

If a patient feels thirsty, likes to drink cold water, and feels dry in mouth and tongue, use Baihu Jia Renshen Tang as the primary treatment.[424]

---

[416] If the Yangming Fire is mostly in the body surface (muscles), use Baihu Tang. Some doctors believed that the Zhizi Chi Tang condition belongs to Yangming (body surface) Qi stage.

Dr. Du Yumao: The Yangming Qi phase includes Zhizi Chi Tang, Baihu Tang (Baihu with Ginseng Tang), Zhuling Tang (and Huangqin Tang?).

[417] When the Wind pathogenic Qi penetrates from the Taiyang stage into the Yangming stage of the body, it becomes Yang pathogenic Qi. Yang means warm and hot, to cause fever but not cold in the Yangming stage.

[418] If there is no sweat, there will be an itchy feeling. This is because the body condition is weak and the body has insufficient energy to produce sweat (the body is dry inside).

[419] In the textbook, it says the patient has a fever, profuse sweating, and thirst. When the body has a fever, it is rare to have profuse sweating at the same time. With heavy sweating, the body cannot retain a high body temperature.

[420] Big pulse: The pulse feels broader than usual.

[421] *Floating pulse*: Body surface is hot; *Slippery pulse*: inner hot condition. The pulse has to be felt very carefully.

Dr. Hao Wanshan: Floating pulse here means Fire. This has been introduced in Dahuang Huanglian Xiexin Tang condition (floating pulse in Guan position), in Xiao Xianxiong Tang condition (floating-slippery pulse) and Zhuling Tang condition (floating pulse). The pulse for Baihu Tang is not floating-big (not as the TCM textbook says).

[422] The text in parenthesis does not exist in the Kangping version of *Shanghan Lun.*

[423] The Baihu Tang condition belongs to Yangming (body surface) Qi stage.

Dr. Ni Haixia: In Baihu Tang, the herb Shigao (gupse gesso) is a very Cold herbal ingredient, and it works to nourish, to supply water to the blood, to reduce Fire, and fever. Herb Zhimu works to clear the annoyed feeling, stop thirst and supply liquid to the body. So it can work to solve the big thirst and dry mouth and throat. Herb Zhigancao nourishes Stomach Yang and Spleen Yang. When the Spleen Yang is not sufficient, e.g., the spleen is large and compresses the stomach, resulting in reduced appetite, Zhigancao can restore Spleen Yang, and restore function to the Stomach and appetite. Genmi (Glutinous rice) works to protect the mucus inside the branchi. During fever, the mucus of the branchi is very dry. Ginseng works to improve the function of the digestive system and supply more liquid to the body. It also works to protect the heart.

Dr. Ni Haixia: Baihu Tang can occur in the Taiyang, Shaoyang, Yangming, and Jueyin stages, whenever the water part in the blood is lost, and the blood has Fire in it.

Dr. Liao Houze: This is actually outer-fever and inner-cold condition. The mouth temperature is high, but the armpit temperature is low. Using Baihu Tang is the reverse way to treat the patient. Another such reverse treatment is seen when treating fever in a cancer patient: the body temperature is high but inner is Weakness-Coldness. Whenever Fire-clearing therapy does not work, change to Hotness-creating (Warm) therapy. It is also an example of the reverse treatment to treat patients who feel annoyed, who cannot sleep during the day, but generally sleep at night (there is no annoyed feeling at night), and who have a deep and weak pulse.

[424] The pulse feels big but weak if pressed harder. This condition can occur after a prolonged time of fever or constant sweating, or after diarrhea after the use of Purging therapy.

阳明病，法多汗，反无汗，其身如虫行皮中状者，此以久虚故也。

In the Yangming stage, patients should have profuse sweat. A patient has, however, no sweat, and feels wriggling sensation under the skin as there is worm wriggling. The reason for his situation is that the body condition has been in a weakness condition for a long time.[425]

若脉浮发热，渴欲饮水，小便不利者，猪苓 汤主之。阳明病，汗出多而渴者，不可与 猪苓 汤，以汗多胃中燥，猪苓 汤复利其小便故也。

If a pulse feels floating, the patient has a fever, feels thirsty and wants to drink water, and urinating is difficult, use Zhuling Tang as the primary treatment.[426] If the patient is heavily sweating and feels thirsty, Zhuling Tang should not be used, because with the heavy sweat, the body inside is dry (so that it is easy to develop inner excessive Fullness condition), and Zhuling Tang causes more depletion of water through urine to make the inner Dryness worse.[427]

阳明病，口燥，但欲漱水不欲咽者，此必衄。

In the Yangming stage, if a patient feels dry mouth but only wants to wet the mouth and is

---

Traditional, after the fever stops, if body liquid has not been restored to a reasonable level, the patient feels dry mouth, throat, and lips, is nauseous, hiccups, has an annoying feeling in the chest which causes difficulty falling asleep, the tongue is red in color with little tongue coating, and the pulse feels weak but fast. In this case, use Zhuye Shigao Tang.

[425] No sweat: There is insufficient body liquid supplied from the stomach to the skin, and the patient can not create sweat. Because previous Fire exhausted the body liquid (Yin), there is insufficient water. Note that the body still has Fire.

Dr. Hao Wanshan: In the Yangming stage, there are three disease conditions in which the body has no sweat. The first is Gegen Tang condition (fever, chills, no sweat, pain in the eyes, dryness in the nose and poor sleep). The second is Hotness-Dampness jaundice syndrome (most patients sweat only on the head, and some don't sweat at all). The third is the itchy skin condition noted here (there is inner Fire, but insufficient body liquid to form sweat).

Dr. Hu Xishu: If the patient also has a hard and firm stool, use Maziren Wan for treatment.

Dr. Ni Haixia: For the itch, use Guizhi Jia Huangqi Tang for treatment.

Dr. Wang Hu: Use Gegen Tang for treatment.

[426] Due to depletion of body liquid through Purging therapy, for instance, the stomach Qi becomes weak, and the water in the stomach cannot be shunted into the urine. The body has Fire in both the body surface and in the inside.

Dr. Lao Zhuang: Here we should use Zexie Tang to clear the Fire and deplete accumulated water.

[427] The Zhuling Tang condition is due to Yangming Fire entanglement with water in the urine bladder. The patient had garbage water in the urine bladder before becoming sick this time. Another explanation is that it is due to drinking too much water while in the Baihu Tang condition, which causes garbage water retention in the stomach and the garbage water affects urination.

Dr. Hu Xishu: The Zhizi Chi Tang condition, the Baihu with Ginseng Tang condition and the Zhuling Tang condition here all are the result of using Purging therapy too early.

Dr. Martin Wang: These three formula syndromes can be regarded as three atypical Yangming body surface conditions, due to a previously sick condition of the body. For Zhizi Chi Tang condition, the patient had previous Dampness in the chest (the tongue coating is thick). For Baihu Jia Renshen Tang condition, the patient had Dryness in the stomach before becoming sick this time. For Zhuling Tang condition, the patient has garbage water retention in the urine bladder before becoming sick this time. Therefore, when the Fire moves from the Taiyang body surface into the Yangming stage, the Fire combines with Dampness in the chest to cause Zhizi Chi Tang condition, to exhaust more liquid from the stomach and cause Baihu Jia Renshen Tang condition, and to combine with garbage water in the urine bladder to cause Zhuling Tang condition.

not willing to swallow the water,[428] the patient will have nosebleeds. [429]

(2) Yangming Wind-attack inner stage

If the Yangming body surface condition furthermore develops, the patients will feel bloating in the abdomen, have no bowel movement for several days, have a hardness feeling in the abdomen when touched, dislike being pressed on the belly, have delirious speech, or even lose consciousness. Such a situation is because the Fire in the stomach-intestine has burned off the water, exhausted the body liquid, caused hard, dry and firm stool. Such stool can block the digestive duct, and cause accumulation of toxins in the body.

For treatment, use various Dahuang-containing herbal formulas, depending on the location of the firm stool inside the digestive system. With dry-firm stool in the digestive system, there will be pain from pressure on the abdomen.

(2.1). Tiaowei Chengqi Tang condition

If the firm stool locates in the stomach, the pain will be in the Zhongwan (CV12) point. Use Tiaowei Chengqi Tang[430] for treatment.

太阳病三日，发汗不解，蒸蒸发热者，属胃也，调胃承气汤主之。

In the Taiyang stage for three days, a Sweating therapy was given, the patient starts to feel a constant steaming fever.[431] This situation means that the disease has penetrated in the Yangming stage.[432] Use Tiaowei Chengqi Tang as the primary treatment.[433]

伤寒吐后，腹胀满者，与调胃承气汤。

With a Shanghan disease, after a Vomiting therapy, a patient feels fullness and bloating in the abdomen. [434] For such case, use Tiaowei Chengqi Tang for treatment.[435]

阳明病，不吐，不下，心烦者，可与调胃承气汤。

In the Yangming stage, if a patient has no vomit, no diarrhea, but feels annoyed and

---

[428] Dr. Liu Duzhou: Because the Fire is in the mouth, not in stomach yet, the patient has dry mouth but does not want to swallow the water.

Dr. Liao Houze: A *patient wants to drink water but has no will to swallow* suggests body blood stagnation.

[429] Dr. Liu Duzhou: The nosebleeding here means there is Fire in the Yangming meridian. In the Yangming stage, the Fire in the inner side of the body causes fever, dry mouth, thirst, tidal sweat, difficulty urinating and dry-firm stool.

Dr. Hu Xishu and Dr. Hao Wanshan: The nosebleeding here means there is Fire in the Yangming blood phase. Whenever Fire is in the blood phase, there is s dry mouth and nose, but the patient has no desire to drink water. If the Fire is in the Qi phase, the patient feels dry mouth and throat and wants to drink more water, such as in the Baihu Jia Renshen Tang condition. The Fire disturbs the blood to cause nose bleeding.

Dr. Hao Wanshan: *Floating pulse, fever, dry mouth and throat* belong to Yangming body surface condition. Note that nosebleeding in Taiyang stage may indicate a self-healing of the disease, but it does not mean so in the Yangming stage. In the Yangming stage, the nosebleeding means Fire in the blood, and it is not a sign of self-healing.

Dr. Du Yumao: In the Yangming blood phase, the patient can also have delirious speech, bleeding from the nose, stool or urine, Heat invasion in blood chamber syndrome, poor memory, or even loss of consciousness, and so on.

---

[430] *Tiao* means "to correct", "to adjust". *Wei* means "stomach-intestine". *Chengqi* means "conduct Qi movement".

[431] Dr. Hao Wanshan: The original word for fever should not be translated into a *steam-like* fever.

[432] If the patient has dry mouth, use Baihu Tang. If the patient is thirsty, use Baihu Jia Renshen Tang.

[433] Dr. Liao Houze: Tiaowei Chengqi Tang only solves the Fire, it does not stimulate the bowel movement. Xiao Chengqi Tang only activates the bowel movement, and Da Chengqi Tang causes diarrhea (strong bowel movement).

[434] In this case, there is no pain in the abdomen yet, and the abdomen does not feel hardness when pressed, and bowel movement is normal.

[435] If the bloating and fullness in the abdomen is not developed after the use of Vomiting therapy, Xiao Chengqi Tang needs to be considered.

vexation, use Tiaowei Chengqi Tang for treatment.[436]

(2.2). Xiao Chengqi Tang condition

If a dry-firm stool blocks the small intestine, there will be a pressing pain on the Guanyuan (CV4) and Zhongji points (CV3) points. The tongue coating is yellow, dry and the tongue looks old. The pulse is fast and slippery. Use Xiao Chengqi Tang for treatment.

太阳病，若吐、若下、若发汗，微烦，小便数，大便因硬者，与小承气汤和之愈。

If a Taiyang stage was treated with a Vomiting therapy, or a Purging therapy, or a Sweating therapy, a patient feels mild annoyance, has frequent urination, and has firm stool (not the dry-firm stool yet),[437] use Xiao Chengqi Tang conciliate the digestive system.[438]

阳明病，其人多汗，以津液外出，胃中燥，大便必硬，硬则谵语，小承气汤主之。若一服谵语止者，更莫复服。

In the Yangming sage, a patient has profuse sweating, which causes loss of body liquid and makes stomach in dry status, so there is dry-firm stool in the bowels. Such a firm stool causes delirious speech. For such case, use Xiao Chengqi Tang as the primary treatment. If one drink of the herbal tea stops the delirious speech, do not continue to drink more.[439]

阳明病，谵语，发潮热，脉滑而疾者，小承气汤主之。因与承气汤一升，腹中转失气者，更服一升，若不转失气者，勿更与之。明日又不大便，脉反微涩者，虚也，为难治，不可更与承气汤也。

In the Yangming stage, if a patient has delirious speech, has a tidal fever and the pulse is slippery and fast,[440] use Xiao Chengqi Tang for treatment. After drinking the herbal tea and if there is farting, the herbal tea can be drunk again. If there is no farting, stop using the formula,[441] wait until the next day, and if the pulse becomes slightly rough, the condition suggests that the body is weak and the disease condition is difficult to treat. (Xiao) Chengqi Tang should no longer be used.

(2.3). Da Chengqi Tang condition

---

[436] For people with constipation and annoyance, depression or anxiety or similar emotional disorders, pay attention to the Tiaowei Chengqi Tang condition. Previously we have introduced the following: (1) When the patient feels hot, annoyed, and fullness and pressing feeling in the chest after Sweating therapy or Purging therapy, Zhizi Chi Tang should be used mostly. (2) After Purging therapy, if the patient feels more annoyed, if the stomach area is soft when pressed, and the annoyed feeling is deficient annoyed, then Zhizi Chi Tang should be used.
[437] Frequent urination and hard-firm stool: The disease has progressed into the Yangming stage. If the Yangming stage is developed from body liquid depletion, the inner Fire is not very strong.
[438] If the patient has no annoyed feeling, use Maziren Wan for treatment.

   Dr. Ni Haixia: The herb Dahuang works to remove the stool. If the body condition is Hotness-fullness, Dahuang is used together with Fire-clearing herbs, such as with Xiao Chengqi Tang. If the constipation is due to Coldness-fullness, Dahuang can also be used, but with Wam herbs, such as with Dahuang Fuzi Xixin Tang.

[439] The hard-firm stool, in this case, is not due to high fever, but because the patient usually sweats easily and in the Yangming stage there is furthermore sweating (the fever is not very high). The sweat can exhaust the inner liquid to cause delirious speech. In such inner Fullness condition, use Xiao Chengqi Tang, not Da Chengqi Tang. Similarly, if a patient was given Sweating therapy, had profuse sweating, then Sweating therapy was used again, if the patient has a fullness feeling in the abdomen, and has delirious speech, also use this Xiao Chengqi Tang, not Da Chengqi Tang for treatment.
[440] Dr. Hao Wanshan: If the pulse is deep-hard, this disease condition belongs to Da Chengqi Tang condition. This is a fast-slippery pulse.
[441] Dr. Hao Wanshan: No matter the patient typically has Da Chengqi Tang condition or it is a normal person, after taking Xiao Chengqi Tang, there should be farting. No farting may suggest a special condition during the Yangming stage which can be understood as a paralytic ileus condition. In such paralytic ileus, there may be no farting because the bowel does not respond to the herbal formula.

If there is a dry-firm stool in the large intestine, the pain will be on Tianshu point (ST25, about 5 to 6 cm beside the navel). If it is in the rectum, the pain will be in the right lower part of the abdomen, and the patient will want to lie down, face up, with the right leg bent. The patient has no bowel movement, has much gas, or has awful body odor and water-like stool[442] (with a very firm and big abdomen and strong pressure pain in the belly). There is heavy sweating on the palms and feet. The patient has delirious speech or loses consciousness. The tongue is dry or cracked. The tongue coating is yellow, black as coke and thick. The pulse feels deep but strong or fast and slippery. Use Da Chengqi Tang for treatment.[443]

阳明病，谵语有潮热，反不能食者，胃中必有燥屎五六枚也。若能食者，但硬耳，宜大承气汤下之。

In the Yangming stage, a patient has a tidal fever,[444] delirious speech, and however cannot eat. Such a condition suggests that there is dry stool in the bowels. If the patient still can eat, it means that the stool is indeed firm.[445] Use Da Chengqi Tang to deplete it.[446]

汗出谵语者，以有燥屎在胃中，此为风也，须下者，过经乃可下之。下之若早，语言必乱，以表虚里实故也。下之愈，宜大承气汤

If a patient has sweating and delirious speech, it means that there is dry-firm stool in the bowels.[447] This is Wind-attack condition. Purging therapy (Da Chengqi Tang) should be used for treatment, but it must be used after the body surface condition no longer exists. If the therapy is used too early, the patient will have cluttered speech,[448] because the body condition is deficient in body surface but excess in inner side. For the Purging therapy, use Da Chengqi Tang.

---

[442] Usually, the stool is blue or dark color.

[443] If the patient has slight fullness in the abdomen, the stool is firm in the beginning part but loose in the later part, and then Da Chengqi Tang should not be used. It can be used when the stool is hard-firm in the intestine. Evidence for firm stool is high fever with heavy sweating; frequent urination, the hands, and feet start to sweat, or there is tidal fever/hot feeling in the afternoon. The tidal hot feeling must be accompanied with a slightly firm stool. The tidal hot feeling with the soft stool still does not indicate firm stool in the large intestine.

If the diagnosis of firm stool is difficult, use Xiao Chengqi Tang for a test. After drinking the herbal tea, if there is farting from the anus, it indicates that there is firm stool in the large intestine.

[444] Dr. Hao Wanshan: From Baihu Jia Rebshen Tang condition to Tiaowei Chengqi Tang condition, then moving to Da Chengqi Tang condition, Fire has shrunk deep into the bowels, and the fever changes from whole body hot to continuous hot, to tidal fever. Similarly, the sweat changes from profuse sweat to less sweat in the Da Chengqi Tang condition. In the latter, the sweat remains only on the hands and feet.

[445] If the stool is only firm, but not dry-firm, use Xiao Chengqi Tang for treatment.

[446] *Tidal fever, delirious speech and cannot eat*, all are common indications of the forming of dry-firm stool in the bowels, and the Da Chengqi Tang should be used. In the early stage of Yangming, the patient can eat because there is Fire in the stomach. Now the patient cannot eat. It means there is dry-firm stool in the bowels and there is also dried and old, not-yet digested food (garbage food) in the stomach. The dirty corrupted air rushes and pushes up to affect appetite and digestion.

[447] The delirious speech suggests that the disease has progressed into the Yangming stage too (the Taiyang stage is not over yet). This is Taiyang-Yangming successive co-existing condition.

[448] Purging therapy will bring body surface Fire into the bowel to make the Dryness condition inside worse.

Dr. Liu Duzhou: Sweat here indicates the Yangming body surface condition. This is a Yangming body surface and Yangming inner Fullness co-existing condition.

Dr. Hu Xishu: Sweat here means the Taiyang Wind-attack condition.

Dr. Martin Wang: Sweat here might be either the Taiyang condition or a Yangming condition. It needs to be clarified. For sweat in the Taiyang stage, it is not heavy and the fever, if any, is not very high for most patients. For sweat in the Yangming stage, the sweat is heavy, wave-like (tidal), the fever is also high and wave-like (tidal), and the fever is mostly higher in the afternoon.

阳明病脉迟, 虽汗出，不恶寒者，其身必重，短气腹满而喘。有潮热者，(此外欲解，可攻里也)。手足戢然而汗出者，(此大便已硬也)，大承气汤主之；若汗多微发热恶寒者，外未解也，其热不潮，未可与承气汤；若腹满不通者，可与小承气汤，微和胃气，勿令大泄下。

In the Yangming stage, a pulse feels slow,[449] though there is sweat, the patient has no aversion to cold.[450] For such case, the patient will feel generalized heaviness,[451] feels shortness of breath,[452] fullness in the abdomen, and has panting.[453]

If the patient has a tidal fever (suggesting that the body surface condition is to be dissolved, a Purging therapy can be used) and there is sweat on the hands and feet (now the stool is firm),[454] use Da Chengqi Tang as the primary treatment.[455]

If the patient has profuse sweating, and slight fever with an aversion to cold, (it means the body surface condition remains.[456]) and if the fever is not as tidal, Purging therapy should not be used.

If the patient feels mostly fullness, use Xiao Chengqi Tang to calm the Stomach Qi. Do not create massive diarrhea.

阳明病，潮热，大便微硬者，可与大承气汤，不硬者，不与之。若不大便六七日，恐有燥屎，欲知之法，少与小承气汤，汤入腹中，转矢气者，此有燥屎，乃可攻之；若不转矢气者，此但初头硬，后必溏，(不可攻之)，攻之，必胀满不能食也。欲饮水者，与水则哕。其后发热者，必大便复硬而少也，以小承气汤和之。不转矢气者，慎不可攻也。

In the Yangming stage, there is a tidal fever, and the stool is slightly firm,[457] Da Chengqi Tang can be used. If the stool is not firm, it should not be used.

If there is no bowel movement for six to seven days and if it is suspected that there is firm stool inside, use Xiao Chengqi Tang to test. If there is farting, it means that there is firm stool inside the intestine and the Da Chengqi Tang can be used.

If there is no farting,[458] and if the stool is only firm in the beginning part but loose in the latter part, the Da Chengqi Tang should not be used. Otherwise, the patient will feel more bloated and cannot eat. In such a case, if the patient wants to drink water, the water will cause hiccups.[459] If the patient has a

---

[449] Slow pulse usually suggests that the body is in a weak condition, so Purging therapy should be used carefully.

[450] *Sweat and no chills*: Yangming body Surface condition is fully present. Due to the slow pulse, the inner Fire should not be intense.

[451] *Heavy feeling in the body*: There is Dampness in the body. This also indicates that the Fire inside the body is not intense.

[452] *Short of breath*: This is due to the presence of retained water in the stomach.

[453] *Panting*: This is due to inner Fire rushing up.

[454] Dr. Liu Duzhou: This means there is whole body sweat plus sweat on the hands and feet.

Dr. Ni Haixia: If the sweat is on the whole body, it means that the liquid in the digestive system has not been depleted entirely yet. If the whole body has no sweat except for the hands and feet, it means that the liquid in the digestive system has been depleted completely.

[455] *Wave-like fever and sweat on the hands and feet* suggest that the inner side of the bowel is full of firm stool that needs to be depleted using Purging therapy. Da Chengqi Tang and Xiao Chengqi Tang belong to Purging therapy.

[456] It can be either Taiyang body surface condition or Yangming body surface condition.

---

[457] Dr. Hao Wanshan: The stool should be firm, not slightly hard. The original text is "slightly firm".

[458] Dr. Hao Wanshan: Whether for a healthy person or a patient with old-firm stool, there should be farting after the use of Xiao Chengqi Tang. If there is no farting after the use of the herbal formula, it is most likely a paralytic ileus in which the bowel cannot move to produce farts. After the bowel recovers from the paralytic condition, there will be a beginning-firm and latter-soft stool.

Dr. Hu Xishu: After the use of Xiao Chengqi Tang, there is no farting, but the stool passes out as beginning-firm and latter-soft stool. The use of Xiao Chengqi Tang is correct.

[459] Dr. Hao Wanshan: Only with the paralytic ileus should the patient have hiccups after drinking water. This is because the air in the bowel does not move down and the water could stimulate the diaphragm to cause the hiccups.

fever later, the stool will become firm again and less in volume. In such cases, use Xiao Chengqi Tang to conciliate the bowel. If there is no farting, the intense Purging therapy (Da Chengqi Tang) should not be used.

得病二三日，脉弱，无太阳 柴胡 证，烦躁，心下硬，至四五日，虽能食，以小承气汤少少与，微和之，令小安，至六日，与承气汤一升。若不大便六七日，小便少者，虽不能食，但初头硬，后必溏，未定成硬，攻之必溏，须小便利，屎定硬，乃可攻之，宜大承气汤。

With a Shanghan disease for two to three days, the pulse feels faint. No conditions are indicating the Taiyang or Shaoyang (Chaihu syndrome) conditions. The patient feels annoyed, restless, and hardness in the upper abdomen. On the fourth and fifth day, the patient can eat. Use a small dose of Xiao Chengqi Tang to harmonize the stomach slightly. On the sixth day, use the full treatment of this formula.

If there is no bowel movent for six to seven days, the volume of urination is small; the patient cannot eat, the stool is firm in the beginning but loose in the latter part, the condition means the stool is not firm yet. [460] Intensive Purging therapy (Da Chengqi Tang) should not be used. Wait until the urination is smooth, then the stool can be confirmed being firm. Use intensive Purging therapy, such as Da Chengqi Tang as the primary treatment. [461]

阳明少阳合病，必下利。(其脉不负者，顺也；负者，失也。互相克贼，名为负也)。脉滑而数者，有宿食也，当下之，宜大承气汤。

In the Yangming-Shaoyang concurrent stages, there should have diarrhea. [462] … If the pulse

is slippery and frequent, the body condition suggests that there is retained food in the bowel. Purging therapy should be used. Use Da Chengqi Tang for treatment. [463]

二阳并病，太阳证罢，但发潮热，手足絷絷汗出，大便难而谵语者，下之则愈，宜大承气。

In the Taiyang-Yangming successive stages, once the Taiyang stage is over, the patient has a tidal fever, has mild but continuous sweating on the hands and feet, the bowel movement is difficult, the patient has delirious speech, Purging therapy can solve the disease situation. Use Da Chengqi Tang for treatment. [464]

病人烦热，汗出则解，又(复)如疟状，日晡所发热者，属阳明也。脉实者宜下之，脉浮虚者，宜发汗，下之宜大承气汤。发汗宜 桂枝 汤。

A patient has an annoyingly hot feeling. The patient has a sweat (after being treated with a Sweating therapy), the body condition seems improved after the sweat. Later, however, the patient has alternating hot and cold as having malaria. If the patient has a fever in the later afternoon, the disease belongs to the Yangming. If the pulse feels strong, [465] use Purging therapy for treatment. If the pulse feels floating and weak, [466] Sweating therapy

---

[460] If Da Chengqi Tang is used when the stool is firm in the beginning part but soft in the later part, there will be constant diarrhea.

[461] Dr. Hu Xishu: This paragraph reminds the doctor to cautious wait for concrete evidence for the use of Da Chengqi Tang, especially when the pulse feels slow or weak.

[462] The original texts "其脉不负者，顺也；负者，失也。互相克贼，名为负也" is hard to understand and to translate.

[463] In this case, if the Shaoyang disease condition is much stronger than the Yangming, use Da Chaihu Tang.

Dr. Liu Duzhou: There are different ideas about this paragraph. Does it have two separate meanings or is it one condition? If two meanings, then *In the Yangming and Shaoyang concurrent condition, there will be diarrhea* is one meaning, and *If the pulse is slippery and frequent, it suggests that there is retained food in the* bowel is the other meaning.

[464] In this case, the Taiyang stage is over, so that Purging therapy can be considered. This means that the disease condition now no longer belongs to the Taiyang-Yangming concurrent condition.

[465] *Fever at a fixed time in the later afternoon and if the pulse feels strong* belongs to Yangming.

[466] *Fever at a fixed time in the later afternoon and if the pulse feels floating and weak* belongs to Taiyang Wind-attack.

is needed.[467] For Purging therapy, use Da Chengqi Tang; for Sweating therapy, use Guizhi Tang.[468]

伤寒若吐、若下后，不解，不大便五六日，上至十余日，日晡所发潮热，不恶寒，独语如见鬼状。若剧者，发则不识人，循衣摸床，惕而不安，微喘直视，脉弦者生，涩者死，微者但发热谵语者，大承气汤主之。若一服利，止后服。

With a Shanghan disease, Vomiting therapy or Purging therapy failed to improve the disease condition. The patient has no bowel movement for five to six days, or even up to ten days. The patient also has a tidal fever in the evening (sunset time), has no aversion to cold. The patient chatters as if seeing a ghost. In severe cases, the patient may loss recognition of people, try to touch surrounding material (bed-sheet), appears irritable and restless, has mild shortness of breath, and eyes stare straight ahead.[469] If the pulse feels string,[470] the patient can still be alive. If the pulse is rough, the patient will die. For mild cases, if the patient only has a fever and has delirious speech, use Da Chengqi Tang as the primary treatment. If there is bowel movement, stop using it.[471]

伤寒六七日，目中不了了，睛不和，无表里证，大便难，身微热者，此为实也。急下之，宜大承气汤。

With a Shanghan disease for six or seven days, a patient stares and the eyes do not move.[472] There is no evidence for the body surface condition, the bowel movement is difficult, and the patient has a mild fever.[473] Such a situation is an excess disease condition.[474] Urgent Purging therapy should be applied. Use Da Chengqi Tang.[475]

汗不解，腹满痛者，急下之，宜大承气汤。腹满不减，减不足言，当下之，宜大承气汤。

After Sweating therapy, the body surface condition remains not improved, and a patient has severe bloating along with fullness and pain in the abdomen. Use Da Chengqi Tang for urgent treatment.[476] After the treatment, if the extent of the bloating and fullness in the belly is only slightly improved (or the reduction is neglectable), use the Da Chengqi Tang again.[477]

---

[467] If either of the treatments still cannot improve the fever, check if there is garbage water retention or dead blood condition in the body, especially the latter. With dead blood condition, the patient feels very annoyed or exhibits mad-like behavior or craving to eat. Use Di Dang Tang.

Dr. Liu Duzhou: The floating-weak pulse, the fever, and sweating indicate that there is Yangming body surface condition (not Taiyang body surface condition).

[468] Here again, the Guizhi Tang is used to create "sweat".

[469] *Chattering as if seeing a ghost, losing recognition of people, touching surrounding material, being irritable and restless, mild asthma, and eyes staring straight ahead* all suggest a severe condition. The Yang Qi in the body is floating out of the body and is not bound to the Yin.

[470] In one book version, it is string pulse.

[471] In TCM, once a patient has problems with consciousness, the doctor should check the bowel movement to see if the disease is in the Yangming stage. The Yangming stage is associated with

disorders in the abdomen region, which is believed to be the second "brain" of the body. This concept has only recently been accepted by Western medicine.

[472] Dr. Hao Wanshan: The Liver liquid (Yin) has been exhausted.

[473] Dr. Hao Wanshan: This is a severe condition in which the body Yin liquid has been largely exhausted, and the body has insufficient energy to struggle against the pathogenic Qi so that the body reaction seems less intense. The patient has no apparent tidal fever and no sharp pain around the navel.

[474] Excess condition: This is not a weak condition. It means that there is some disease mass in the body. Mass here means firm stool.

[475] If a patient with Shanghan disease has had such an eye problem and difficulty in bowel movement, the disease condition suggests that there is firm stool in the bowel now, even though the bowel movement is only difficult and the fever is only mild.

[476] This is a disease condition in which solid and firm stool is formed in the bowel, and the Fire inside the body is severe, which could exhaust the body liquid very quickly so that urgent treatment with Da Chengqi Tang is needed to stop the Fire.

[477] For a patient with bloating and fullness, if the bloating and fullness subside for a while, then the feeling comes back again, or the patient does not feel

阳明病，发热，汗多者，急下之，宜大承气汤。

In the Yangming stage, when there are fever and profuse sweating, urgent Purging therapy is needed. Use Da Chengqi Tang.[478]

病人不大便五六日，绕脐痛，烦躁，发作有时者，此有燥屎，故使不大便也。

A patient has had no bowel movement for five to six days, has pain around the naval, feels annoyed. Such symptoms occurred with fixed time. These conditions suggest that the patient has a dry-firm stool in the bowel,[479] which blocks bowel movement.[480]

大下后，六七日不大便，烦不解，腹满痛者，此有燥屎也。所以然者，本有宿食故也，宜大承气汤。

A patient was treated with intensive Purging therapy (and had a significant bowel

movement), there was no bowel movement again for six to seven days. The patient feels continuously annoyed and has fullness and pain in the abdomen. These conditions indicate a dry-firm stool in bowels, which is caused by earlier retained food in the intestines. For treatment, use Da Chengqi Tang.

阳明病，下之，心中懊恼而烦，胃中有燥屎者，可攻。腹微满，初头硬，后必溏，不可攻之。若有燥屎者，宜大承气汤。

In the Yangming stage, a Purging therapy was used. A patient feels annoyed, and there is a dry-firm stool in the bowel. In such case, the Purging therapy can be used again. If the patient only feels slight fullness in the abdomen, and the stool is firm just in the beginning part but soft in the latter part,[481] then the Purging therapy should not be used. If there is a dry-firm stool, use Da Chengqi Tang for treatment.

病人小便不利，大便乍难乍易，时有微热，喘冒不能卧者，有燥屎也，宜大承气汤。

A patient has difficulty urinating. The bowel movement is sometimes easy but sometimes tricky,[482] sometimes has a mild fever, has panting or dizziness or drunk-like feelings (cloudy mind) that prevent lying down. Such disease conditions indicate a dry-firm stool in the bowel. Try to use Da Chengqi Tang.[483]

---

bloated in the morning but does in the afternoon, or they feel bloated during the day, but less so at night, such bloating and fullness belong to a Weakness condition. This requires a Warm and nourishing therapy, such as the use of Hou Jiang Xia Cao Renshen Tang.

[478] Clearing the Fire through stool is one of the most important ways to remove significant Fever. A patient in the Yangming stage with profuse sweating can experience that the disease progress very fast and that the disease condition exhaust the body liquid, resulting in death.

Dr. Du Yumao: There are several explanations for the three Purging therapies used in the Shaoyin stage: (1) this is severe Shaoyin Hotness condition; (2) the Shaoyin stage develops into Yangming stage; (3) the Shaoyin Cold-manifestation suddenly changes into Shaoyin Hotness condition; (4) Yangming inner stage shows false Coldness, which is similar to the Shaoyin stage.

This condition can also be treated with Da Chaihu Tang. Its usage (to replace the Da Chengqi Tang) is introduced in the book Jin Kui Yao Luo (金匮要略).

[479] Old, solid and firm stool: The stool formed in the bowel before becoming sick this time. The patient must have eaten a lot and then had constipation. Such firm and solid stool are different from the firm stool that is formed while being sick this time. The recently formed firm stool is relatively easier to be depleted with proper Purging therapy.

[480] In this case, try Da Chengqi Tang.

---

[481] For such a case, use Zhizi Chi Tang for treatment.

[482] Dr. Hao Wanshan: The body has three ways to expel Fire: sweat, urine, and water-diarrhea (The Fire presses body liquid into the bowel). When the body Fire presses the body liquid to the bowel, the stool is always to come down.

[483] In the Yangming stage, if urination is natural, the stool tends to be firm. If urination is abnormal, the stool tends to be soft. However, if urination is abnormal but the stool is not always firm if the patient has asthma that causes difficulty sleeping, if the patient has an up-rushing feeling, all suggest that there is Fire inside the body. In this case, even if the patient has not lost conscience yet, it suggests a firm stool ready in the abdomen. So, urgent Purging therapy should be used.

Da Chengqi Tang is very powerful for removing dry-firm stool from the large intestine and colon. However, it may also easily cause terrible diarrhea and deplete body liquid, causing

(2.4). Maziren Wan[484]

趺阳脉浮而涩，浮则胃气强，涩则小便数，浮涩相搏，大便则难，其脾为约，麻子仁丸主之。

The pulse on the back of foot feels floating and rough (not slippery). The floating pulse suggests that Stomach Qi is strong.[485] The rough pulse suggests that the urination is frequent.[486] With the floating and the rough entanglement in the body, the bowel movement would be difficult. The function of Spleen is restrained. This disease condition is called Spleen-restrained syndrome.[487] Use Maziren Wan as the primary treatment.

(With the Spleen-restrained syndrome, the patient can have no bowel movement for several days, or even more than ten days, without apparent discomfort. This syndrome is mostly caused by depletion of body liquid by various means (such as heavy sweating due to Sweating therapy, or frequent urination, and so on.) With this syndrome, the pulse can also feel floating when lightly touched[488] but feels hollow when pressed harder.[489])

(Among the three Chengqi Tang, Tiaowei Chengqi Tang is the mildest in function. It works for patients with Hotness (Fire) and blockage (no bowel movement), but not for intensive bloating or big-size abdomen. Xiao Chengqi Tang is stronger in function. It is used for obstruction, bloating, big belly, but only if the fire and dryness are not intense. Da Chengqi Tang is the strongest in function. It is used for strong Hotness, Dryness, blockage, bloating, big-sized abdomen, hardness in the abdomen and abdominal pain.[490])

2.2 Yangming Cold-attack stage [491]

Cold-attack Yangming body surface stage

If Cold pathogenic Qi penetrates the digestive system, the disease is in the Cold-attack Yangming stage. Patients in this stage have different symptoms and body signs from the Wind-attack Yangming stage. The Cold-attack Yangming stage can be caused by drinking a large volume of cold or ice water, or eating a large amount of cold food or hardly digesting food, especially if the digestive system is in a weak condition, or if the disease occurs during a hot summer.[492]

---

death. It is very important to make sure that the stool is indeed firm in the large intestine and that Da Chengqi Tang is the only choice for solving the problem. It is recommended to give the patient Xiao Chengqi Tang as a test. If the patient has frequent gas (farting), the farting indicates that Da Chengqi Tang can be tried.

[484] Here *wan* means pill.

[485] Dr. Hao Wanshan: Here again the floating pulse indicates the Fire.

[486] Dr. Hao Wanshang: With Spleen Yin deficiency, the Spleen can absorb liquid from the digestive system and distribute it to the body tissue, but cannot bring the liquid back to the digestive system to wet or to lubricate the stool now. For this reason, the urine is large in volume, but the stool is firm.

[487] The Spleen-restrain syndrome was translated as "splenic constipation" in WHO terminology glossary.

Dr. Liao Houze: Patients with the Spleen-restrain syndrome tend to have a high bone on the top of the nose.

[488] Such floating pulse suggests Fire in body surface.

[489] Such hollow pulse suggests insufficient blood inside.

[490] There is another Chengqi Tang that is used in clinics. It is called complemented Da Chengqi Tang. It uses herb Zhiqiao (the shell of herb Zhishi) to replace herb Zhishi, with the addition of fried Laifu seeds, peal kernel, and Chishao. It increases the function of the original Da Chengqi Tang to conduct Qi movement in the bowel, to release blood stagnation in the bowel. It is used for simple intestine obstruction.

[491] Many doctors who took part in the study of *Shang Han Lun* did not mention or discuss the Yangming Cold-attack condition.

[492] Because the Yangming Cold-attack stage is usually not caused by the invasion of exogenous pathogenic Qi, many TCM doctors who deal with the *Shanghan Lun* do not mention or discuss this Cold-attack stage of the Yangming disease. They may regard such

阳明病若能食，名中风；不能食，名中寒。

In the Yangming stage, if a patient can eat, the disease condition belongs to the Wind-attack Yangming; if a patient cannot eat, [493] (There is no appetite and eating makes the patient feel pain or bloated in the abdomen.) the disease condition belongs to the Cold-attack Yangming.

阳明病，若中寒，不能食，小便不利，手足戢然汗出，(此欲作固瘕)，必大便初硬后溏。(所以然者，以胃中冷，水谷不别故也)

In Cold-attack Yangming stage, patients cannot eat, urination is difficult, [494] there is mildly sweat on the hands and feet [495] (Such condition is to develop into Gujia (固瘕) syndrome.[496]), the stool will be firm in the

beginning part, but looser (shapeless) in the latter part.[497]

(The reason for the Gujia syndrome is the Coldness in Stomach/Spleen, the water in the digestive system cannot be shunted to the urinary system.) [498]

伤寒，脉浮而缓，手足自温者，是系在太阴；太阴者，身当发黄，若小便自利者，

---

disease as a miscellaneous disease, rather than a Shanghan disease.

In the summer, the inside of the body has Coldness, though the body's outside has Hotness. This is similar to the earth in summer: the outside is hot, but the underground is cold. Therefore, it is easier to cause Cold-attack Yangming disease in the summer when consuming lots of cold food or drink.

Dr. Kang Cangping: Yangming Cold-attack is a Coldness-Weakness disease condition in the Stomach (Yangming), while the Taiyin stage is Coldness-Weakness in the Spleen system. (Kang Cangping: Discussion about the Yangming Wind-attack and Cold-attack in the book *Shanghan Lun*. Gansu J TCM. 2008, 21(7):4)

[493] Digestion needs warm energy, but if the inner side of the digestive system is cold, the patient cannot eat.

[494] Dr. Hao Wanshan: One of the functions of the Spleen is to separate water into the urine. With insufficient Spleen Yang, the Spleen cannot change water into the urine, so urination is less frequent.

[495] Dr. Liu Duzhou: Sweat on the hands and feet in the Cold-attack and the Wind-attack Yangming stages are different. In the former, the hands and feet are cold. In the latter, the hands and feet are warm. In the former, the sweat is due to weak Yang Qi which is unable to fold and seal the sweat. In the latter, the sweat is due to inner Fire, which presses the body liquid out of the body (reducing Fire).

[496] Gujia syndrome (固瘕) is a clinical syndrome, in which the stool is firm in the beginning but loose in the latter part, or the stool is the mixture firm and loose stool.

Cold-attack Yangming can develop into Dietary jaundice syndrome (谷疸).
[497] Due to insufficient Spleen Yang Qi, stool movement in the bowel is slow, which causes the stool to be firm in the beginning part. The latter loose stool reflects the Coldness and Weakness in the digestive system (the Spleen system).

Dr. Ni Haixia: Due to Coldness in the stomach, the stomach fails to evaporate water to create enough urine. The extra water "spills" into the hands and feet. Due to the Coldness, food cannot be digested and it becomes corrupted. The corrupted food mixes with non-evaporated cold water to form Cold diarrhea (no strong lousy odor). This disease condition can be treated with either Gancao Ganjiang Tang or Wuzhuyu Tang.

Dr. Liao Houze: The patient has a bloating in the abdomen, has stool which is firm in the beginning but loose in the latter part. Such a disease condition is more commonly seen in patients with hepatitis. The pulse for such patients is strong, long and straight. For treatment, use Chaihui Guizhi Tang with Xiao Chengqi Tang, or with Tiaowei Chengqi Tang.

[498] Dr. Du Yumao: With Gujia syndrome, the stool is very loose but is not diarrhea. The stool is a mixture of stool and water. For treatment, use Hou Jiang Xia Cao Renshen Tang (厚姜夏草人参汤). With Gudan syndrome, there is Coldness-jaundice. For treatment, use Yinchen Lizhong Tang.

Dr. Dai Wen: There are entirely different opinions about how to understand this paragraph. We believe that this is Cold-attack Yangming condition, in which the stomach is weak, and there is solid stool in the bowel which blocks the food movement in it. The stool can be as loose or mixed with firm stool. For treatment, the principle is to warm the digestive system. It is also necessary to move the entangled firm stool from the bowel by using Dahuang. (Dai Wen and Jiang Jianguo. Discussion of undigested diarrhea syndrome with the internal cold of Yang brightness syndrome. Shandong J TCM. 2010, 29(10:659-660)

不能发黄；至七八日，大便鞕者，为阳明病也。

With a Shanghan disease, if the pulse is floating-soft,[499] there are warm or hot only on the hands and feet (not in other parts of the body), the disease is ready in the Taiyin stage. In this stage, if the urination is difficult, there will be jaundice. If it is normal, there will be no jaundice.[500] If the disease exists for eight to nine days, and the stool becomes like a firm ball, the disease is in the Yangming stage.

阳明病脉迟，食难用饱，饱则微烦，头眩，必小便难，此欲作谷疸，虽下之，腹满如故，(所以然者，脉迟故也)。

In the Yangming stage, the pulse feels slow.[501] The patient cannot eat to satiation. If so, the patient will feel dizzy and feels annoyed slightly,[502] and the urination will be difficult,[503] (and the abdomen will feel bloated). In such a case, the patient would tend to have Dietary jaundice (谷疸)

syndrome.[504] If a Purging therapy is used (because the bloated and fullness in the abdomen), the bloated feeling will remain unchanged (because the pulse is slow).

食谷欲呕，属阳明也，吴茱萸汤主之，(得汤反剧者，属上焦也。小半夏汤主之。)

If a patient tends to vomit after eating, his disease is in Yangming stage, use Wuzhuyu Tang as the primary treatment[505] (If the condition becomes worse after drinking this herbal tea, it means that the disease is in the Upper Jiao. In such a case, use Xiao Banxia Tang as the primary treatment.[506])

若胃中虚冷，不能食者，饮水则哕。

If the Stomach is in deficient and cold condition and the patient cannot eat, water drinking can cause a hiccup.[507]

2.3 Atypical Yangming body surface condition

阳明病，反无汗，而小便利，二三日，呕而咳，手足厥者，必苦头痛；若不咳不呕，手足不厥者，头不痛。

In the Yangming stage, patients should sweat, but a patient does not sweat, and his urination is normal. On the second or third day, if the patient is nauseous, coughs, and has Jue syndrome, the patient will have an annoying headache. If there is no cough and no nausea, no Jue syndrome, there will be no headache.[508]

---

[499] In the original text, the pulse is 浮而缓. It is supposed to be translated into floating and slow. However, here it can also be understood as floating-soft.

[500] The Taiyin stage is associated with Spleen. The Spleen dominates Dampness. If the Cold pathogenic Qi moves into the Taiyin stage, it will entangle with the Dampness to form jaundice. However, if urination is regular, the Dampness will be expelled out of the body, and jaundice cannot occur.

Dr. Liu Duzhou: Jaundice in the Taiyin is Hotness-Dampness jaundice.

[501] Dr. Liu Duzhou: The slow pulse is Taiyin pulse. Ths slow pulse suggests the presence of Dampness in the body.

[502] The stomach is in Weakness and Coldness condition and cannot digest food. The remaining water in the stomach causes dizziness and difficulty in urination.

Dr. Ni Haixia: The undigested food stalls in the stomach and causes the annoyed feeling. With poor digestion, there is insufficient nutrition supplied to the brain, causing dizziness and cloudy mind.

[503] Because of the Coldness and Dampness, urination is abnormal. Due to difficulty in urination, jaundice can occur.

[504] The Gudan (谷疸) was translated as "dietary jaundice" in WHO terminology glossary. It should be treated with Weidan Tang.

[505] Dr. Hu Xishu: This disease condition should not be listed here in the Yangming stage. It should belong to the Taiyin stage.

[506] This condition can also be treated with Zhizi Chi Tang or Xiao Chaihu Tang.

[507] This is because of Weakness and Coldness in the stomach. The stomach cannot evaporate the drunken water. The water becomes accumulated in the stomach. Therefore, drinking more water causes hiccups.

For such hiccup, use formula Lizhong Tang plus herb Dingxiang and Wuzhuyu for treatment.

[508] This is an early stage of Yangming that developed from Shaoyang. Nausea and coughing indicate the

阳明病，但头眩，不恶寒，故能食而咳，其人咽必痛，若不咳者，咽不痛。

In the Yangming stage, a patient feels dizzy only and has no aversion to cold. Such a patient can eat but has a cough and a sore throat. If no coughing, there will be no sore throat.[509]

阳明病，脉浮而紧者，必潮热，发作有时，但浮者，必盗汗出。

In the Yangming stage, if the pulse feels floating and tight, the patient will have a tidal fever at a fixed time during the day.[510] If the pulse feels floating only, the patient will have night sweats.[511]

阳明中风，口苦咽干，腹满微喘，发热恶风，脉浮而紧，若下之，则腹满，小便难也。

In Wind-attack Yangming stage, a patient experiences bitterness in the mouth, dryness in the throat, bloating in the abdomen, slight panting; has a fever and an aversion to wind. The pulse is floating-tight. In such a case, if a Purging therapy is used, the patient will have stronger fullness in the abdomen and urination will be difficult.[512]

2.4 Special types of Yangming stage

(1)   Heat invasion in blood chamber syndrome

阳明病，下血谵语者，此为热入血室；但头汗出者，刺 期门，随其实而泻之，濈然汗出则愈。

In the Yangming stage, if a patient has bleeding (from urine, stool, uterus or vagina) and has delirious speech, this situation is Fire

---

Shaoyang stage. The cold hands and feet indicate Shaoyang Jue syndrome (Si Ni San syndrome). The Hotness in the Yangming is not strong yet. Due to Fire inside the stomach, urination is normal. This is the early stage of Yangming, so there is no sweating yet.

   Dr. Liu Duzhou: For treatment, I recommend using Wuzhuyu Tang.

[509] *No aversion to cold and can eat* suggest that it is Yangming Wind-attack stage. In Cold-attack stage, the patient has headaches, while in Wind-attack, the patient feels dizzy. Because it is Wind-attack, the body's inside experiences Hotness. The coughing and the sore throat are due to accumulated Fire inside the body. The sore throat is also due to intense coughing that hurts the throat.

[510] The Yangming tidal fever easily happens in the later afternoon (about 3 pm). The time zone from 3 pm to 5 pm is the Yangming zone in Chinese medicine.

[511] Dr. Hu Xishu: This is the early phase of the Yangming stage. The floating-tight pulse is the Taiyang stage. The tidal fever is an indication of the Yangming stage. The Yangming stage has not fully developed yet. Night sweats in most cases are due to inner Fire.

   Dr. Liu Duzhou: The floating-tight and floating pulses indicate the Yangming stage because the Yangming stage can also have these types of the pulse. The night sweat is a sign of the presence of Fire in the Yangming body surface condition. If the Fire is in the Yangming inner part, the sweat will be tidal sweat during the daytime.

[512] Dr. Hu Xishu: *Fever and aversion to wind* indicate the Taiyang stage. The patient does not sweat and should feel annoyed. Together with *shortness of breath, bitter taste in the mouth and dryness in the throat,* there is Fire inside. This is Da Qinglong Tang condition. The inner side of the digestive system is not full yet, e.g., the firm stool has not formed yet, so Purging therapy should not be used. *Bitter taste in mouth and dryness in the throat* is the indication of inner Fire. The use of Purging therapy will cause the body water goes to the bowel, no sufficient water to the urine.

   Dr. Liu Duzhou: The *fever and aversion to wind* indicate Yangming body surface/meridian condition. *Bitter taste in mouth and dryness* is the indication of inner strong Fire. The *floating-tight pulse* means that there is pathogenic Qi in body surface and there is fullness inside. This means that the disease is in both the body surface and inner side of the Yangming stage. The body Surface condition should be cured first. The use of Purging therapy will deplete body liquid and cause difficulty in urination.

   Dr. Martin Wang: The *fever, aversion to wind, and floating-tight pulse* indicate the Taiyang stage; the *bitter taste in mouth and dryness in throat* indicate the Shaoyang stage; the *fullness and shortness of breath* should be the Yangming stage. This is three Yang co-existing condition. Should try Xiao Chaihu Tang?

invasion in blood chamber syndrome.[513] If the patient sweats on the head, use acupuncture on the Qimen (期门 , LV14) point (with depleting or bleeding technique). [514] The disease condition would be dissolved after having sweat.

(2)   Jaundice

阳明病，发热汗出，此为热越，不能发黄也。但头汗出，身无汗，剂颈而还，小便不利，渴饮水浆者，此为瘀热在里，身必发黄，茵陈蒿汤主之。

In the Yangming stage, there is a fever and sweating. This situation is called Fever-escape syndrome, which means that (the Fire will be depleted from the body and) there will be no chance of jaundice. If the patient sweats only on the head (not below the neck), has difficulty urinating, feels thirsty and wants to drink water, such a condition indicates entangled Hotness and Dampness inside the body, and there will be jaundice.[515] Use Yinchenhao Tang as the primary treatment. [516]

伤寒七八日，身黄如橘子色，小便不利，腹微满者，茵陈 蒿汤主之。

With a Shanghan disease for seven to eight days,[517] a patient has bright yellow jaundice, difficulty urinating, and mild fullness in the abdomen. Use Yinchenhao Tang as the primary treatment.[518]

伤寒瘀热在里，身必发黄，麻黄 连轺赤小豆汤主之。

With a Shanghan disease and with stagnated Fire inside the body, there will be jaundice.

---

[513] There are different opinions about the location of the Blood chamber. Basically it refers to the uterus and its surrounding cavity. Here the Hotness in the Blood chamber is due to the invasion of the Yangming Fire in the uterus.

Dr. Hao Wanshan: The bleeding here should mean bleeding from the uterus, not from bowel or colon. Delirious speech in the Yangming stage occurs in the afternoon (3 pm to 5 pm). Delirious speech due to Hotness in Blood chamber occurs in the evening, in which the patient should also have pain and tightness in the flank region of the abdomen.

[514] For women, the accumulated Fire could release through menstrual blood, causing recovery. For men, the Fire may accumulate in the Lower Jiao cavity. The Fire cannot deplete from the body so it steams up in the head as sweat. So, Dr. Zhang Zhongjing used acupuncture to solve this problem. This disease condition can also be treated with herbal therapy, such as using Guizhi Fuling Wan, or Di Dang Tang. In summary, the Fire-in-blood chamber condition can occur in the Taiyang, Shaoyang and Yangming stages. Patient with this condition usually has inner bleeding history (from the uterus, ovary, bowel, stomach, and so on.).

Dr. Liu Duzhou: Here the delirious speech is due to Fire in the bloodstream. It is different from the deliriousness in typical Fire in the bowel.

[515] If a patient had Dampness body constitution before becoming sick this time, the invading Fire would be entangled with the Dampness. If the patient has no sweat or has difficulty in urination, the Fire-Dampness will cause jaundice. If there is sufficient sweat or frequent/normal urination, jaundice cannot be formed.

[516] There are two kinds of jaundice: Yang jaundice and Yin jaundice. Yang jaundice is caused by entangled Fire and Dampness, in which the skin color is fresh yellow. Yin jaundice is caused by entangled Cold and Dampness, in which the skin color is dark yellow (or dirty yellow). Jaundice in the Yangming stage is mostly Yang jaundice. Jaundice in the Taiyin stage is mostly Yin jaundice. Acute jaundice tends to be Yang jaundice, and chronic jaundice tends to be Yin jaundice. The treatment of Fire-Dampness condition is usually challenging. To deplete the Fire (with Cold herbs) may increase the Dampness and to remove the Dampness may increase Fire (and with depletion of water may cause Yin deficiency). Therefore the Fire and the Dampness need to be depleted at the same time with a proper ratio of herbs. Depending on the relative intensity of the Fire and the Dampness, the herbal formula used for the treatment of jaundice is different. Yinchenhao Tang works for jaundice with relatively more Dampness than the Fire.

[517] The seventh to the eighth day of a Shanghan disease is the time when the disease will penetrate the Yangming stage (either from Taiyang to Yangming or from Shaoyang to Yangming).

[518] Yinchenhao Tang is used for Fire-Dampness jaundice (Fire is more than the Dampness). It removes the Dampness and Fire via urine and stool.

Dr. Hu Xishu: Yinchen Wu Ling San is used to treat Cold-Dampness jaundice.

Use formula Mahuang Lianqiao Chixiaodou Tang as the primary treatment.[519]

伤寒，身黄，发热者，栀子 柏皮汤主之。

With a Shanghan disease, jaundice and fever, use Zhizi Bopi Tang as the primary treatment.[520]

阳明病被火，额上微汗出，而小便不利者，必发黄。

If a disease in Yangming stage is treated with Fire therapy, there is mild sweating on the front of the head (but not in other parts of the body) and difficulty urinating, there will be jaundice.[521]

阳明病，无汗，小便不利，心中懊憹者，身必发黄。

In the Yangming stage, if there is no sweat, but there is difficulty urinating and annoyance feeling, there will be jaundice.[522]

2.5 Conditions in which Purging therapy should not be used

伤寒呕多，虽有阳明证不可攻之。

With a Shanghan disease, with frequent nausea,[523] Purging therapy should not be used even if there is clear evidence for the Yangming stage.[524]

阳明病，心下硬满者，不可攻之。攻之，利遂不止者死，利止者愈。

In the Yangming stage, with fullness and hardness in the upper abdomen, Purging therapy should not be used. Otherwise, there will be diarrhea. If diarrhea continues, the

---

[519] The formula Mahuang Lianqiao Chixiaodou Tang works to cure the body surface Cold-attack condition (by sweating) and to deplete Dampness. If the body surface condition is Wind-attack condition (with jaundice), use Guizhi with Huangqi Tang. If jaundice occurs in the Shaoyang stage, use Xiao Chaihu Tang, with or without a combination of other herbal formulas, such as Wu Ling San, or Yinchenhao Tang. If jaundice occurs in Shaoyang-Yangming co-existing condition, use Da Chaihu Tang with Yinchenhao Tang. Therefore, the treatment of jaundice depends on the disease stages and the nature of jaundice too (Dampness-Hotness or Coldness-Dampness).

[520] In this jaundice condition, the patient has more fever and annoyed feeling, and fewer symptoms inside the abdomen. The stool is not firm. All suggest more Fire than the Dampness in the body. The patient has no strong body Surface condition or inner condition (e.g., no stomach bloating, no thirst) either.

[521] In Yangming body surface condition, the patient typically has fever and sweating. For Yangming inner condition, such as the Stomach Fullness syndrome, the patient may have no sweat. For early Yangming stage in the meridian level, a patient may have no sweat either. If there is no sweat, Gegen Tang should be used to create sweat to deplete pathogenic Qi from the body. If the patient is exposed to fire, the exogenous fire will stimulate Fire inside the body. The double Fire makes jaundice hard to deplete from the urine.

[522] Dr. Liu Duzhou: This is Fire-Dampness condition. The Dampness holds the Fire to cause *no sweat,* or the sweat is restricted to the head. The Fire holds wetness, so urination is also difficult. The accumulation of the Fire and Dampness causes jaundice and annoyance. In the Coldness-Dampness jaundice condition, there is no such annoyance.

[523] Dr. Hao Wanshan: Nausea could be due to the Shaoyang stage (gallbladder Fire). The Shaoyang stage should not be treated with Purging therapy. It could also be due to the Fire in the upper chest part of the body (Yangming Fire condition), and it should be treated with Zhizi Chi Tang. In clinics, such typical Da Chengqi Tang condition with nausea can be seen in strangulated intestinal obstructions. Patients with such obstructions can also have no bowel movement, pain around navel, fullness, bloating and pain in the abdomen, high fever (toxic condition), loss of consciousness, and nausea (especially when the blockage is in the upper part of the intestine). With such disease conditions, the use of Da Chengqi Tang could cause breaking of the intestine wall to cause severe infectious, toxic shock and death.

Dr. Ni Haixia: If the patient has nausea, frequent acid reflux, and is now in the Yangming stage, use Da Chaihu Tang, instead of Chengqi Tang.

[524] Frequent nausea suggests the presence of the Shaoyang stage. This is Shaoyang-Yangming co-existing condition. In the Shaoyang stage, Sweating therapy, Vomiting therapy, and Purging therapy should not be used. Treat the Shaoyang condition first.

patient will die. If it can stop, the disease can be improved.[525]

阳明病，面合赤色，不可攻之，必发热色黄，小便不利也。

In the Yangming stage, with pink color on the face, Purging therapy should not be used. Otherwise, there will be fever, jaundice and difficult urination.[526]

阳明病，不能食，攻其热必哕，(所以然者，胃中虚冷故也)，以其人本虚，攻其热必哕。

In the Yangming stage, if a patient cannot eat, Purging therapy should not be used.[527] Otherwise, the patient will have a hiccup. (This is because the stomach is weak and cold before sick this time.) The body is already in a deficient situation, to use Purging therapy to deplete more heat will cause hiccups.[528]

2.6 Changes after Purging therapy

阳明病，下之，其外有热，手足温，不结胸，心中懊侬，饥不能食，但头汗出者，栀子豉汤主之。

In the Yangming stage, after Purging therapy treatment, there is a fever in body surface, the patient has warm hands and feet,[529] has no Chest-bind syndrome,[530] feels annoyed, feels hungry but cannot eat,[531] and there is sweat only on the head. For such a case, use Zhizi Chi Tang as the primary treatment.[532]

---

[525] Fullness and hardness feeling in the upper abdomen suggest Weakness condition in the stomach. Purging therapy will deplete the stomach Yang Qi and cause diarrhea.

Dr. Liu Duzhou: The fullness and hardness in the upper abdomen indicate Pi syndrome. It is a Weakness condition in the stomach. It is not the Excess condition in the bowel. Therefore, Purging therapy should not be used.

Dr. Hao Wanshan: The fullness and hardness feeling in the upper abdomen could be due either to the higher position (such as in the stomach) of the Yangming inner stage or a Pi syndrome. The former condition is not the typical Yangming inner condition that has firm-stool in the bowel. The latter condition is a Weakness condition, so Purging therapy should not be used.

[526] The pink face suggests that this is Taiyang body surface condition. The body will sweat but not yet. Purging therapy will make the inner body weaker and cause difficulty in urination. It will also cause the Fire and water (Dampness) to shrink into the inner side of the body to cause jaundice.

Dr. Liu Duzhou: The red color in the whole face suggests Fire in the Yangming body surface. Purging therapy will bring the Fire into the body to entangle with Dampness, and cause jaundice.

[527] In the Yangming stage, a *patient cannot eat* suggests that the disease belongs to the Cold-attack stage. If *cannot eat* is due to Yangming inner Wind-attack condition, the patient should also have tidal sweat.

[528] Dr. Ni Haixia: For mild Coldness in the stomach, use Wuzhuyu Tang for the treatment. For a little bit more severe condition, use Lizhong Tang, and for severe cases, use Fuling Si Ni Tang for the treatment. The presence of hiccups after the use of Fire-clearing therapy can tell if the inner condition is Coldness or Hotness in the digestive system.

[529] *Feels heat in the body and has warm hands and feet*: There is Fire in the body surface and inside. Here, the inner Fire is mostly in the esophagus, not in the stomach.

Dr. Hao Wanshan: *Warm hands and feet* can be an indication for both the Yangming and the Taiyin stages.

Dr. Liao Houze: In Yangming stage, hands and feet both are warm or hot. In Shaoyang stage, only the palm is hot.

[530] The patient had no garbage water accumulation in the middle part of the body before becoming sick this time, so the Purging therapy does not cause Chest-bind syndrome, it causes Zhizi Chi Tang condition instead.

[531] In clinics, not all people who feel hungry can eat. A hungry feeling and eating are different things. Also, to feel dry mouth and to feel thirsty are also different clinic phenomenon. To feel thirsty and to drink is a different thing too. TCM doctors must distinguish them clearly.

[532] The *annoyed feeling, hunger but cannot eat, sweat only on the head*, all indicate Yangming hot steaming in the upper part of the body (mostly in the esophagus). It is not an indication for dry-firm stool in the bowel. It indicates a Yangming surface level disorder, not an organ level disorder. In this case, the Purging therapy was used too early.

2.7 Wrong treatment of the Yangming stage

病人脉数，数为热，当消谷引食，而反吐者，此以发汗令阳气微，膈气虚，脉乃数也，数为客热，不能消谷，以胃中虚冷，故吐也。

The pulse feels fast, fast pulse suggest Fire, the patient should feel hungry, but the patient, however, vomits after eating.[533] This condition indicates that a previous Sweating therapy [534] resulted in depletion of body Yang Qi and weakness in diaphragm Qi, so the pulse becomes fast. The fast pulse represents the exogenous Fire, which cannot function to digest food. The Stomach is in Weakness and Coldness condition so that the patient vomits.

寸口脉浮大，而医反下之，此为大逆。浮则无血，大则为寒，寒气相搏，则为肠鸣。医乃不知，而反饮冷水，令汗大出，水得寒气，冷必相搏，其人必哕。

The pulse feels floating and big on the wrist. Purging therapy is, however, used. Such treatment is a big mistake. *Floating* pulse suggests lack of blood and a *big* pulse suggests Coldness. Cold and Qi entangled each other to cause intestine rumbling. The doctor did not know this, and let the patient drink cold water with the aim to create profuse sweat. The water so entangled with Cold to cause hiccups.

伤寒四五日，脉沉而喘满，沉为在里，而反发其汗，津液越出，大便为难，表虚里实，久则谵语。

With a Shanghan disease for four to five days, the pulse feels deep,[535] the patient has panting and feels bloating and fullness in the abdomen. Deep pulse suggests that the disease is on the inner side of the body. In this case, if a Sweating therapy is used however to create more sweat, there would be more exhaustion of body liquid, the bowel movement will become difficult. The body condition turns into surface weakness and inside an excess situation, and the patient will have delirious speech later.

伤寒十三日，过经谵语者，以有热也，当以汤下之。若小便利者，大便当硬，而反下利，脉调和者，知医以丸药下之，非其治也。若自下利者，脉当微厥；今反和者，此为内实也。调胃承气汤主之。

With a Shanghan disease for thirteen days, a patient has delirious speech.[536] This condition suggests a Fire inside the body. Such a situation should be treated with a Purging therapy.[537] If urination is frequent, the stool should be firm, but now there is however diarrhea. The pulse feels pretty reasonable. Such a condition is caused by previous Purging therapy.[538] This process is a wrong treatment. If the diarrhea is the result of the natural development of the disease, the pulse should be faint, and the body should have Jue syndrome. Now the pulse is harmonized, not faint, suggesting that there currently is an Excess condition on the inner side of the body. Use Tiaowei Chengqi Tang as the primary treatment.

阳明病。本自汗出。医更重发汗。病已差，尚微烦不了者。以亡津液胃中干燥。故令大便鞭。○（注当问其小便日几行。若本小便日三四行。今日再行。故知大便不久出。今为小便数少。以津液当还入胃中。故知不久必大便也。）

---

[533] Or has no desire to eat, or does not want to eat for fear of pain in the stomach.
[534] The use of Sweating therapy in such case was because of the fever and fast pulse. The doctor misdiagnosed the condition as body surface Fire condition.
[535] The deep pulse means that the disease is an inner condition, not in body surface condition, so that Sweating therapy should not be used.

[536] Delirious speech indicates the presence of Yangming Fire in the stomach. The Stomach meridian links to the Heart, so stomach fire affects the Heart and causes delirious speech (the coma condition). (The Heart dominates the mind.)
[537] Here, Tiaowei Chengqi Tang should be used to clear the Stomach Fire. Do not use Da Chengqi Tang.
[538] In this book, Purging therapy means the use of various Chengqi Tang. They are Cold type Purging therapy, and these formulas work to cleanse inner Fire. *Warm type cleansing therapy* means to use Badou pills to cleanse Cold-type constipation. It was commonly used in ancient times.

In the Yangming stage, patients should sweat.[539] A patient was however treated with a Sweating therapy again to create even more sweat. The disease seems to have subsided for the most part[540] but the patient still feels slightly annoyed. This situation is because the Sweating therapy depleted water from the body, and there is Dryness in the stomach, which created dry-firm stool.[541] (Note: Doctor needs to know the urination of the patient. If the patient usually has three to four times per day, and now the urination is the same pattern, it is known that the bowel movement would need some time to occur. If the urination becomes less in frequency, it is known that the body liquid would return to bowels and the bowel movement would happen soon.)

阳明病，自汗出，若发汗，小便自利者，此为津液内竭，虽硬不可攻之，当须自欲大便，宜蜜煎导而通之。若土瓜根及与大猪胆汁，皆可为导。

In the Yangming stage, patient sweats. A Sweating therapy is used, however, and the patient has frequent urination. This case means that the liquid inside the body will be depleted. In this case, Purging therapy should not be used even if there may be strong evidence for the existence of firm stool in the bowel.[542] Wait until the patient has a desire to pass the stool, then try a Conducting therapy by using Mijian Dao. Tuguagen or pig gallbladder juice can also be used as a conductor.

太阳病，寸缓关浮尺弱，其人发热汗出，复恶寒，不呕，但心下痞者，此以医下之也。如其不下者，病人不恶寒而渴者，而转属阳明也。小便数者，大便必硬，不更衣十日，无所苦也。渴欲饮水，少少与之，但以法救之。渴者，亦五苓散。

In the Taiyang stage, a patient has the pulse feels slow on the Cun position, floating on the Guan position and faint on the Chi position. The Patient feels feverish and sweats and feels an aversion to cold again. There is no nausea but fullness in the upper abdomen (i.e., Pi syndrome). Such body condition is due to a misuse of a Purging therapy.[543] If the Purging treatment was not used, the patient feels no aversion to cold, but is thirsty and feels fullness in the upper abdomen (and has difficulty urinating),[544] the disease condition belongs to Yangming. If urination is frequent, the stool will become firm. The patient has no bowel movement for ten or more days but no discomfort. [545] If the patient feels thirsty, let the patient drink water little by little. Do not let the patient

---

[539] The *sweat* might be the sweat in the Taiyang or in the Yangming stage. Here it should be the sweat that indicates the Taiyang stage. Sweating therapy can improve most of the symptoms. (If the sweat belongs to the Yangming stage, then the Sweating therapy cannot improve the symptoms; it will make the body condition worse).

Dr. Hu Xishu: This disease condition should not be regarded as Yangming stage. It is listed here for the distinguishment. Firm stool may not always belong to Yangming and may not always need treatment.

[540] The Sweating therapy depleted body liquid, so the amount of sweat, therefore, becomes less, and it seems as the body condition has been "improved".

[541] For such patients, check the urination. If the frequency and volume of the urine now are less than before, the stool will become soft and be more comfortable to pass out, because there will be more water in the bowel, rather than in urine. For this reason, Purging therapy should not be used.

Dr. Liu Duzhou: Here the dry-firm stool is caused by insufficiency body liquid, not due to the inner Fire.

[542] Sweating therapy and the person's frequent urine will cause the formation of firm stool in the bowel. The case here has no strong fever. The firm stool in the bowel becomes dry due to the depletion of water, not due to inner Fire. Therefore, conventional Purging therapy should not be used. The patient here has no fullness and pain in the abdomen, no tidal fever or delirious speech, no such evidence for the presence of dry-firm stool in the bowel.

[543] The Pi syndrome caused by the use of Purging therapy should be treated with either Guizhi Tang (if the body surface condition is not over yet), then various Xiexin Tang (depending on clinical conditions).

[544] The thirst, the fullness feeling in the upper abdomen, and the difficulty urinating suggest garbage water retention in the stomach.

[545] This is atypical Taiyang inner stage. Purging therapy should not be used. Use Maziren Wan or Mijian Dao for treatment. If there is a sign of inner Fire, use Maziren Wan.

drink too much water once.[546] With thirst, use Wu Ling San for treatment.

2.8 *Differentiation in the Yangming stage*

夫实则谵语，虚则郑声。郑声重语也。

An Excess condition is associated with delirious speech (谵语). A deficient condition is with repeated speech (郑声).[547]

阳明病欲食，小便反不利，大便自调，其人骨节疼，翕翕如有热状，奄然发狂，戢然汗出而解 (者)。(此水不胜谷气，与汗共并，脉紧则愈。)[548]

In the Yangming stage, a patient can eat (e.g., the Yangming Wind-attack stage). The patient should have regular or frequent urination, but now the urination is difficult, while bowel movement remains normal. With pain in the joints, mildly generalized hot (on the body surface, but not on the inside of the body) and an unexpected madness behavior, the disease condition will subside after the body has sweat.[549]

阳明中风，口苦咽干，腹满微喘，发热恶寒，脉浮而紧；若下之，则腹满、小便难也。

In the Wind-attack Yangming, a patient has a bitter taste in the mouth and dryness in the throat, feels abdominal bloat and fullness, has slight panting, and has a fever and an aversion to cold. The pulse feels floating and tight.[550] For such disease conditions, if Purging therapy is used, the patient will feel more bloating and fullness in the abdomen and have difficulty urinating.[551] (This is three Yang co-existing condition.)

阳明证，其人喜忘者，必有蓄血。(所以然者，本有久瘀血，故令喜忘)，屎虽硬，大便反易，其色必黑者，宜抵当汤下之。

In the Yangming stage, a patient forgets things (forgetfulness) easily.[552] There must have retained blood amassment in the body. (There is a long-term of blood amassment, which causes the forgetfulness.) In such a case, though stool is firm too, the bowel movement is normal,[553] but the stool color must be black. Use Di Dang Tang to clear away the dead blood.[554]

---

[546] Drinking too much water will cause garbage water accumulation in the stomach, so to create Wu Ling San syndrome.

[547] Delirious speech means that a patient speaks loudly and about strange things, but not logical things. Repeated speech means that a patient speaks silently and with a weak voice, with repeated words or sentences.

[548] Here there are original texts"此水不胜谷气，与汗共并，脉紧则愈。" It is hard to translate.

[549] Here, the joint pain and hot feeling suggest the Taiyang stage. This is a Taiyang-Yangming successive condition, though the disease condition for Yangming is not strong yet. The madness and the sweat can be regarded as a healing crisis. There is a hot debate about the meaning of this paragraph.

[550] *Bitter taste in mouth and dryness in throat*: This is Shaoyang stage. *Fever and aversion to cold, panting, floating and tight pulse*: This is Taiyang stage. *Bloating and fullness feeling in the abdomen*: Yangming stage.

[551] There is no sign indicating the Excessiveness condition inside the bowel yet, so the Purging therapy will make the stomach even weaker so that the stomach cannot shunt water from the digestive system to the urinary system to form urine.

[552] With dead blood accumulated in the blood, new blood is difficult to be produced, and the Heart loses nourishment from fresh blood, causing the patient to have a poor memory.

[553] Due to the presence of blood in the stool to lubricate the stool, the stool does not quickly become dry and is easy to pass out.

[554] Dr. Liu Duzhou: In the blood amassment syndrome, the pulse could be deep-slippery. Due to the firm stool in this syndrome, it is necessary to distinguish the Maziren Wan syndrome and Mijian Dao syndrome. If the Yangming condition occurs in patients with such chronic blood amassment syndrome, it is also necessary to distinguish Xiao Chengqi Tang condition. Here, the dead blood is inside and as part of the bowel. According to the book *Huangdi Nei Jing*, the dead blood in the lower part of the body will cause madness.

For people with dementia, always check the bowel movement and the color. If there is accumulated dead blood (blood amassment) in the Taiyang stage, the patient tends to be mad, so Taohe Chengqi Tang is used. If it is the Yangming stage, the patient tends to have a poor memory, and Di Dang

病人无表里证，发热七、八日，虽脉浮数者，可下之。假令已下，脉数不解，合热则消谷善饥，至六、七日，不大便者，有瘀血，宜抵当汤。若脉数不解，而下不止，必协热便脓血也。

A patient has no body surface symptoms but has a fever for seven to eight days. Even if the pulse feels floating and fast, Purging therapy can still be used.[555] After a bowel movement, if the pulse remains fast and the disease condition remained not improved, the patient will have a strong appetite and craves food.[556] If there is no further bowel movement until the sixth to the seventh day, the disease condition indicates an accumulated dead blood inside the body.[557] Use Di Dang Tang for treatment. After such treatment and if the pulse remains fast, and there is constant diarrhea, there will be pus and blood in the stool. (Di Dang Tang is not to be used furthermore.)

Tang is used. Di Dang Tang is stronger than the Taohe Chengqi Tang since the Taiyang meridian is associated with a lesser amount of blood, while the Yangming meridian is rich in both blood and Qi.

Dr. Hao Wanshan: Such conditions tend to be seen in the bleeding of the upper digestive system. If the bleeding continues, the treatment should focus on the stopping of bleeding. Use Sanqi, Ginseng, and Baiji (powder form). After stopping the bleeding (hemoglobin stops to drop down), and if there is Hotness condition in the body, use Taohe Chengqi Tang to clear the Fire and dissolve the dead blood. If there is no Hotness condition, then use Di Dang Tang to dissolve the old dead blood.

[555] In clinics, if a patient has a high fever for several days, if the pulse feels floating and fast, and there is no bowel movement for several days, usually use Da Chaihu Tang with Shigao for the treatment. If the patient also has nausea and vomits, use Xiao Chaihu Tang with Shigao and Dahuang.

[556] *Crave food*: This is due to the Fire in the stomach.

[557] This paragraph introduces other symptoms for blood amassment syndrome: the pulse feels floating-fast, the patient has a good appetite but no bowel movement for several days with a mild fever. This condition needs to be distinguished from Spleen-restrain syndrome. In the latter, the patient can also eat and can have no bowel movement for several days without any discomfort.

2.9 Turnover of the Yangming stage

直视谵语，喘满者死。下利者亦死。

If a patient's eyes stare straight without movement, and the patient has delirious speech, and if the patient has panting and fullness in the abdomen, the patient is going to die. If such a case is with diarrhea, the patient is also going to die.[558]

发汗多，若重发汗者，亡其阳，谵语脉短者死；脉自和者不死。

With profuse sweating, a Sweating therapy is used again. This treatment will deplete the body Yang. If the patient has delirious speech and the pulse is short, the patient will die. If the pulse matches the disease condition, the patient may not die.[559]

3. *Shaoyang stage*

If pathogenic Qi invades the body space between the hollow organs (such as stomach, intestine, urine bladder, gallbladder, pericardium), and solid organs (such as heart, lung, liver, spleen, kidney), and it affects gallbladder, uterus, various glands, lymph system, chest cavity, abdomen cavity, then the disease in most cases belongs to the Shaoyang stage.[560]

---

[558] Dr. Liu Duzhou: *Staring straight* happens because the inside Fire is so severe that the body liquid is exhausted and the body has insufficient liquid (Liver Yin) to nourish the eyes. Therefore the patient will die. *Delirious speech with diarrhea* happens because the Fire is too intense to press the body liquid (Yin liquid) downwards in the body. Therefore the patient is also going to die.

[559] Dr. Liu Duzhou: In Yangming inner stage, there is strong Fire inside. This is an Excess syndrome, and the pulse should be deep-tight (feels strong too). If the pulse is short and weak, it means that the pulse does not match the disease condition and the outcome of the disease is not hopeful. An Excess condition should see a Yang pulse (fast, floating, big, slippery, strong), and a Weakness (Deficiency) condition should see a Yin pulse (such as weak, deep, short, faint, thin pulse).

[560] Dr. Tan Jiezhong: Shaoyang might be understood as also involving the parasympathetic nerve and endocrine system. It involves the signal connection among organs, and switch functions such as the

The Shaoyang stage can be caused by a direct attack of pathogenic Qi in the Shaoyang region of the body, or it could have developed from the Taiyang stage, or from the Jueyin stage.[561]

Diseases in the Shaoyang stage are not like diseases in the Taiyang stage, in which patients like warmth (with an aversion to cold and with a floating pulse). Neither are they like those in the Yangming stage, in which patients hate warmth (with hatred of heat and a big and a strong pulse). The patient does not like those in the three Yin stages (see below) either, which include a deep and weak pulse. The symptoms and clinical manifestations of the diseases in the Shaoyang stage are between them.

The Shaoyang stage has a body surface stage and an inner stage too. Both stages are usually present at the same time[562] and they are treated with the same herbal formula.

Diseases in the Shaoyang stage tend to be a Qi stagnation condition, which also tends to develop into a Fire condition. Therefore the herbs used for the treatment of Shaoyang diseases are in most cases Fire-cleansing herbs (such as Chaihu, Shaoyao, Zhishi). Because the Shaoyang dominates the transport of body Qi and water, a disorder in the Shaoyang stage tends to cause accumulation of water, fluid,[563] and phlegm in the body.

Diseases in the Shaoyang stage does not locate in the body surface or the inner organs, so for the treatment of them, it is improper to use Sweating therapy, Vomiting therapy, Purging therapy and Diuretic therapy.[564] Instead, the treatment of them should include Conciliating, Balancing, and Harmonizing therapies.

The Shaoyang stage also tends to co-exist with other stages at the same time, such as the Shaoyang-Taiyang co-existing stage, the Shaoyang-Yangming co-existing stage, and the Shaoyang-Taiyin co-existing stage.[565] In

---

switch for body temperature, for hormone secretion, for a bowel movement, for the sympathetic nerve to the parasympathetic nerve, and so on.

There is an opinion that the Hand Shaoyang meridian involves the esophagus, the duodenum, pancreatic duct, and ureter. Diseases in these locations can be treated from the Hand Shaoyang meridian and belong to the Shaoyang disease. (丹易甘生的博客.传统手少阳三焦的腑归类混乱及发展. http://blog.sina.com.cn/s/blog_6c32ebff0102vfum.html)

[561] The Jueyin meridian and the Shaoyang meridian have an Exterior-Interior relationship. When the disease in the Jueyin stage becomes better, the pathogenic Qi could pass into the Shaoyang, where it can be further expelled out of the body. For the same reason, if the Shaoyin stage is not cured, the pathogenic Qi can further penetrate the deeper Jueyin stage.

Dr. Tan Jiezhong: According to the development sequence of diseases in book *Shanghan Lun*, the Shaoyang stage can also be developed from the Yangming stage.

[562] The body surface conditions and the inner conditions in the Taiyang or Yangming stages can present separately.

Dr. Tan Jiezhong: According to the Song version of the book *Shanghan Lun*, it can be summarized that the Shaoyang meridian and inner organ diseases usually co-exist. However, according to the Gui

version of the book *Shanghan Lun*, the inner gallbladder disease can exist alone (use Da Chaihu Tang, Chaihu Shaoyao Zhishi Gancao Tang, or Xiao Chaihu with Mangxiao Tang for the treatment of gallstone).

[563] The *fluid* can be understood as less condensed phlegm. It is also translated as "rheum", "thin mucus" in some books.

[564] This is because the Yang Qi in the Shaoyang is very mild. Such therapies could exhaust body Yang Qi to make Shaoyang stage diseases worse.

[565] The Shaoyang meridian is associated with Gallbladder and triple Jiao system. They work pretty much as lubricants for the smooth function of Yang Qi movement and for body liquid transportation between the organs and body systems. Therefore, if the pathogenic Qi hurts the Shaoyang, Yang Qi production and transportation in the body surface (Taiyang) is damaged. Digestion and bowel movement (the Yangming and Taiyin) are also retarded. For this reason, if the Shaoyang is sick, the body tends to have an accumulation of water, phlegm or have compression and stagnation of Qi. The stagnated Qi further develops into Fire.

Because the *Triple Jia* has such multiple functions, we believe that the current translation of this term as

this case, treatment must target all of the co-existing stages at the same time.

3.1 Shaoyang body surface stage

少阳之为病，口苦、咽干、目眩也。

The diseases in the Shaoyang stage mean that patients have a bitter taste in the mouth,[566] dryness in the throat,[567] dizziness and blurry vision.[568] (For treatment, use Xiao Chaihu Tang.)

少阳中风，两耳无所闻，目赤，胸中满而烦者，不可吐下，吐下则悸而惊。

In Wind-attack Shaoyang stage, patients have reduced hearing ability,[569] have red eyes,[570] feel bloated in the chest, and feel irritated.[571] (For treatment, use Xiao Chaihu Tang.) Do not use Vomiting therapy or Purging therapy.

"Triple Burner", "Triple Energizer", "Triple Heater", and "Triple Warmer" is not proper.

Dr. Tan Jiezhong: Because the Shaoyang is easy to confuse with other stages, if the clinical condition point to these other stages but the treatment of these stages does not work, pay attention that there might be a Shaoyang disease hidden in the symptoms.
[566] It can be any particular and strong taste in mouth, such as bitter, sweat, metal, sour, astringent, salty, spicy, and sticky, and so on.

Dr. Tan Jiezhong: If the bitter taste in mouth occurs in the morning, it may be Shaoyang disease. If it occurs in the later afternoon, it might be Yangming disease.

Dr. Gong Shicheng: The bitter taste can also be seen in other clinical conditions, such as in Weakness in Spleen, where Heart Fire cannot meet Kidney Water; in Stomach and Lung Yin deficiency in Warm diseases; in Dampness accumulation in Spleen; in people who smoke cigarettes; and in people who takes some medicines, such as Chloroquine.
[567] The throat is dry, but there is still saliva in the mouth (the tongue is not dry). The dryness feeling can be tingling, blocking, foreign puncturing, tightness, and so on.

Dr. Hao Wanshan: Fire in any organs can cause a bitter taste and dry mouth, but they are mostly seen in gallbladder Fire and Stomach Fire. If they are due to Shaoyang gallbladder Fire, there should also be other symptoms of the Shaoyang diseases, and if they are due to Yangming stomach Fire, the patient could also have stomach pain, bloating, or gum swelling or bleeding. With Shaoyang Fire, the bitter taste and dry throat occur mostly in the early morning, and with Yangming stomach Fire, they occur mostly in the afternoon (especially after a nap at or afternoon).

Dr. Tan Jiezhong: Dry throat is not substantial evidence to diagnose Shaoyang diseases.

[568] The dizziness here means that such a feeling happens when opening or closing the eyes. It does not mean the dizziness that happens when the body posture changes (such as from lying down to sitting up, or from bending to standing up). It does not mean the dizziness after eating to one's full either. The feeling can be slightly cloudy mind, slightly dark in the eyes, or blurring vision such as flashes.

Dr. Tan Jiezhong: Dizziness alone cannot be diagnosed as Shaoyang disease. We need some other evidence to make the diagnosis of Shaoyang disease. Even if the dizziness belongs to the Shaoyang, the herbal formula Wen Dan Tang works better than Xiao Chaihu Tang. If there is the dizziness and string pulse, the pulse should not be deep-string. The pulse should be deep. The deep-string pulse points to the use of Ling Gui Zhu Gan Tang. For the blurred vision, check if there are blood vessels growing in the eyes. If blood vessels are growing from the outside of the eye towards the pupil, it is Shaoyang. If they grow from the upper side down to the pupil, it is Taiyang. If they grow from the bottom to the pupil, it is Yangming. However, if the pulse is very deep, pay attention if the eye diseases are due to Liver Coldness condition (Wuzhuyu Tang condition), which may suggest liver cancer, especially for those people who drink lots of Cold tea, or eat lots of cold food or drink beverage that is too cold (with ice).

Dr. Tan Jiezhong: If there is no evidence for Taiyang stage diseases, and the bitter taste, dry mouth and throat, dizziness and blurred vision all are present at the same time, Xiao Chaihu Tang can be tried.
[569] It can be a reduced hearing ability, just a blocked feeling, or only itchy ears.
[570] It can be red color, or itchiness, or dryness, or pain, or bloating, or some tears in the eyes.
[571] The *reduced hearing ability and red color in the eyes* indicate Shaoyang body surface condition. The *fullness feeling and annoyed* indicates Shaoyang inner condition.

Otherwise, the patients will have palpitations and become easily scared or frighted.[572]

伤寒，脉弦细，头痛发热者，属少阳。少阳不可发汗，发汗则谵语，此属胃，胃和则愈，胃不和，则烦而悸。

With a Shanghan disease, if the pulse feels string and thin,[573] there are fever and headache,[574] the disease condition belongs to Shaoyang.[575] For treatment of the Shaoyang stage, Sweating therapy should not be used,[576] because it will cause delirious speech.

---

[572] The gallbladder dominates the braveness of a person. After using Vomiting therapy and Purging therapy the Yang Qi of the gallbladder and heart (the gallbladder meridian has a branch to the Heart meridian) are damaged so that the patient easily feels scared and has palpitations.

[573] Stringy pulse: The pulse feels like a string when pressed not lightly or hard. If the pulse feels like floating-string (when pressed very lightly), the pulse indicates Taiyang condition (the floating-tight and the floating-string are not easy to distinguish). If it feels deep-string (when pressed hard), the pulse indicates the Shaoyin stage (acute pain condition). Here the pulse is stringy and thin in the Shaoyang stage. The thin pulse occurs because, in the Shaoyang stage, the body Qi and blood become less sufficient (compared to how they are in the Taiyang stage).

[574] Dr. Hao Wanshan: The headache here means a migraine. The fever here is a continuous fever. This is stagnated Fire in the gallbladder. The *fever in the alternating fever-cold feeling* belongs to Shaoyang body surface condition.

[575] Fever and headache can be seen in the Taiyang, Shaoyang and Yangming stages. In the Taiyang stage, the pulse feels floating-tight or floating-weak. In Shaoyang, it is string-thin. In the Yangming, it is big (in the Yangming body surface condition). The pattern of the fever is also different in the three stages. In the Taiyang, the patient feels a fever and chills or an aversion to wind; in the Shaoyang, there is alternating fever and cold feeling. In the Yangming, there is only fever, no chills, and the patient has an aversion to heat.

[576] Sweating therapy will deplete body liquid and push the disease deep into the Yangming stage. The delirious speech means that Fire has been brought into the Stomach.

Dr. Hu Xishu: For the treatment of the fever and headache in the Shaoyang stage, use Xiao Chaihu

The delirious speech belongs to the Stomach (Yangming stage). If the Stomach is in harmonized status, the disease will get improved. If not, the patient will feel annoyance and palpitation.[577]

3.2 Shaoyang inner stage

伤寒五六日，中风，往来寒热，胸胁苦满，默默不欲饮食，心烦喜呕，或胸中烦而不呕，或渴，或腹中痛，或胁下痞硬，或心下悸，小便不利，或不渴，身有微热，或咳者，与小 柴胡 汤主之。

In Shanghan Wind-attack condition for five to six days, a patient feels an alternating cold and hot,[578] an intense and annoying bloating

---

Tang with Shigao. If the tongue coating is also yellow, use Da Chaihu Tang with Shigao.

[577] For the Yangming stage as such, use Tiaowei Chengqi Tang, or Xiao Chengqi Tang, to calm the Stomach.

[578] The cold and hot feelings happen on the same day. If the patient feels hot some days (one or two days or more) but cold (one or two days or more) on some other days, the condition may belong to Jueyin stage, or to malaria.

Dr. Hao Wanshan: There are three ways to explain the alternating fever-cold feeling in the Shaoyang stage. The first explanation is that it is because the pathogenic Qi locates in between the body surface (the cold layer of the body) and the body's deeper part (the hot compartment of the body). If the body defense force is strong enough to push the pathogenic Qi out, the body feels cold. If the pathogenic Qi is strong enough to invade deeply, the body feels hot. The second explanation is that if the pathogenic Qi is in the three Yang stages, the body feels hot and if it stays in the three Yin stages, the body feels cold. This is because Shaoyang is the pivot between the three Yang stages and the three Yin stages. My own, third, explanation is that the pathogenic Qi is still within the Shaoyang stage. When the pathogenic Qi is stronger, the body feels cold, and when the body defense energy is stronger, the body feels hot.

The *alternating hot and cold feeling* belongs to Shaoyang body surface condition. Other symptoms belong to Shaoyang inner condition.

Dr. Tan Jiezhong: In the Shaoyang stage, the cold is mild, and the intensity of the cold feeling is much less than the fever or warm feeling. It is not like

101

in the chest,[579] has no appetite at all,[580] feels irritated and annoyed,[581] and tends to have frequent nausea.[582] The patient with this syndrome could have many other symptoms, such as an irritated feeling in the chest without nausea, feeling thirsty, feeling pain in the belly, sticky bloating and a hard feeling in the flank region, palpitations in the upper stomach, difficulty urinating, a slightly hot sensation in the body without feeling thirsty, or a cough. For all of such cases, use Xiao Chaihu Tang as the primary treatment.eatment.[583]

血弱气尽，腠理开，邪气因入，与正气相搏，结于胁下，正邪分争，往来寒热，休作有时，默默不欲饮食。藏府相连，其痛必下，邪高痛下，故使呕也。小柴胡汤主之。

Blood is weak, and Qi is exhausted, body tissue is loosened, pathogenic Qi so can penetrate in and entangles with health-maintaining Qi. The entanglement bounds in the flank region. Due to the struggle between these two Qi, the patient has an alternating fever and chills sensation which occurs in a fixed time pattern, is nauseous and has no appetite.[584] In the body, the solid organs and the hollow organs are connected or associated structurally or functionally. The pain will move to other organs below the original organ. Pathogenic Qi is high, and the pain is bellow, so there is nausea. For such case, use Xiao Chaihu Tang as the primary treatment. [585]

---

malaria, in which the fever and cold both are very strong. In the Shaoyang stage, the patient might feel hot from time to time, and only slightly fear the cold. The hot feeling occurs in most cases once every day, not several times per day. It can occur as the patient feels much better in the morning after a common cold or flu, so the person goes to work, but he or she feels slight feverish in the afternoon again. (If the fever occurs two to three times per day, it might be Mahuang Guizhi Half-half Tang condition, where the pulse feels floating.) However, if the fever occurs five to six times per day, it may belong to the Shaoyang stage again (pulse feels thin-string).

Dr. Liao Houze: In the Shaoyang stage, it can be the alternating Hot-chilly, or only cold feeling, or only hot feeling, or cold feeling with slightly hot feeling.
[579] The main stem and the main branch of the Shaoyang meridian distribute through the chest.
[580] One of the functions of the Shaoyang Gallbladder is to improve the digestion of food in the Stomach-Spleen system. With the stagnation of Shaoyang Yang Qi, the desire to eat is reduced. The patient has no appetite, but can still eat. After eating, there is no discomfort in the stomach.
[581] A branch of the Shaoyang meridian connects to the Heart. The Fire in the Shaoyang can, therefore, bother the Heart and cause irritation and an annoyed feeling.
[582] Dr. Hu Xishu, Dr. Hao Wanshan, and Dr. Liu Duzhou: This does not mean that the patient likes to have nausea. It means that the patient tends to have frequent nausea. No one likes nausea.
[583] There are four groups of symptoms here. With any one of the four groups of the symptoms, plus other evidence for the presence of the Shaoyang stage, Xiao Chaihu Tang can be considered (e.g., there is no need to wait for all of the four groups of symptoms to be present at the same time). The mention of Wind-attack Shaoyang means that this Shaoyang stage

developed from the Taiyang Wind-attack stage. A patient who has such symptoms is a person who usually sweats easily. The body condition is relatively weak.

The principle of the treatment of the Shaoyang stage is to conciliate the body condition by supporting body inner defense ability and by expelling invaded Fire. Vomiting therapy and Purging therapy should not be used, because these therapies could bring the pathogenic Qi deeper into the Yangming stage. Similarly, these therapies should not be used in the Taiyang stage either.

Dr. Ni Haixia: There are several recommendations to modify Xiao Chaihu Tang according to variations of the original Xiao Chaihu Tang conditions. These modifications have been added by later doctors, and are not in the original text of the book *Shanghan Lun*. The Xiao Chaihu Tang principly treats the common cold or flu that occurs during menstruation. For the treatment of breast cancer, the basic formula is also Xiao Chaihu Tang. Add Guizhi to it. The Guizhi brings the milk down to the uterus.
[584] The Fire in the Gallbladder bothers the Stomach to cause Stomach Qi up-rushing.
[585] This paragraph is hard to understand and to translate. Pathogenic Qi directly invades the Shaoyang stage because the blood is insufficient and Qi is weak. The body defense system is less able to struggle against the pathogenic Qi and fails to prevent the invasion. The health-

本太阳病不解，转入少阳者，胁下硬满，干呕不能食，往来寒热，尚未吐下，脉沉紧者，与小 柴胡 汤。

If a disease is originally in Taiyang stage (either Cold-attack or Wind-attack), is not dissolved and it moves into the Shaoyang stage, patients feel hardness and fullness in the flank region,[586] feel retch and cannot eat, have an alternating hot-cold sensation. Vomiting therapy or Purging therapy has not been used, and the pulse feels deep-tight.[587] In such case, use Xiao Chaihu Tang as the primary treatment.[588]

---

maintaining Qi and the pathogenic Qi entangled and struggled with each other in the flank region, resuing in the alternating hot-cold with a fixed time of onset and stop, and poor appetite. Because the Gallbladder and the Liver are connected functionally, the disease in the Gallbladder can pass to the Liver too. The disease in the Liver can also affect the function of Stomach-Spleen, causing nausea and pain in the stomach.

In the Five-element theory, the cycle is from Wood to Fire, to Soil, to Metal, to Water and then returns to the Wood again. Therefore the position of the Wood (Gallbladder-Liver) is higher than the Soil (Stomach-Spleen).

[586] The *hardness and fullness feeling in the flank region and the alternating hot-cold feeling* indicate Shaoyang body surface condition.

[587] The deep-tight pulse suggests there is an Excess condition inside the body.

Dr. Hao Wanshan: The deep-tight pulse is difficult to distinguish from deep-string. Here the pulse can be understood as a deep-string pulse. If the Shaoyang Yang Qi stagnates in a short time, the pulse usually feels like a string. After a long time of stagnation, the pulse feels deep-string. For such patients, the face is less bright, the hands are cold to touch, and the primary emotion is depression. Such patient tends to have low stamina, easily get upset and depressed or anxious. With deep-string pulse, it is known that the Shaoyang Yang Qi stagnation has been there for a long time. The deep pulse or the deep-string pulse also suggests Qi stagnation.

[588] Dr. Hu Xishu: This is Taiyang-Shaoyang successive condition. The condition in both stages should be treated at the same time. Use formula Chaihu Guizhi Tang, Chaihu Guizhi Fanjiang Tang, Chaihu Tang with

伤寒四五日，身热恶风，颈项强，胁下满，手足温而渴者,小柴胡汤主之。

With a Shanghan disease for four to five days, a patient feels hot and an aversion to wind, feels tightness on the back and the nape, feels fullness in the flank region, has warm hands and feet and feels thirsty. For such case, use Xiao Chaihu Tang as the primary treatment.[589]

伤寒，阳脉涩，阴脉弦，法当腹中急痛，先与小建中汤，不差者，小柴胡汤主之。

With a Shanghan disease, if Yang pulse feels rough (when pressed lightly) and Yin pulse is string (when pressed harder), the patient should have acute pain in the abdomen. If so, try Xiao Jianzhong Tang first. If this formula does not work, use Xiao Chaihu Tang as the primary treatment.[590]

Gegen Tang, or Chaihu Tang with Ma Xin Shi Gan Tang, or others, depending on clinical conditions.

[589] In this case, *the hot and an aversion to wind and tightness on the nape* indicate the Taiyang stage. The *fullness feeling on the flank region and the tightness feeling in the side of neck* indicate the Shaoyang stage. The *hot, thirsty* and *warm hands and feet* indicate the Yangming stage. In the three Yang concurrent conditions, because there is no water retention or water-reversing condition, use Xiao Chaihu Tang for the treatment.

Dr. Hu Xishu: For this case, it is better to use Xiao Chaihu Tang plus Shigao.

Dr. Liu Duzhou: Because there is thirst, it is better to use Xiao Chaihu Tang without Banxia but with Tianhuangfeng for the treatment.

[590] Such a pulse can be felt in both the Taiyin and Shaoyang stages. Try Xiao Jianzhong Tang first, because it works to warm inner side of the body, and also could improve the body surface condition (Xiao Jianzhong Tang is modified from Guizhi Tang). When the Taiyin and Shaoyang stages co-existing, warm the Taiyin with the Xiao Jianzhong Tang first, then conciliate the Shaoyang with Xiao Chaihu Tang.

Dr. Liu Duzhou: Even if the acute pain locates on the flank region, try Xiao Jiangzhong Tang first, then the Xiao Chaihu Tang.

Dr. Ni Haixia: The Yang pulse here should mean the Cun position and the Yin pulse means the Chi position. Such pulses suggest inner Coldness condition. For children with inner Coldness condition,

少阳病，气上逆，今胁下痛，甚则呕逆，此为胆气不降也，柴胡芍药枳实甘草汤主之。

In the Shaoyang stage, there is Qi up-rising which causes pain in the flank region. In severe cases, the patient feels nauseous or vomits. This situation is because the gallbladder Qi does not fall downwards. Use Chaihu Shaoyao Zhishi Gancao Tang as the primary treatment.[591]

伤寒中风，有柴胡证，但见一证便是，不必悉具。

In Wind-attack Shanghan disease, if there are physical manifestations that suggest Chaihu Tang condition,[592] then the Chaihu Tang can be used even if there is only one symptom (indication).[593]

伤寒五六日，头汗出，微恶寒，手足冷，心下满，口不欲食，大便鞭，脉细者，此为阳微结。假令纯阴结，不得复有外证，悉入在里，此为半在里半在外也，脉虽沉紧，不得为少阴病，所以然者，阴不得有汗，今头汗出，故知非少阴也。可与小柴胡汤，设不了了者，得屎而解。

With a Shanghan disease for five to six days, a patient sweats, but the sweat is only on the head.[594] The patient has a slight aversion to cold,[595] has cold hands and feet,[596] is bloated

---

the color on the root of the nose is blue. Xiao Jianzhong Tang can warm up the inner digestive system, to cure the abdominal pain and to increase appetite. After the use of Xiao Chaihu Tang, if there is still a pain in the abdomen, the disease condition suggests that the blood is returning from the veins beneath the small intestine and is not blocked. For the treatment, remove Huangqin from Xiao Chaihu Tang but add Saoyao.

Dr. Hao Wanshan: This should be understood as: after the treatment with Xiao Jianzhong Tang and the acute abdominal pain subsides, if the Shaoyang condition remains, use Xiao Chaihu Tang. In the Shaoyang-Taiyin co-existing condition, treat the Taiyin first, then the Shaoyang.

Dr. Hu Xishu: The deep-string pulse can be seen in both the Taiyin and Shaoyin stages. It indicates weakness and pain. It may not be easy to distinguish the two conditions, so, better to use Xiao Jianzhong Tang first. After the treatment, if the pain subsides somewhat, but not completely, use Xiao Chaihu Tang.

[591] Dr. Tan Jiezhong: The Qi uprising feeling may not only be coughing. Usually, the Gallbladder Qi should move downwards, and the Liver Qi moves upwards. If the upwards Qi (Liver Qi) is inhibited, there would be pain under the left rib arch (use Chaihu-containing herbal formulas for the treatment). If the downwards Qi (gallbladder Qi) is inhibited, there would be pain under the right rib arch (use Zhishi-containing formulas).

[592] This is a Taiyang-Shaoyang co-existing condition. Treat the Shaoyang first. After the Shaoyang functions well, the body defense Yang Qi can work better to struggle against the pathogenic Qi in the Taiyang stage.

[593] The typical clinic manifestations indicating the Shaoyang stage include a bitter taste in mouth, dry throat, blurred vision; alternating hot-cold feeling, fullness-bloated feeling in the flank region, low appetite, annoyed feeling and frequent nausea. The pulse is string or deep-string, and the tongue coating is white. The original text in *Shanghan Lun* says that if there is even one of these symptoms, the Xiao Chaihu Tang can be used for the treatment.

Dr. Hao Wanshan: it is better to have two or more symptoms that indicate the Shaoyang stage disease, then the Xiao Chaihu Tang can be used. One single symptom may not be sufficient to indicate the use of Xiao Chaihu Tang.

Dr. Hu Xishu: If there is one of the typical symptoms, with typical string pulse, then Xiao Chaihu Tang can be used.

Dr. Tan Jiezhong: With the previous Taiyang disease and then having a symptom such as bitter taste, dry mouth, dizziness, alternating hot-cold feeling, annoyed feeling, and frequent nausea, no appetite, bloating or discomfort under the rib arch, then the Shaoyang diagnosis can be set up. Otherwise, the diagnosis for Shaoyang disease is very difficult actually, because the evidence for the Shaoyang disease is scattered. One of the characteristics of Shaoyang is that it mixes, or occurs together, with the Taiyang, or Yangming, or Taiyin stage. We need to pay attention to finding the primary evidence for the Shaoyang disease. It is difficult to tell which body constitution the Xiao Chaihu Tang is suitable for treatment.

[594] The Fire is entangled in the triple Jiao cavity, so the sweat can only occur on the head, not on the whole body.

[595] *Aversion to cold*: body surface condition.

in the upper abdomen, has no desire to eat,[597] has a firm and ball-like stool [598] and the pulse feels thin.[599] This situation is Yang mild-entanglement syndrome. If the condition were pure Yin entanglement condition, there would be no body surface condition and no sweating. The condition here means that the disease is half in body exterior and another half in the interior. Even if the pulse here feels deep-tight, it should not be regarded as the Shaoyin stage, because the disease of Yin nature has no sweating. Now the patient has sweat on head, so the disease is not in the Shaoyin stage. For such condition, use Xiao Chaihu Tang for treatment. After drinking the herbal tea, if the situation has not improved dramatically, wait for several days. The disease will get improved after a bowel movement.[600]

阳明病，发潮热，大便溏，小便自可，胸胁满不去者，与小柴胡汤.

In the Yangming stage, if there is a tidal fever, loose bowel movements, regular urination,[601] and a consistent bloating feeling in the chest and the flank region, use Xiao Chaihu Tang for treatment.[602]

阳明病，胁下硬满，不大便而呕，舌上白苔者，可与小 柴胡 汤。上焦得通，津液得下，胃气因和，身濈然汗出而解也。

In the Yangming stage, a patient feels hardness and bloating-fullness in the flank region, has no bowel movement, is nauseous,[603] and the tongue coating is white. Give Xiao Chaihu Tang for treatment.[604] Once the Upper Jiao functions normally, body liquid can transport smoothly downwards, the Stomach Qi becomes harmonized, the body would have mild sweat and the disease condition can be released.

伤寒发热，汗出不解，心下痞硬，呕而下利者，大柴胡汤主之。

With a Shanghan disease, a patient has a fever and sweats. The sweat does not reduce the Heat. The patient feels bloated, has an extreme hardness in the upper abdomen, is nauseous and has diarrhea.[605] In such case, use Da Chaihu Tang as the primary treatment.[606]

---

[596] *Cold hands and feet*: The Fire is entangled inside the body and the Fire cannot pass to the end of the arms and legs to warm the hands and feet.
[597] *Bloating feeling in the flank region and has no desire to eat*: Shaoyang Fire entanglement.
[598] *Firm and ball-like stool*: Fire entangles in the Yangming stage.
[599] The pulse should be deep-thin. It suggests Qi entanglement in the deep part of the body.
[600] Dr. Hao Wanshan: This is Taiyang, Shaoyang and Yangming co-existing condition.
[601] The tidal fever indicates Yangming restrained Fire. It is not the Yangming inner stage condition, because there still is bowel movement, the stool is loose, and urination is not frequent.
[602] This condition is often seen in acute dysentery. Here, *tidal fever* belongs to Yangming, while *bloating and fullness feeling in the chest and in the flank region* suggest the Shaoyang stage. This is a Shaoyang-Yangming co-existing condition.

[603] *Nauseous*: Gallbladder Fire bothers the Stomach.
[604] Dr. Liu Duzhou: This condition is the Shaoyang stage, not the Yangming stage. The *no bowel movement* is due to entanglement of Fire in the upper middle part of the body, which blocks the body liquid from moving down to the lower part of the body so that the bowel becomes dry. Xiao Chaihu Tang releases the block and cures the difficulty in bowel movement. In the Yangming inner stage, the tongue coating should be dry and yellow. *No bowel movement* here is necessary to distinguish from the Yangming inner organ condition. If the condition is really the Shaoyang-Yangming co-existing condition, then Da Chaihu Tang, not Xiao Chaihu Tang, is needed for treatment.
[605] Dr. Hao Wanshan: This is Shaoyang organ Fire and Shaoyang Hardness-Fullness condition (the Fire and gallbladder are entangled as a firm mass in the gallbladder). Nausea occurs because the gallbladder fire bothers the stomach. Diarrhea occurs because the gallbladder Fire presses the bowel.
[606] The *fever and sweat* is not a body surface condition but a Yangming condition. The *bloating, fullness and pain in the upper abdomen* are Shaoyang condition. Therefore, use Da Chaihu Tang to cure the Shaoyang first. This is typical acute dysenteritis. If the patient also has an odor from the mouth, add herb Shigao to the formula. If the upper abdomen is firm and the pain is mild, and the vomiting is very severe, use Xiao Chaihu Tang plus Shigao.

(With a Shanghan disease, a patient may also have Hotness Jue syndrome. There is a hardness-fullness and hurried sensation in the flank region. The patient has continuous nausea and diarrhea and has Jue syndrome. Use Da Chaihu Tang as the primary treatment.[607])

伤寒胸中有热，胃中有邪气，腹中痛，欲呕吐者，黄连汤主之。

With a Shanghan disease, a patient has Hotness in the chest and water in the stomach,[608] has abdominal pain and tends to be nauseous.[609] For such condition, use Huanglian Tang as the primary treatment.[610]

In clinics, the Da Chaihu Tang condition needs to be distinguished from formula Gegen with Qin Lian Tang and Lizhong Tang (Guizhi Renshen Tang).
[607] If there is Hotness-jue condition but no inner Hardness-fullness condition, typically use Baihu Tang for the treatment.
[608] Original text in *Shanghan Lun* here said: "there is pathogenic Qi in the stomach".
[609] Dr. Hao Wanshan: The original word *chest* here should mean the stomach. The original word *stomach* should mean the spleen. This is a Stomach Fire and Spleen Coldness condition.

Dr. Huang Huang: This means that the patient feels annoyed; has palpitations; has insomnia; has discomfort in the stomach, such as feeling air running, pushing or punching in the abdomen; pain around navel or under the navel; pressing, bloating, falling; or feels water movement in the bowel, and so on.
[610] The Fire in the chest stimulates the water in the stomach to cause annoyed feeling and nausea and pain in the abdomen. If there is no water in the stomach, there will be the annoyed feeling alone but not nausea. This patient can also have diarrhea, but the diarrhea is not as strong as in Huang Qin Tang condition. The Huanglian Tang condition here is more similar to Gancao Xiexin Tang condition. Due to Fire that tends to rise, the face of the patient tends to be red. Because the Fire is in the chest cavity, this syndrome is included into the Shaoyang stage.

Dr. Ni Haixia: The stomach Deficient-Fire rises and meets the water and Dampness in the chest and in the mediastinum to form phlegm. With the burning of the Deficient-fire in the chest, the patient vomits after eating or drinking. The tongue coating is yellow. At the same time, the patient has diarrhea (the lower Coldness condition). So, this is an upper-Hotness and

3.3 *Wrong treatment of the Shaoyang stage*

凡柴胡汤病证而下之，若柴胡证不罢者，复与柴胡汤，必蒸蒸而振，却发热汗出而解。

If clinical conditions indicate the use of Chaihu-containing formula, but a Purging therapy is however used.[611] If the Chaihu condition remains, the Chaihu Tang can still be used. The disease condition will be dissolved after the patient experiences strong body shakes, then fever and sweating.[612]

太阳病，过经十馀日，反二、三下之，後四、五日，柴胡证仍在者，先与小柴胡汤。呕不止，心下急，郁郁微烦者，为未解也，与大柴胡汤下之则愈。

In the Taiyang stage for ten or more days (there is evidence indicating Shaoyang stage too). Purging therapy was used two or three times, however.[613] During additional four to five day, if the Chaihu condition remained (such as an alternating hot and cold feeling, bitter mouth, and so on), try Xiao Chaihu Tang for treatment. If most of the symptoms

---

lower Coldness condition. Huanglian Tang is used for the treatment of cholera (together with acupuncture treatment on Weizhong (UB40) and Waiguan (SJ5) points).
[611] It is wrong to use Purging therapy in the Shaoyang stage.
[612] Dr. Hu Xishu: The *hot feeling, shaking, fever and sweat* are a healing crisis. It happens more often with the use of the Chaihu-containing formulas, and if the patient is weak and did not get treatment for a long time. The patient needs to be informed about this healing crisis, to avoid the fear of the consequences. Sweat here does not mean that Xiao Chaihu Tang can create sweat.

Dr. Hao Wanshan: Do not misdiagnose the intravenous infusion reaction as a healing crisis.

Dr. Tan Jiezhong: Such healing crises can occur as a sudden blackout and the body falling. After several seconds, the patient will get better and then will recover completely. This phenomenon may scare the people around the patient and people may be eager to call an ambulance.
[613] In the Shaoyang stage, Purging therapy should not be used, otherwise, the pathogenic Qi will be brought deep into the Yangming stage.

pass, but the patient still has constant nausea, feels tightness and a hurried sensation in the upper abdomen,[614] and feels slightly annoyed, the body condition as such indicates that the disease has not been fully improved. Use Da Chaihu Tang to conduct the pathogenic Qi out of the body through bowel movement.[615]

伤寒五六日，呕而发热者，柴胡 汤证具，而以他药下之，柴胡 证仍在者，复与 柴 胡 汤。此虽已下之，不为逆，必蒸蒸而振，却发热汗出而解。若心下满而硬痛者，此 为结胸也，大陷胸汤主之。但满而不痛者，此为痞，柴胡 不中与之，宜 半夏 泻心汤。

With a Shanghan disease for five to six days, a patient feels nauseous and has a fever. There are other symptoms or signs both indicating the presence of Chaihu Tang condition, but the patient was treated with Purging therapy instead. After the treatment, if there are still indications prompting the use of Chaihu Tang, then use it. It is not a big mistake yet. With Chaihu Tang, the patient will feel the heat from the inner body and shake, feel hot and sweaty, and then the

disease will be over.[616] After the Purging therapy, if the patient feels a hardness, fullness, and pain in the upper abdomen, the disease condition is Hotness Chest-bind syndrome. Use Da Xianxiong Tang as the primary treatment. If the patient feels only fullness and bloating, but no pain, this is Pi syndrome. Chaihu-containing herbal formula will not work. Use Banxia Xiexin Tang for the Pi syndrome.[617]

太阳病，过经十馀日，心中温温欲吐，而 胸中痛，大便反溏，腹微满，郁郁微烦，先此时，自极吐下者，与调胃承气汤，(若 不尔者，不可与。但欲呕，胸中痛，微溏者，此非柴胡证。以呕，故知极吐、下 也。)

In the Taiyang stage for ten or more days, a patient feels nauseous, feels pain in the chest, but the stool is loose, the abdomen feels slightly bloated, and the patient feels somewhat annoyed. If a Vomiting therapy and Purging therapy have been used before, now use Tiaowei Chengqi Tang for treatment (to calm the stomach). If not yet and if the patient feels desires being nauseous (nausea makes him feel better), feels pain in chest and has loose stool, such a condition does not belong to Chaihu Tang condition. Because there is nausea, the situation is the results of aggressive Vomiting or Purging therapy. (For such case, use Huangqin with Banxia Shengjiang Tang.[618])

伤寒十三日不解，胸胁满而呕，日晡所发 潮热，已而微利，此本柴胡证，下之而不 得利。今反利者，知医以丸药下之，非其 治也。潮热者，实也，先宜小柴胡汤以解 外，後以柴胡加芒硝汤主之。

---

[614] The *tightness and hurried feeling in the upper abdomen* suggest that the pathogenic Qi has become entangled in the Yangming inner stage. There is Fire in the stomach that causes continuous nausea. This is a Shaoyang-Yangming successive condition. Da Chaihu Tang works for both the Shaoyang and Yangming stages. We can use Purging therapy too. For Taiyang-Shaoyang successive condition, use Chaihu Guizhi Tang.

Dr. Hao Wanshan: *Constant nausea, fullness and hurried feeling in flank region and the slightly annoyed feeling*, all indicate the Shaoyang stage, not at all the Yangming stage. This is Shaoyang organ Hardness-fullness condition, similar to Yangming inner organ Hardness-fullness condition, but here the disease is in the gallbladder. Da Chaihu Tang is used here to deplete the Hardness-fullness from the gallbladder, a similar aim as using Chengqi Tang to deplete dry-firm stool from the bowel in Yangming inner condition. This Gallbladder Hardness-fullness condition can be seen in acute cholecystitis, acute onset of biliary calculi, and even acute pancreatitis.

[615] Tidal Fire and sweating from the armpits are evidence of Da Chaihu Tang condition. The armpit belongs to the Shaoyang stage.

---

[616] *Feels hot from inner body, shaking, feels hot and sweaty before the patient gets better:* this is healing crisis. It more easily happens in weak patients.

[617] Note: For treatment of Pi syndrome, Banxia Xiexin Tang is needed.

Dr. Du Yumao: The three Xiexin Tang are all Coldness in Spleen but Hotness in the stomach-intestine. They belong to the Yangming-Taiyin stage, not the Shaoyang stage. Therefore they are not Conciliating therapy.

[618] This paragraph reminds us that nausea cannot be regarded as unique to the Shaoyang stage.

With a Shanghan disease for thirteen days without improvement, the patient feels fullness in the chest and flank, [619] has nausea [620] and a tidal fever in the afternoon (around 3 pm). [621] After cessation of the fever, the patient has slight diarrhea (loose stool). The original clinic condition belongs to Chaihu syndrome. A Purging therapy was however used before, [622] which did not result in diarrhea. Now the patient has diarrhea, indicating that the Purging treatment is not the proper treatment. Tidal fever means an Excess condition. The condition should be treated with Xiao Chaihu Tang to release body surface condition first, followed by the use of Chaihu Jia Mangxiao Tang [623] to cure the tidal fever. [624]

伤寒八九日，下之，胸满，烦，惊，小便不利，谵语，一身尽重，不可转侧者，柴胡加龙骨牡蛎汤主之。

With a Shanghan disease for eight to nine days, the disease condition is treated with a Purging therapy. [625] The patient feels fullness in the chest, annoyed, scared, has difficulty urinating, [626] has delirious speech, [627] and feels heaviness in the whole body so much so that patient feels difficulty turning over the body. [628] In this case, use Chaihu Jia Longgu and Muli Tang as the primary treatment. [629]

若已吐、下、发汗、温针，谵语，柴胡汤证罢，此为坏病，知犯何逆，以法治之。

If Vomiting therapy, Purging therapy, Sweating therapy, or Fire-needle acupuncture has been used by mistake for the treatment of a disease in the Shaoyang stage, and if the Chaihu syndrome remains, continue to use a Chaihu-containing herbal formula for treatment. If there is no evidence for the Shaoyang stage, treat the current condition with a proper way needed, depending on the given body conditions. (For example, if the patient has delirious speech, use Tiaowei Chengqi Tang, or Xiao Chengqi Tang).

---

[619] This is a Shaoyang condition.

[620] *Nausea*: the Shaoyang Fire bothers the Stomach.

[621] *Tidal fever*: This is a Yangming condition. The tidal fever occurs around 3 pm in the afternoon. This is the Yangming time zone during the day for the body, and it is also the Yangming time zone of nature. The body Yangming time meets the nature Yangming time. The nature of the Yangming is Dryness and Hotness. So, the patient feels tidal fever at this time.

Dr. Hao Wanshan: The original disease condition is the Shaoyang-Yangming co-existing condition, and it should be treated with Da Chaihu Tang. The patient has a fullness feeling in the flank region, tidal fever in the afternoon, has no bowel movement and the tongue coating should be yellow and dry.

[622] Dr. Hao Wanshan: Purging therapy here mostly means the use of Badou, which belongs to Warm Depleting herbs (e.g., herbs are Warm in nature). With its use, the bowel movement is improved but the Fire was not cured.

[623] Chaihu with Mangxiao Tang is Xiao Chaihu Tang plus herb Mangxiao. It has no strong Purging function. It works to calm the stomach (release the Fire in the stomach).

[624] Dr. Ni Haixia: This paragraph means that the original disease condition is Da Chaihu Tang condition. After treatment with this herbal formula, the stool came out but the condition changes to the Xiao Chaihu Tang condition.

[625] *The disease has already lasted for eight to nine day, and the patient felt fullness in the chest, annoyed and scared after Purging therapy* all suggest that the disease has already in the Shaoyang stage. Therefore treatment with Purging therapy is a mistake.

[626] *Difficulty in urination*: the condition involves the Taiyang stage.

[627] *Delirious speech*: Stomach Fire, Yangming stage.

[628] Purging therapy makes the inner body weak, and the pathogenic Qi invades into the inner part of the body to occupy the weakened inner part (in the stomach and the bowel), and it rushes up to stimulate the brain to cause annoyance, fear, and delirious speech. *Heavy body*: the Fire spreads to the whole of the body and blocks body Qi distribution. *Difficulty in urination*: the Qi of the Triple Jiao stagnates and cannot move smoothly. This is the Shaoyang stage with Heart Qi deficiency (this condition can be understood as Shaoyang-Yangming-Shaoyin co-existing condition).

[629] Dr. Ni Haixia: This herbal formula is good for the treatment of poor sleep in weak patients with sweaty hands and feet. It is not suitable for the patient who has constipation, dry mouth, and sweat on the head at night.

There is an opinion that this condition belongs to three Yang co-existing condition (Li Yuming. The Chaihu Jia Longgu and Muli Tang condition belongs to three Yang co-existing condition. J. Shandong University of TCM. 2011, 35(5):400-403)

3.4 Turnover of the Shaoyang stage

伤寒三日，三阳为尽，三阴当受邪，其人反能食而不呕，此为三阴不受邪也

After three days of the Shanghan disease, usually the three Yang (diseases or stages) should be over, and the pathogenic Qi may penetrate in deeper Yin (diseases or stages). If the patient now has the desire to eat and isn't nauseous, the disease is not going to develop into the Yin stages. [630]

伤寒三日，少阳脉小者，欲已也。

With a Shanghan (disease) for three days, If Shaoyang pulse feels small (not floating or strong, or deep). This pulse suggests that the disease condition is to be over. [631]

服柴胡汤已，渴者，属阳明，以法治之。

After treatment with Chaihu Tang, if the patient feels thirsty, the disease condition belongs to Yangming stage. Treat the situation accordingly. [632]

伤寒六、七日，无大热，其人躁烦者，此为阳去入阴故也。

With a Shanghan disease for six or seven days, there is no strong fever, but the patient feels annoyed and has a restless body. [633] This condition suggests that the disease is going to move into the Yin (inner deep Yangming stage).

3.5 Differentiation of the Shaoyang stage

得病六七日，脉迟浮弱，恶风寒，手足温，医二三下之，不能食，而胁下满痛，面目及身黄，颈项强，小便难者，与柴胡汤，后必下重。本渴饮水而呕者，柴胡不中与也，食谷者哕。

With a Shanghan disease for six to seven days, [634] the pulse feels slow, floating and weak. The patient feels chilly, aversion to cold, [635] and hands and feet are warm. [636] A Purging therapy was used two to three times. [637] The treatment makes the patient unable to eat, and the patient feels bloating and fullness in the flank region. [638] The patient has yellow color on the face, eyes, and body (jaundice), [639] feels tightness on the back and the nape [640] and has difficulty urinating. In such case, if Xiao Chaihu Tang

---

[630] Dr. Hu Xishu: This paragraph mostly does not belong to the original text of *Shanghan Lun*. It was written by Dr. Wang Shuhe.

Dr. Ni Haixia: This should mean that after twenty-one days the disease will pass deeper into the Yin stages (the Taiyin, Shaoyin and Jueyin stages). Disease course in each Yang stage is seven days.

[631] Hu XIshu: This paragraph may also be written by Dr. Wang Shuhe.

[632] If thirst presents during the Shaoyang stage, treatment with Xiao Chaihu Tang should cure it. If there is no thirst during the Shaoyang stage, and after the use of Xiao Chaihu Tang the patient starts to feel thirst, it means that the disease has left the Shaoyang and come into the Yangming stage.

[633] *Annoyed feeling and restless in the body* suggest that there is inner Hotness. The sixth day and the seventh days are the time when the Shanghan disease is moving to the Yangming stage.

[634] Six to seven days is the time when the disease penetrates the Shaoyang stage.

[635] *Floating, slow, and weak pulse and chills, aversion to cold* suggest that the body defense energy became weak. The pulse indicates that there is body surface condition.

[636] *Warm hands and feet*: the disease has also involved the Yangming and Taiyin stages. In Taiyin stage, the hands and feet are warm. The Taiyin is related to the presence of Dampness. Yangming is related to the Fire inside.

[637] For such cases, the use of Purging therapy is wrong, because Purging therapy should not be used with the Taiyang stage, the Shaoyang stage, or the Yangming body surface Stage if the inner side is not dry enough to cause firm stool yet.

[638] The depletion of body liquid (the Yang Qi) through bowel moment makes inner Fire rush up to the diaphragm area to cause a bloated feeling and reduced appetite.

[639] Due to the presence of Dampness, Fire and difficulty in urination, the Fire and the Dampness create jaundice condition. (If the urination is normal, the Dampness can deplete out of the body through urine, so there will be no jaundice.)

[640] This is because there is Dampness in the muscle. The nape belongs to Taiyang meridian, and the side of the neck belongs to Shaoyang meridian.

is used, the patient will have tenesmus sensation. [641]

(Another case is: a patient feels thirsty. After the drink of water, the patient vomits. [642] In this case, Chaihu Tang does not work either. [643] For such patient, eating food can result in hicupp.)

4. Taiyin stage

The Taiyin stage involves the Spleen. [644]

The main function of the Spleen system in the body is to transport water, Dampness, and nutrition absorbed via the digestive system. [645] In the Taiyin stage, Spleen Yang

Qi is deficient, [646] and the function of water transportation is affected so that there is retention of Dampness and Coldness in the body, causing an abdominal fullness and pain, diarrhea, vomiting, from time to time. If the pathogenic Qi invades the Spleen system and only causes disorder of the Qi and Blood movement in the body, the patient might only have pain or a fullness feeling in the abdomen but has no vomiting or diarrhea.

The Taiyin stage also has a body surface condition, which is a muscular pain in the arms and legs. The reason is that the arms and legs are dominated by both the Yangming and the Taiyin (muscle phase).

The Taiyin stage can develop from the Taiyang stage, Shaoyang stage, or Yangming stage due to improper use of Purging therapy. The pathogenic Qi can also directly attack the Spleen system to cause Taiyin stages.

---

[641] This is because Xiao Chaihu Tang can increase the inner Dampness. The *fullness feeling and pain in the flank region and cannot eat* mislead the diagnosis as Shayang stage to Xiao Chaihu Tang.

[642] Due to the depletion of Fire through Purging therapy, the Dampness becomes relatively more in the body, the water is overwhelming and the stomach and cannot accept any more, so that we have water reversing condition.

[643] The whole condition seems to indicate the use of Xiao Chaihu Tang for the treatment, but due to the presence of Dampness and Fire in the body, Xiao Chaihu Tang is not powerful enough to solve the whole condition. If Xiao Chaihu Tang alone is used, with the depletion of Fire with this herbal formula, the Dampness in the body will be relatively more, and cause water-reverse condition. In this case, the best way is to use the Xiao Chaihu Tang together with Yinchen Wu Ling San. The Wu Ling San works to cure the Dampness (water reversing condition, Yinchen works to reduce both Fire and Dampness (jaundice) and Xiao Chaihu Tang works to solve the whole Shaoyang condition.

This paragraph tells us that Xiao Chaihu Tang should not be used for Dampness-Fire condition or garbage water retention condition.

Dr. Ni Haixia: Use Fuling Si Ni Tang for the treatment.

[644] The foot Taiyin meridian is part of the Spleen system. The hand Taiyin meridian is in the Lung system. But diseases in the Lung system are mostly described in the Taiyang stage.

[645] The Taiyin Spleen system also controls the complexity of the blood vessels, and holds the blood inside the vessels. Theoretically, if the Spleen is

deficient, there will be bleeding. However, such a function of the Spleen was not involved in the Taiyin stage in the Shanghan disease.

The Spleen system governs most of the body's liquid parts so, in the book *Huangdi Nei Jing*, it is the strongest Yin in the body (triple Yin). However, in the book *Shanghan Lun*, the severity of the Taiyin is the least among the three Yin stages. This suggests that the concept of Taiyin in *Shanghan Lun* and *Nei Jing* may not be the same.

Dr. Hao Wanshan: The *Huangdi Nei Jing* describes mostly physiology, but the *Shanghan Lun* describes pathology.

[646] Dr. Liao Houze: In the body, Spleen governs thinking. Patients with Spleen deficiency are not good for their own family, have low enthusiasm for outsiders and strong self-esteem. There are many contradictory things and the logic is not strict. This is also a Spleen disease. A person with the wrong teeth has congenital Spleen deficiency. Those with vertical stripes on the tip of the nose also have Spleen deficiency. The brain functions are normal, the thinking and analysis of things are immature, a mess, or contradictory. The Spleen determines how much and where to distribute absorbed food. With Splenectomy, the patient has a poor appetite, has swelling, has shortened life. On the other hand, patients with Hypersplenism tend to eat a lot, but have a little bowel movement. Use Maren and jujube to slow and soften the Spleen.

4.1 Taiyin body surface condition

太阴中风，四肢烦痛，脉浮者，可发汗，
宜 桂枝 汤。 阳微阴涩而长者，为欲愈。

In Wind-attack Taiyin stage, if a patient feels annoying pain on the arms and legs,[647] the pulse feels floating, Sweating therapy can be used. Use Guizhi Tang. If Yang pulse feels faint (when the pulse is pressed slightly) and Yin pulse feels rough and long (when it is pressed hard), these disease conditions will get better without help.[648]

太阴病，脉浮者，可发汗，宜 桂枝 汤。

In the Taiyin stage, if the pulse feels floating, Sweating therapy can be used. Use Guizhi Tang for treatment. [649]

4.2 Taiyin inner condition

本太阳病，医反下之，因而腹满时痛者，
属太阴也，桂枝 加芍药汤主之。大实痛
者，桂枝 加 大黄 汤主之。太阴为病脉弱，
其人续自便利，设当行 大黄 芍药者，宜
减之，以其人胃气弱，易动故也。

A Shanghan disease is initially in the Taiyang stage, a Purging therapy was, however, used. The patient feels bloating and pain in the abdomen from time to time, such a situation means that the disease has changed into the

Taiyin stage. In this case, use Guizhi Jia Shaoyao Tang as the primary treatment. [650] If

---

[647] Dr. Liu Duzhou: The *annoying pain on the arms and legs* belongs to the Taiyin stage. Taiyin dominates the arms and legs.

Dr. Hu Xishu: The *annoying pain on the arms and legs* here should belong to the Taiyang stage. It is hard to understand why it is listed in the Taiyin stage.

[648] Note: Taiyin Wind-attack condition can get better by itself.

[649] Dr. Hu Xishu: The condition here is similar to Gegen Tang for the treatment of Taiyang-Yangming concurrent co-existing condition, in which the Taiyang is Cold-attack Taiyang. While here it is Taiyang-Taiyin successive condition. Guizhi Tang can cure the body Surface condition as well as the inner weak condition too (Ginseng, Gancao, and jujube in Guizhi Tang can nourish the inner condition). If the condition is really the Shaoyin stage with Taiyang body surface, then Sweating therapy (with Mahuang Tang) cannot be used first (the treatment of the Shaoyin stage should be the first).

[650] There is a hot debate about this paragraph, about the reason to use Guizhi Jia Shaoyao Tang, and for the difference between this formula and Xiao Jianzhong Tang.

Dr. Liu Duzhou: The case here is not due to Taiyin Cold-Dampness or Yangming Hotness-Dampness or Hotness-Dryness condition. There is no Taiyang condition either. It is a disorder of Qi and Blood in the digestive system or the disorder between the Liver (blood) and Spleen (Qi).

Dr. Hu Xishu: The words *"belongs to Taiyin"* are wrong. This is not a Taiyin condition at all. This is not a Weakness condition in the typical Taiyin stage. If it is Taiyin Coldness-Weakness condition, how dare we use Dahuang (Dahuang is Cold in herbal nature) and Shaoyao? (Shaoyao is also mild-cold in herbal nature. It treats hot conditions, not cold conditions.) The pain here is a fullness pain (not a weakness pain) and the abdominal bloating is also a fullness bloating (not a weakness bloating). For a typical Taiyin disease, the use of Shaoyao or Dahuang will cause death. This paragraph is for the distinguish aim. It is Taiyang body Surface condition with bowel spasm.

Dr. Hao Wanshan: The case here belongs to the Taiyin stage. If there are acute and strong spasms in the stomach, use Xiao Jianzhong Tang for the treatment.

Dr. Du Yumao: This is the Taiyang-Taiyin stage. The Taiyin is Spleen-mild-Yang deficiency. The patient has no diarrhea. If the Spleen Yang deficiency is severe, and the patient has diarrhea, use Guizhi Jia Renshen Tang.

Dr. Martin Wang: This condition can be understood as Taiyang-Yangming progressive condition. The Yangming is Yangming inner condition. It is a disorder of the Qi and Blood in the bowel. The Guizhi Jia Shaoyao Tang deals with both the related Taiyang and Yangming conditions. It is the principle in the successive condition that the herbal formula needs to deal with all the related stages. (For concurrent co-existing condition, the herbal formula needs to focus on one stage each time.) If there is no body surface condition, the pain and the bloating in the abdomen from time to time may be treated with Xiao Jianzhong Tang, Lizhong Tang or Fuzi Lizhong Tang.

The Guizhi Jia Shaoyao Tang condition and the Guizhi Jia Dahuang Tang condition can be seen in intestine spasms, adenomesenteritis or atrophia infantum.

the abdominal pain is intense, the patient feels abdominal bloating, use Guizhi Jia Dahuang [651] as the primary treatment. In the Taiyin stage, the pulse is weak, (suggesting that the body condition is weak), whenever the Shaoyao and Dahuang are needed, they should be used in low dosage. [652]

太阴之为病，腹满而吐，食不下，自利益甚，时腹自痛。若下之，必胸下结硬。

The Taiyin stage is characterized by abdominal bloating, [653] vomiting, [654] poor appetite, [655] diarrhea, which can be worse and worse, and abdominal pain from time to time. [656] If a Purging therapy is used for

treatment, the patient will have Pi syndrome in the upper abdomen. [657]

自利不渴者，属太阴，以其脏有寒故也，当温之，宜服四逆辈。

If a patient has diarrhea but is not thirsty, [658] the disease belongs to the Taiyin. This situation is due to the Weakness and Coldness condition inside the body. [659] For treatment, use various Inner-warming therapies (such as Lizhong Tang, Si Ni Tang,

---

[651] Dr. Hao Wanshan: The addition of Dahuang here is not to improve bowel movement or to expel the retained stool, it is used to activate blood circulation and to dissolve stagnated blood.

Dr. Du Yumao: This is Taiyang-Taiyin successive condition. The pathogenic Qi causes Hotness in the intestine and exhausts liquid. There is constipation but no delirious speech and no wave-fever.

[652] This is because both herbs belong to Cold nature, and using too much may make the Taiyin cold-weakness condition worse.

[653] The abdominal bloating feeling in the Taiyin stage is true Weakness condition. It means that the patient likes to press and warm the abdomen. There is no solid mass inside the abdomen. In comparison with the Hou Jiang Xia Cao Renshen Tang condition, the bloating in the latter is a mixture of Weakness and solid garbage material inside the abdomen. The bloating occurs from time to time. When it occurs, the patient does not want to press or to warm the abdomen. When the bloating subsides, the patient does not care about pressing or to warming the abdomen. Furthermore, in the Yangming inner organ condition, in which there is solid stool garbage inside the bowel, the bloating is consistent. The patient does not want to press or to warm the abdomen at all.

[654] Due to Stomach deficiency, the Stomach cannot evaporate water and cannot distribute water to lungs and to urine bladder. There will be garbage water accumulation that causes bloating and vomiting. The bloating in the Taiyin stage is soft-bloating feeling. The bloating is solid-bloating in Yangming inner condition.

[655] Dr. Liao Houze: Poor appetite is a common characteristic of the Taiyin and Shaoyin stages.

[656] Due to Weakness and Coldness inside, the bowel cannot hold the garbage water, causing diarrhea. The

---

abdominal pain and diarrhea can become less severe after warming with a hot water bag, and so on.

The principle in the treatment is Warm therapy. The main herbal formula used is Lizhong Tang or various Si Ni Tang.

[657] Dr. Ni Haixia: Normally, the food coming into the stomach enlarges the stomach, which compresses the spleen to let the spleen passes blood to the pancreas. The pancreas gets warmer and warms the stomach and starts pushing the stomach to move, so the stomach starts to digest food. If the blood from the spleen is reduced for some reasons, the digestive function of the stomach will be affected too. The food becomes corrupted into white color liquid. It cannot be absorbed and so it remains in the stomach to prevent further intake of food, resulting in poor appetite. The white clolor liquid accumulates more and more, meaning that the Dampness of the spleen is growing and the spleen becomes large. The enlarged spleen compresses the stomach to reduce the ability of the stomach to accept food. Patients with the enlarged spleen can spit white liquid and the stool also has mucus.

Dr. Liao Houze: The main formula used in the Taiyin stage should be Yuebi Jia Zhu Tang.

[658] *Has no thirst* means the diarrhea is not due to Fire or Shaoyin Coldness-Weakness condition. In the Fire condition, the Fire exhausts body liquid to cause thirst. In the Shaoyin stage, the water cannot be evaporated into vapor to distribute to other parts of the body, so the patient can also feel thirsty. However, in the latter case, the thirst is not strong. The patient wants to drink warm water and wants to drink a small amount of warm water each time.

[659] In the Taiyin stage, the more diarrhea, the more abdominal bloating feeling, but the patient has no thirst. The disease is in the Spleen. In the Shaoyin stage, the diarrhea is due to lower Kidney Yang deficiency, which cannot evaporate water up, so there is thirst.

and so on.) depending on actual clinic conditions.[660]

(If vomiting is severe in the Taiyin stage, or if vomiting happens as soon as food enters the mouth, use Ganjiang Huangqin Huanglian Ginseng Tang.)

4.3 Differentiation diagnosis in Taiyin stage

The Taiyin stage should be distinguished from Yangming stage:

In Cold-attack Yangming stage, the patient cannot eat (i.e., has poor digestion). Eating worsens the stomach bloating, dizziness, irritation, sweating on the hands and feet, difficulty urinating, and diarrhea. In the Taiyin stage, the patient can still eat, but the appetite is poor. Eating does not make the condition worse.

In Wind-attack Yangming stage, the patient also feels bloating in the abdomen, but has difficulty in bowel movement, and is thirsty with the desire to drink much cold water.

The Taiyin stage should also be distinguished from Shaoyin and Jueyin stages, as all the three can have diarrhea.

In the Taiyin stage, diarrhea does not cause thirst, the pulse is floating and slow, and the hands and feet are warm. In the Shaoyin stage, diarrhea occurs along with thirst, there could be undigested food or blood in the stool, the pulse is deep and thin and faint, and the hands and feet are cold. In the Jueyin stage, the cold feeling in the hands and feet is much stronger, and there could be both blood and pus in the stool.

4.4 Special types of Taiyin stage

Jaundice

伤寒脉浮而缓，手足自温者，系在太阴。太阴当发身黄；若小便自利者，不能发黄。至七八日，虽暴烦，下利日十余行，必自止 (以脾家实，腐秽去故也。)。

With a Shanghan disease, if the pulse is floating and soft, and if the hands and feet feel warm,[661] the disease is in the Taiyin stage. In this stage, it is easy to have jaundice. If the urination is regular, jaundice will not

---

[660] Dr. Liu Duzhou: For inner Taiyin Coldness-Weakness condition, if the vomiting is severe, use Lizhong Tang plus Dingxiang and Wuzhuyu. If the diarrhea is more severe and the patient even feels heavy and cold on the lower back, use Lizhong Tang plus Cangzhu and Fuzi. If there is also Dampness together with the Coldness and Weakness, the patient has diarrhea and difficulty in urination, use Lizhong Tang plus Fuling and Zexie.

Dr. She De: The original Chinese text here is "use the Si Ni herbal formula group for the treatment", but did not indicate the exact name of the herbal formula. Many doctors believe that this formula should be Lizhong Tang. However, in Shanghan diseases, a Taiyin disease can easily change into a Shaoyin disease, which is deadly. To prevent the change, using Si Ni Tang should be the correct way. The use of Lizhong Tang is not proper. Only in the miscellaneous diseases showing the Taiyin syndrome, should Lizhong Tang be used. (She De. The Taiyin disease should be treated with Si Ni Tang. http://aaaaaa2307a.lofter.com/post/1ccdcdd1_6dfa3aa)

[661] Dr. Liu Duzhou: The *pulse changes from floating-tight in the Taiyang stage into floating-soft* suggests that the Cold moved into the inside of the body and became Hotness. The warm hands and feet here mean that the body has a fever. In the Yangming stage, the fever is in the whole body and, in the Taiyin stage, the fever is only in the hands and feet.

Dr. Hao Wanshan: The warm hands and feet can be seen in both the Yangming and the Taiyin stage. In the Yangming, the patient is thirsty but in the Taiyin, is not. The reason is that the arms and legs are dominated by the Stomach-Spleen system of the body.

Dr. Ni Haixia: If the pulse feels floating-soft, the disease is Taiyang Wind-attack. If it feels floating-tight, it is in Cold-attack Taiyang stage. In either condition, the hands and feet are cold. If the hands and feet become warm, it indicates that the disease has moved into the Taiyin stage. The warmth means the outflow of the Stomach Qi. Normally the Stomach Qi should remain inside to digest food.

Dr. Cai Changfu: It is not normal if a patient feels very cold in the hands and feet, neither so if a patient feels very warm in the hands and feet. It does not mean that the warm hands and feet are better for health.

occur. [662] In the Taiyin stage for seven to eight days, even if the patient feels very much annoyed, and has diarrhea ten or more times per day, diarrhea can stop naturally. [663] (The reason is that the body condition has been improved and the body defense ability struggles to expel the Dampness, causing the annoyed feeling and frequent diarrhea to expel garbage stool).

5. Shaoyin stage

If a patient has the following symptoms or signs, the disease is in the Shaoyin stage:

(1) The pulse is tiny-thin (faint), [664] the patient desires to lie down for rest again and again (no energy and no desire to do things);

(2) With above, and there are diarrhea [665] and thirst;

(3) With the (1), and the urine is as pure as clear water.

The Shaoyin stage involves Heart (Fire) [666] and Kidney (Water). [667] It is characterized as the Coldness-Weakness condition in the body, or as Yang Deficiency with Yin Excess. The body condition is colder and weaker than in the Taiyin stage. The excessive Yin in the Shaoyin stage tends to refuse the Yang Qi and make the Yang Qi float or escape from the body in severe cases.

The Heart and the Kidney are the essential organs in the body. Therefore, in the Shaoyin stage, these diseases can have a greater chance of cause death.

The Shaoyin stage can develop from the Taiyang stage (naturally or via wrong treatment), or the pathogenic Qi can directly attack in the Shaoyin stage. Those patients who are easily attacked by Cold pathogenic Qi are those who had Kidney Yang Deficiency before becoming sick this time. [668] The Shaoyin stage can also occur in some special conditions, such as if a person was attacked suddenly by extreme cold. [669] The Shaoyin stage can also develop from the Taiyin stage when diseases in the Taiyin stage are not treated properly or had no treatment at all.

The Shaoyin stage can also be separated into Shaoyin body surface condition and inner condition. Shaoyin body surface condition manifests mostly as a sore throat. Shaoyin inner condition can be either a Hotness

---

[662] The pulse becomes floating while still slow (weak), and the hands and feet become warm. The disease condition suggests that the body starts to have more Yang Qi to evaporate the inner Dampness through urination. Therefore, if urination is normal, the Dampness can be expelled out and there won't be jaundice. If the urination is difficult, the Dampness and the Hotness will be entangled inside the body to form jaundice.

[663] Frequent diarrhea, together with a floating pulse and warm hands and feet suggests the restoration of body Yang Qi. The sudden annoyed feeling and frequent diarrhea here can be regarded as a healing crisis.

Note: Only with the overwhelming of Dampness in the Taiyin stage could there be such a healing crisis. If the Taiyin is mostly the Coldness-Weakness condition, the condition must be treated to get better.

If, after eight to nine days, the stool becomes firm, this change means that the Dampness has been depleted and the fever remains, so the Taiyin stage (Coldness and Dampness) moves into the Yangming stage (Dryness and Hotness).

[664] Tiny pulse: Yang deficiency. Thin pulse: Blood deficiency.

[665] Diarrhea in the Shaoyin stage: the stool is loose, no shape or it is a water-like stool, without too bad odor. Patient has no urgent feeling in the anus.

[666] The hand Shaoyin meridian connects to the Heart.

[667] The feet Shaoyin meridian connects to the Kidney.

[668] Kidney Yang Deficiency can be caused by over sexual activity, use of sexual stimulation drugs, frequent masturbation, frequent fear (such as watching scary film or TV programs), an experience of severely scary events (such as an earthquake, war, murder, business bankruptcy, investment failure, and so on.) and kidney diseases. Elderly with Kidney deficiency can die more easily than most people when attacked by a common cold or flu.

[669] A person is attacked by a sudden cold: covered suddenly in an avalanche, cold water, freezing room, snowstorm, and so on. In such cases, the Kidney Yang Qi and Heart Yang Qi are compressed even if the person has no original Kidney Deficiency. In such cases, the pulse feels deep-tight.

Note: The pulse feels floating-tight in the Taiyang Cold-attack stage.

(Heart)-transformation or a Cold (Kidney)-transformation condition. [670]

There are three types of Coldness-transformation conditions. The first is the Yang Deficiency and Yin Excess condition. Patients with this disease condition feel cold and pain all over the body, have cold-sweat,[671] and tend to lie down with a heavy blanket covering the body. The mind's reactions are slow and clouded. There is diarrhea with undigested food in the stool. Urination can be either frequent [672] or difficult, but the urine is clear in color. The pulse can be deep, or mild and thin, or even very difficult to feel (faint). For treatment, use Si Ni Tang.

The second is the condition of Yin Excess and Yang floating (on body surface). Usually, the Yang should mix with Yin to warm the Yin. If the Yin is too strong, the Yang cannot penetrate the Yin to warm it. The Yang is refused, rejected, and floats on the body surface. Patients with this condition have the same symptoms as the previous Yang Deficiency-Yin Excess condition, but the body feels warm,[673] and no longer feels cold. For treatment, use Tongmai Si Ni Tang. Increase the amount of Ganjian and Fuzi in the original Si Ni Tang to increase the ability of the herbal formula to improve the body Yang Qi.

The third condition is Yin Excess and Yang floating on the face (Upcast Yang syndrome). Patients with this condition have the same symptoms as in the two disease conditions above, but also have pink color in the cheeks. [674] For treatment, use Baitong Tang. The function of this formula is to connect and conduct the Yin and the Yang, to chase and bring the Yang Qi back to the body.

5.1 Shaoyin body surface condition

(1) 少阴病，始得之，反发热，脉沉者，麻黄附子细辛汤主之。

In the Shaoyin stage for a short time, a patient has a fever (typically there should be no fever in the Shaoyin stage) and the pulse is deep. [675] For such case, use Mahuang Fuzi Xixin Tang as the primary treatment.

(2) 少阴病，得之二、三日，麻黄附子甘草汤微发汗，以二、三日无里证，故微发汗也。

In the Shaoyin stage for two to three days (and has a common cold or flu, e.g., there are body surface conditions, and no symptoms indicating Yangming stage), use Mahuang Fuzi Gancao Tang for treatment (to create a little sweat). To treat as such is because there is no inner condition after two to three days of the disease.

(If the patient has sweat before the treatment, has stiff joints, feels chilly and aversion to wind, use Guizhi Jia Fuzi Tang.[676])

---

[670] Dr. Du Yumao: The cold-transform condition is the main transformation. Hotness-transform is pretty much a variation of the Shaoyin stage.

[671] Cold sweat: the Yang Qi is deficient and cannot seal and protect the body surface.

[672] Frequent urination: the Kidney Yang cannot hold the urination. Difficulty in urination: the Kidney Yang cannot promote the secretion of urine.

[673] The body temperature may or may not be high. The Yang Qi is the warm energy in the body. With the Yang Qi floating in the body surface, the body feels warm. For such patients, even if the body temperature is high, the patient still wants to cover the body with more blankets.

[674] The red cheeks should be distinguished from the red face of the Fire condition in Yangming body surface condition.

[675] Dr. Hu Xishu: *Fever* means the pathogenic Qi is on the body surface. *Deep pulse* means there is garbage water inside of the body. The body surface condition and the inner garbage water need to be treated at the same time. The pulse in the Shaoyin stage should be thin-faint but not deep.

Dr. Hao Wanshan and Dr. Liu Duzhou: This is co-existing Taiyang body surface and Shaoyin body surface condition. For many elderly patients, when they catch a common cold or flu, they suffer from such. The death rate is high.

Dr. Tan Jiezhong: The pulse in the Chi position might be floating. In other words, patients with floating pulse in the Chi position mostly are in the Shaoyin stage.

[676] The pulse in Shaoyin body surface condition should be floating and mildly thin.

(3) 太阳病，发热头痛，脉反沉；若不差，身体疼痛，当救其里，宜四逆汤。

In the Taiyang stage, a patient has a fever and headaches, and pulse is however deep.[677] If the disease condition remains, and if the patient feels generalized pain, improve the inner body condition first. Use Si Ni Tang.

(4) 少阴病，身体痛，手足寒，骨节痛，脉沉者，附子汤主之。

In the Shaoyin stage, a patient feels generalized pain, feels cold in hands and feet, pain in joints, and has a deep pulse. In such case, use Fuzi Tang as the primary treatment.[678]

(5) 少阴病，得之一、二日，口中和，其背恶寒者，当灸之，附子汤主之。

In the Shaoyin stage for one to two days, there is no particular taste in the mouth,[679] but the patient feels an aversion to cold on the back,[680] such conditions should be treated with moxibustion[681] or formula Fuzi Tang as the primary treatment. [682]

(6) 少阴病二、三日，咽痛者，可与甘草汤，不差，与桔梗汤。

In the Shaoyin stage for two to three days, a patient has pain in the throat, [683] try Gancao Tang for treatment. If it does not work, try Jigen Tang (or Banxia Powder or Banxia Tang). [684]

Dr. Hu Xishu: Shaoyin body surface condition with sweating requires the use of Guizhi Jia Fuzi Tang.
[677] This disease condition can be understood as co-existing Taiyang and Shaoyin stages. The deep pulse indicates the Shaoyin stage.
[678] The deep pulse indicates the presence of garbage water inside the body. The pain in the body and joints suggests that this is Coldness and Dampness in the muscles and joints. This is Bi syndrome. In the body surface condition of Shaoyin (Mahuang Fuzi Xixin Tang condition), the pulse is also deep, but the body has a fever.
    Dr. Ni Haixia: In the shaoyin stage, the inner side is Coldness. The Coldness is due to too much water in the blood. The water is cold. Such blood cannot bring enough warmth to the body, resulting in cold and pain in the body.
[679] *No special taste in mouth*: the mouth does not feel dry or bitter; the tongue coating is not yellow or white.
[680] *Aversion to cold on the back*: there is garbage water in the stomach. The garbage water should be cured soon, to prevent the Shaoyin stage moving into the Taiyin stage (with vomiting and diarrhea).
    Dr. Hao Wanshan: TCM says that the back belongs to Yang. With Yang deficiency, the back feels cold. It is known that in early pregnancy, the body Yin and Yang move to the uterus to nourish the fetus. The female, therefore, feels a short period of cold on the back, dizziness or ache in the head and constipation. All of these symptoms can happen before the change of pulse that indicates the pregancy.
    Dr. Hao Wanshan: Note that there is also cold feeling on the back in Baihu Jia Renshen Tang, which belongs to Yangming Fire condition. In this condition, the patient has a very dry mouth and wants to drink heavy amounts of cold water. Here in the Shaoyin stage, and in the early stage of the pregnancy, the patient does not feel very thirsty and has no strong willingness to drink lots of water.
[681] Use Moxibustion on Geguan (BL46) and Guanyuan (CV4) points.
    Dr. Ni Haixia: Wherever on the body feels cold, just do the moxibustion there. There's no need to stick to fixed acupuncture points for moxibustion.
[682] In this case, there is no apparent body surface condition, so Mahuang Fuzi Gancao Tang is not used. In Baihu Tang condition, the patient can also feel cold on the back, but the patient feels dry mouth.
[683] Dr. Xu Chenghe: The dry throat and the sore throat can be seen in both Cold-attack and Wind-Hotness-attack (such as in Warm diseases) diseases. It is not at all an absolute condition for the diagnosis of Wind-Hotness diseases. It is wrong to use a sore throat as gold evidence to make a diagnosis of Wind-Hotness disease.
[684] Dr. Hu Xishu: A sore throat in the Shaoyin stage should belong to the Shaoyang. Diseases in the Shaoyang stage involve the eyes, ears, mouth, and should also involve the throat here. The sore throat here also means tonsillitis. In clinics, we may use Xiao Chaihu Tang plus herb Shigao and Jiegen. If the inflamed tonsil has pus, we need to use a stronger herbal formula, such as Baihu Zengye Tang (白虎增液汤) or Yunu Jian (玉女煎).
    Dr. Liu Duzhou: If there is no very much depletion of body liquid via diarrhea, the isolated Fire can also result from very strong Coldness in the body. Such isolated Fire can also float up to affect the throat and cause a sore throat. Patients with Shaoyin sore throat

116

(7) 少阴病，咽中伤，生疮，不能语言，声不出者，苦酒汤主之。

In the Shaoyin stage, a patient has pain and an ulcer in the throat, has difficulty speaking or loss of voice, use Kujiu Tang [685] as the primary treatment.

(8) 少阴病，咽中痛，半夏散及汤主之。

In the Shaoyin stage, a patient has a sore throat. [686] Use Banxia San or Banxia Tang as the primary treatment.

---

have less swelling in the throat; the tongue is red and dry, the tongue coating is small, urination is a little bit difficult and a little yellow, and the pulse feels thin, faint and fast.

Dr. Tan Jiezhong: The sore throat in the Shaoyin stage must be distinguished from those in the Ma Xing Shi Gan Tang condition, Yinqiao San (银翘散) or Sang Ju Yin (桑菊饮) syndrome. In the latter ones, the pulse feels floating, but the pulse in the Shaoyin stage is deep, faint and thin. A sore throat in the Shaoyin stage can also be treated with Mahuang Fuzi Xixin Tang. The dose of herb Fuzi should be more than the Mahuang and Xixin. It can also be treated using Fuzi Xixin Qin Lian Tang (附子细辛芩连汤).

Dr. Martin Wang: Either due to the depletion of body liquid (insufficient Yin liquid), or to too much Coldness (too much Yin), the Yang Qi cannot bind to the Yin (to mix with Yin), so the Yang Qi is isolated alone and floats up to cause a various problem. Here the sore throat is one of many disorders. For comparison, the Fire in the Taiyang, Shaoyang and Yangming stages mostly are not such isolated Fire, because, in these three stages, the body liquid is not depleted very much yet. Such Fire can be cleared with Cold herbs. The isolated Fire, however, needs to be calmed down with Yin-nourishing, or body Liquid-nourishing herbs or herbal ingredients, such as Gancao.

Dr. Liao Houze: For a sore throat (tonsil swelling), use Xiao Qinglong Tang plus herb Xuanshen, Maidong, Gancao and Jiegen. Also, use Yudan (玉丹) on the surface of the tonsils.

[685] The Kujiu is the vinegar.

[686] The sore throat here means the whole throat becomes swollen. This is a very dangerous acute condition and can cause death.

Dr. Liu Duzhou: This condition is caused by Cold attack on the throat.

5.2 Shaoyin body inner condition

少阴之为病，脉微细，但欲寐也。

The Shaoyin stage is characterized as that the pulse feels faint and thin and the patient has a desire to lie down. [687]

少阴病，脉沉者，急温之，宜四逆汤。

In the Shaoyin stage, if the pulse feels deep, the body condition should be warmed up urgently. Use Si Ni Tang for treatment. [688]

少阴病，欲吐不吐，心烦，但欲寐，五六日，自利而渴者，(属少阴也)，虚故引水自救。若小便色白者，少阴病形悉具。(小便白者，以下焦虚有寒，不能制水，故令色白也。)

In the Shaoyin stage, a patient feels a desire to vomit but cannot, feels annoyed, and desires to lie down for a break. [689] After five

---

[687] Dr. Tan Jiezhong: The patient does not want to get up from the bed, has no desire to do things, is lazy or negative in dealing with challenges in life or in work. In the Shaoyin stage, when the Heart Yang Qi is affected, the body can become insensitive. For example, the patient may have a fever but does not feel hot. At the beginning of the Shaoyin stage, the emotion and personality change first. Because of the "lazy" feelings, the patient is easily scolded at work and may lose their job and become depressed. For dementia patients, be careful that the patient might be in the Shaoyin stage.

[688] *Deep pulse* can indicate that the disease is on the inner side of the body and also that there is water accumulation inside the body. The pulse is not floating, thin, or faint, so there is no Shaoyin body surface condition. With the inner garbage water, the Shaoyin condition can easily pass into the Taiyin stage to cause nausea and diarrhea.

Dr. Hao Wanshan: Once the pulse feels deep, treatment is urgently needed, even if there are no more symptoms yet. The treatment would become more difficult once typical symptoms for the Shaoyin stage occur.

[689] The *annoyed feeling and the desire to vomit* are due to the accumulation of garbage water in the stomach. Patients with Shaoyin body constitution and with accumulated water in the stomach before becoming sick this time can easily have diarrhea after a Cold-attack.

to six days, the patient has diarrhea and feels thirsty. [690] If the urine is clear as water, the evidence for the diagnosis of the Shaoyin stage is concretely set up. (The clear color of urine means that the Lower Jiao of the body is with Weakness and Coldness, both of which make the body fail to govern the water, so the urine is clear as water). [691]

传少阴，脉沉细而数，手足时厥时热，咽中痛，小便难，宜附子细辛黄连黄芩汤。

After a disease passed into the Shaoyin stage, If the pulse feels deep, thin and fast, and the hands and feet feel cold but also hot sometimes, the patient has a sore throat and has difficulty urinating, use Fuzi Xixin Huanglian Huangqin Tang for treatment. [692]

脉浮而迟，表热里寒，下利清谷者，四逆汤主之。

The pulse is floating-slow. The body has Hotness in the body surface, but Coldness in the inner side. The patient has diarrhea with undigested food in the stool. Use Si Ni Tang as the main formula. [693]

少阴病，下利，脉微涩，呕而汗出，必数更衣；反少者，当温其上灸之。

In the Shaoyin stage, a patient has diarrhea. The pulse feels faint and rough, and there are nausea and sweating. Diarrhea will be more in frequency and in volume too. If diarrhea is, however, less, the treatment should focus on warming the Stomach (to allow the body to build up more body liquid) with moxibustion (on the Stomach meridian, such as Zusanli point). [694]

少阴病，得之二、三日以上，心中烦，不得卧，黄连阿胶汤主之。

In the Shaoyin stage for more than two to three days, the patient feels annoyed in the chest, so much so that there is difficulty falling asleep, [695] use Huanglian Ajiao Tang as the primary treatment.

Dr. Tan Jiezhong: The patient may just not want to get up from the bed, have no desire to act for life or work. The patient becomes actually "lazy".
[690] Dr. Hao Wanshan: Diarrhea should contain undigested food, because there is insufficient "Fire" to digest eaten food (just like there's no fire to cook food). Once there is undigested food in the stool, the disease belongs to the Shaoyin stage. The thirsty feeling is due to insufficient Fire to evaporate water to distribute to the body (including the throat). The patient feels thirsty and wants to drink water, but the patient only wants to drink warm water and wants to drink only a little amount each time.
[691] The coldness and the body liquid depletion are more apparent in the Shaoyin stage than in the Taiyin stage. Diarrhea with clear-water-like urine and thirst are absolute evidence for the Shaoyin stage. The desire-to-vomit and the annoyed feeling are due to the rejection of the Yang Qi by the deep Coldness in the lower part of the body (the overwhelming of the Yin).
[692] Dr. Tan Jiezhong: This is Shaoyin Kidney Yang deficiency (Cold) with Heart Yin deficiency (Fire). The herbal formula is, therefore, a mixture of Warm herbs (Fuzi and Xixin) and Cold herbs (Huanglian and Huangqin). Alternatively, use Mahuang Fuzi Xixin Tang plus Yinqiao San. If the patient has constipation, use Mahuang Fuzi Dahuang Tang.

[693] This paragraph is initially listed as the Yangming stage. This condition should be Taiyang-Shaoyin co-existing condition. The principle for the treatment is to cure the inner Coldness-Weakness condition first, then to cure the body surface condition.
   Dr. Hu Xishu: The herbal formula Baitong Tang might be better than the Si Ni Tang here.
   Dr. Liu Duzhou: This condition is inner Coldness that presses Yang Qi to the body surface. The *fever and sweating, and floating pulse* is floating Yang Qi.
[694] Dr. Hu Xishu: Use Si Ni Tang to warm the Stomach. Use moxibustion on Zusanli point (ST36), not on Baihui (GV20) point. Regular Yin-nourishing herbs, such as Shengdi and Maidong, should not be used.
   Dr. Liu Duzhou: This disease condition can be treated with Fuzi Tang and/or by using moxibustion on Baihui (GV20) and Guanyuan points (CV4).
[695] Dr. Hu Xishu: The *annoyed feeling and hard to fall asleep* means that the pathogenic Qi has penetrated into the Shaoyang stage. The Fire is in the chest. This condition is similar to Zhizi Chi Tang condition. However, Huanlian Ajiao Tang has more insufficient body liquid (Fire with insufficient body liquid). Zhizi Chi Tang condition has relatively more Fire. If the Taiyin body surface condition moves to the inner part of the body, in most case, it moves into the Taiyin or Jueyin stage, less in the Shaoyang stage.
   Dr. Liu Duzhou: This condition is due to the Fire-transformation of the Shaoyin stage (the Cold-water

118

少阴病，下利咽痛，胸满心烦，猪肤汤主之。

In the Shaoyin stage, a patient has diarrhea, a sore throat, feels fullness in the chest and is annoyed in the heart. Use Zhufu Tang as the primary treatment. [696]

少阴病，下利，(脉不微者)，白通汤主之。

In the Shaoyin stage, a patient has diarrhea (and the pulse does not feel faint). Use Bai Tong Tang as the primary treatment. [697]

少阴病，下利，白通汤主之。利不止，厥逆无脉，干呕烦者，白通加猪胆汁汤主之。服汤脉暴出者死，微续者生。

In the Shaoyin stage, a patient has diarrhea, use Bai Tong Tang as the primary treatment. After such treatment, if diarrhea continues, there is Jue syndrome, [698] the pulse is hard to detect, and the patient belches and feels annoyed, then use Tong Mai Si Ni Tang Jia

---

transformation of the Shaoyin stage is Zhenwu Tang condition). This means that the Shaoyin stage can manifest as either Fire (the Heart) syndrome or as Cold water (Kidney) syndrome.

Dr. Hao Wanshan: This is a Yin deficiency and Fire excess condition. It is Fire-transformation of the Shaoyin stage. This formula is not proper for the treatment of long-term Neurasthenia but is useful for patients who have more difficulty falling asleep after a common cold.

Dr. Martin Wang: This condition may be understood as the Yang Qi floating and rushing up to the heart to disturb the Heart. The floating of the Yang Qi is due to too much Coldness in the lower part of the body (Kidney). The Yang Qi is refused by the Cold. It floats to the Heart (the Upper Jiao, the chest), but not to the body surface yet. An alternative way to understand this condition is that, normally, Heart Fire needs Kidney Water to balance (to harmonize), to make the Fire warm but not burning. Now in the Shaoyin stage, the body liquid (the water) is insufficient (such as thirst along with diarrhea), the Heart Fire is not kept at the normal warm level and is not calm-warm (which shows as an annoyed feeling). This is understood as a disconnection between the Fire and the Water (Cold) inside the body. In either way, it is difficult to understand the condition as the Shaoyang stage. Patients who suffer from this condition may be ones who had Weakness in the Heart before becoming sick this time.

[696] Dr. Hu Xishu: All the symptoms here suggest that the Shaoyin stage has moved to the Shaoyang stage. This is Shaoyin-Shaoyang co-existing condition. Diarrhea here is not Weakness-Coldness diarrhea, but Hotness diarrhea. The Zhufu Tang here works to nourish the body liquid and to clear Hotness, not to clear Coldness.

Dr. Liu Duzhou: In this condition, diarrhea causes depletion of body liquid (the Yin), the body Yang Qi has insufficient Yin to be held, the body Yang Qi that is so floating and becomes isolated Fire or an escaped Fire. Due to the nature of Fire being to float up, the isolated inner Fire floats up to attack the throat and cause a sore throat, fullness in the chest, and an

annoyed feeling. The herb Zhufu in Zhufu Tang is pigskin. It should not include oil or muscle of the meat.

Dr. Du Yumao: The sore throat here belongs to Shaoyin Hotness-transformation condition.

Dr. Martin Wang: The reason for the Zhufu Tang is similar to that for Huanglian Ajiao Tang condition in which the floating Fire affects the Heart.

[697] Dr. Hu Xishu: This paragraph means that the patient has body surface condition (such as chills, fever, headache) and also diarrhea. The pulse is weak and thin. It is Shaoyin body surface condition with Taiyin inner condition (the Shaoyin-Taiyin co-existing condition). The herbal formula Bai Tong Tang works to create a little sweat to cure the body surface condition and to warm the body inner weakness condition too. If there is no body surface condition and if the pulse is weak, then Bai Tong Tang should not be used. Note that the shallot works to create sweat. It works for body surface condition.

Dr. Hao Wanshan: This should be Yin Excessiveness and Yang-floating (on face) condition. This is evidenced by the ingredients of the herbal formula Bai Tong Tang used. In the use of formula Tong Mai Si Ni Tang, it is said that if there is a pink color on the cheek, then add shallot, suggesting that the shallot treats the Yang-floating condition. Here in Bai Tong Tang, the shallot is the main ingredient, so the condition here should belong to Yin Excessiveness and Yang-floating condition.

Dr. Ni Haixia: This is the upper Hotness and lower Coldness condition. The Fire in the chest and the Coldness in the lower abdomen cannot mix.

[698] Jue syndrome: the cold feeling develops from the toes to the ankle and to the knee; from fingertips to the wrist and to the elbow.

pig gallbladder juice for the treatment. [699] After drinking the herbal tea, if the pulse starts to become mild, the patient will be saved for life. If the pulse becomes strong quickly, the patient will die. [700]

少阴病，下利清谷，里寒外热，手足厥逆，脉微欲绝，身反不恶寒，其人面色赤，或腹痛，或干呕，或咽痛，或利止脉不出者，通脉四逆汤主之。

In the Shaoyin stage, a patient has diarrhea with undigested food in the stool. The body is Coldness inside but Hotness outside. The patient has Jue syndrome. The pulse feels faint, which is near hard to feel. The patient has no aversion to cold, however, and has pink color in the cheeks. [701] The patient may have abdominal pain, or nausea, or a sore throat, [702] or the diarrhea stops but the pulse

is still very difficult to detect. [703] In this case, use Tong Mai Si Ni Tang as the primary treatment. [704]

少阴病，二三日至四五日，腹痛，小便不利，下利不止便脓血者，桃花汤主之。少阴病，下利便脓血者，桃花汤主之。

In the Shaoyin stage for two, three, four or five days, a patient feels abdominal pain, [705] and has difficulty urinating. [706] If there is constant diarrhea, [707] and if there are pus and

---

[699] Dr. Hu Xishu: This means the use of Bai Tong Tang is a mistake because it is Sweating therapy and it has been used when the pulse is weak. In the original text, it says to use Bai Tong Tang Jia pig gallbladder juice. This is the wrong herbal formula. It should be Tong Mai Si Ni Tang. If Bai Tong Tang has been used by mistake, how can it be used again? The amount of warm herbs in the Bai Tong is very small, and not sufficient to cure this severe condition.

Dr. Liu Duzhou: Bai Tong Tang here is insufficient to cure the severe condition because the diarrhea has caused depletion of Yang Qi and Yin liquid in the body (hardly felt pulse). The human urine and the pig gallbladder juice both are liquid parts of the animal body, so they can supply Yin liquid without further increasing Yin Coldness to the body.

Dr. Hao Wanshan: The worsening of the condition after the use of Bei Tong Tang is a disturbing result of the treatment. It means that the herbal tea was not powerful enough to cure the disease. For this reason it is recommended to add pig gallbladder juice.

Dr. Ni Haixa explained this paragraph as using Bai Tong Tang with pig gallbladder juice.

[700] The meaning of the sudden stronger pulse is like a sudden brightening of a candle's light before the flame dies. It can be called *bright-light-before-death (last radiation and stem counterflow)*.

[701] *Pink color on the cheek*: the Yang Qi is rejected and floats on the cheek.

[702] *Pain in abdomen and sore throat*: the Kidney meridian goes to the abdomen and the throat.

[703] The *stopping of diarrhea*: there is no more body liquid to be passed out as a stool. The cessation of diarrhea is accompanied with almost-stopping of the pulse.

[704] In this case, the inner Weakness and Coldness condition is very severe, so much so that food cannot be digested at all, the pulse is hard to feel, the cold feeling in hands and feet is developing more towards the elbow and knee (Jue syndrome), and the Coldness refuses the body Yang Qi to float on the face (the Yang Qi escapes). It looks like there is inner Coldness and outer Hotness, but the Hotness is a false phenomenon.

Dr. Hu Xishu: This is also a Shaoyin-Taiyin co-exist stage too.

Dr. Liu Duzhou: Tongmai Si Ni Tang here should have Ginseng in the formula. It is an increased dose of Si Ni Tang with Ginseng.

Dr. Hao Wanshan: Be careful in the treatment even with acupuncture, for such patients with a pulse that is very difficult to feel. After acupuncture, if the pulse suddenly or very quickly becomes stronger, it may be *bright-light-before-death*.

[705] *Pain in abdomen*: due to Coldness in the abdomen.

[706] Dr. Liu Duzhou: *Difficulty in urination* is due to the depletion of body liquid after long-term diarrhea.

Dr. Hao Wanshan: *Difficulty in urination* is due to Kidney Yang deficiency.

[707] Dr. Hu Xishu: This diarrhea belongs to slippery diarrhea (the anus cannot contract properly) and should have no tenesmus. The diarrhea has blood in the stool, but the body has no signs of Hotness. The diarrhea means that the Shaoyin stage involves the Taiyin stage too. Whenever the Shaoyin stage is accompanied by diarrhea, it usually means that the disease does not leave the Shaoyin stage yet, but also comes into the Taiyin stage.

Dr. Martin Wang: According to Dr. Hu Xishu, this is, therefore, a Shaoyin-Taiyin successive condition. The reason for the blood in the stool is Yang deficiency after a long period of diarrhea. There's blood in the stool, [708] use Taohua (Peach blossom) Tang for the treatment. [709]

少阴病，下痢便脓血者，可刺。

In the Shaoyin stage, a patient has diarrhea with pus and blood in the stool. Use acupuncture for the treatment. [710]

少阴病，二、三日不已，至四、五日，腹痛，小便不利，四肢沉重疼痛，自下利者，此为有水气。其人或咳，或小便 （不）利，或（不）下利，或呕者，真武汤主之。

In the Shaoyin stage for two to three days without getting better, then upon the fourth or fifth day, a patient feels abdominal pain and has difficulty urinating, has pain and heaviness in the arms and legs, and has diarrhea. Such conditions suggest water retention in the body. The patient may have a cough, or normal urination, or no diarrhea or nausea. In any case, use Zhenwu Tang for the treatment. [711]

---

insufficient Yang Qi to seal (to hold) the blood vessels in the colon. Alternatively, the condition can be understood according to Five-element theory: overwhelming of the Cold in the Kidney, which bullies the Heart to cause the bleeding (the red blood belongs to Heart. Normally the Kidney Water bullies the Heart Fire and affects Lung to cause pus (the pus is white; white color body material belongs to the Lung). Usually, the Lung (Metal) is the mother element of the kidney (Water). Now it is the son disease that affects its mother element. The *pus* here may not be the resulting product of an infection in the bowel.

Dr. Liu Duzhou: The reason for the pus and blood in the stool is that Yang deficiency will finally also affect the Yin and the disorder in the body Qi will also eventually affect the blood. This is Cold-slippery diarrhea.

Dr. Hao Wanshan: The diarrhea is without tenesmus. The blood in the stool is dark red, and the stool has no strong bad odor. The bleeding is due to the Spleen Yang deficiency, in which the Yang cannot seal and protect the blood vessels in the colon. If the diarrhea is caused by Hotness-Dampness, the diarrhea is with tenesmus, and the blood should be fresh red. The stool has a terrible odor.

Dr. Du Yumao: The blood and pus in the stool are due to Spleen Yang deficiency. The Spleen Yang Qi cannot hold the blood inside the blood vessels. Diarrhea with bleeding is often caused by Hotness in the intestine and for the treatment, use Gegen Qin Lian Tang or Baitouwen Tang.

[708] The bleeding and pus in stool are due to longtime Weakness and Coldness that erode the mucus of the bowel.

[709] Taohua Tang works to warm the inner side and to improve the contracting ability of the anus to stop diarrhea.

[710] Dr. Liu Duzhou: In the Shaoyin stage, there can also be Hotness-retention diarrhea, which occurs in the early stage of the Shaoyin disease. The patient has diarrhea with heat and stool-retention feeling inside the anus and also has blood and pus in the stool. Cold-slippery diarrhea and the Hotness-retention

diarrhea need to be distinguished. For treatment with acupuncture, it has been recommended by other doctors to use the Youmen (KD21), and Jiaoxin (KD8) points to release the Shaoyin Fire. Others recommend the use of the herbal formula Baitouwen Tang for the treatment. Anyway, in such Hot-retention diarrhea in the Shaoyin stage, it is no longer proper to use Taohua Tang.

Dr. Hao Wanshan: For the acupuncture treatment, if the diarrhea is due to Coldness-Weakness, do acupuncture on Qihai (CV6), Guanyuan (CV4) and Zusanli (ST36) (with moxibustion). If the diarrhea is due to Hotness-Dampness, do acupuncture on Zusanli (ST36), Tianshu (ST25) and Qihai (CV6).

Dr. Ni Haixia: Acupuncture on Guanyuan (CV4) point can stop diarrhea.

[711] This condition is similar to Xiao Qinglong Tang condition, in which the body surface condition is not easy to improve because there is garbage water accumulated in the body. Because of the garbage water in both syndromes, the urine is abnormal, the water goes to the bowel and causes diarrhea. If the urination is normal, there will be no diarrhea. The water can also rush up to cause nausea. The water is Dampness, which accumulates in the muscles to cause muscle pain and heaviness. The body's inside is weak and cold, so there is a pain in the abdomen. To cure the body surface condition, the accumulated water should be cured at the same time. Otherwise, Mahuang Fuzi Gancao Tang will not work properly. The diarrhea in the Zhenwu Tang condition is not due to the involvement of the Taiyin stage.

Dr. Hao Wanshan: There are two reasons for the Zhenwu Tang condition. First, in the Taiyang stage, the treatment is improper, and the treatment damages the Kidney Yang Qi. Second, the Cold

少阴病，下利六、七日，咳而呕渴，心烦不得眠者，猪苓汤主之。

In the Shaoyin stage, a patient has diarrhea for six to seven days, has coughing, nausea, feels thirsty, has an annoyed feeling and has difficulty falling asleep. Use Zhuling Tang as the primary treatment.[712]

少阴病二三日，至四五日腹痛小便不利，八、九日，一身手足尽热者，以热在膀胱，必便血.

In the Shaoyin stage for two to three days, upon the fourth or fifth day, a patient has abdominal pain and has difficulty urinating. Upon the eighth or ninth day, the patient feels hot in the whole body, including the hands and feet.[713] This situation is Heat in Urine bladder[714] syndrome. There will be blood in the urine (or in the stool).[715]

病人脉阴阳俱紧，反汗出者，亡阳也，此属少阴，法当咽痛，而复吐利。

The Pulse feels tight on both the Cun and Chi positions and the patient has unexpected sweating.[716] These conditions suggest that the

---

pathogenic Qi invades and hurts the Kidney Yang Qi in patients who have had Kidney Yang deficiency before becoming sick this time.

Note: In the Taiyin stage, the pain is in the arm and legs, and the hands and feet are warm. In the Shaoyin stage, the pain is in the whole body, and the hands, feet, or back, feel cold.

[712] Dr. Hu Xishu: The Zhuling Tang condition here should not belong to the Shaoyin at all. This herbal formula is used for an infection in the urine bladder (Fire in the urine bladder).

Dr. Liu Duzhou: This condition belongs to the Shaoyin stage. Due to depletion of body liquid via diarrhea in the patient who has had garbage water retention before becoming sick this time, the isolated Fire entangles with the garbage water to cause difficulty in urination. The water is pushed by the isolated Fire to the throat to cause dry throat and coughing, to the chest to cause an annoyed feeling and difficulty falling asleep, and to the stomach to cause nausea. Due to the garbage water, fresh water cannot come into the body for functional use, so the patient feels thirsty. The Zhengwu Tang condition is a Cold-water condition in the Shaoyin stage. The Zhuling Tang condition is a Hotness-water condition in the Shaoyin stage. A patient with Zhuling Tang condition usually has red color on the tongue with water-slippery tongue cover. The pulse feels thin and fast.

Dr. Hao Wanshan: This condition is Yin deficiency with Fire in the urine bladder. There are two things that cause this condition. First, in the Yangming stage, improper Purging therapy brings the Fire into the uine bladder and causes the Hotness-water to entangle in the urine bladder. Second, in the Shaoyin stage, the body is in Yin deficiency and Fire entangled with water in the urine bladder. The patient feels pain and a burning sensation in the urine duct, an urgent feeling for urination, and has frequent urination.

---

[713] If the patient feels hot in the body but cold in the hands and feet, be careful. This might be Yang-floating condition (the Yang Qi is refused by too much Yin Qi (cold) in the body). When the hands and feet are also warm, it suggests that the warmth is true warmth. It is the restoration of Yang Qi in the body, not a false warmth, not the last-warmth-before-death (similar to the sudden bright-light-before-death).

[714] The original text said that this is a Heat in the urine bladder. There are different opinions about this concept.

Dr. Hu Xishu: The heat in the whole body, hands, and feet is the turning of the Shaoyin to Yangming condition. The inner Heat disturbs the blood vessels to cause the bleeding. The Hotness is not inside the urine bladder. It is outside of the urine bladder, so it is *Hotness in the blood chamber syndrome*, not the *Hotness in urine bladder syndrome*. When the disease moves into the *Hotness in the blood chamber*, the disease has a chance to subside by itself.

Dr. Liu Duzhou: We cannot make a final decision for this debate yet. However, for the treatment of Hotness in the urine bladder, it is recommended to use Zhuling Tang.

[715] There is a hot debate about this paragraph. Is the Hotness is in the urine bladder or the blood chamber, and is the bleeding from the urine or the stool?

[716] That *the pulse feels tight in both the Cun and Chi position* suggests that this is a Taiyang Cold-attack condition, in which there should have no sweat. The sweat here suggests that the body is short of Yang Qi to seal the sweat. It is a deficient condition, not body surface Excess condition.

Dr. Hao Wanshan: This condition is a direct attack of Cold to the body, and the disease condition affects Shaoyin. The pulse should be deep-tight, while a Cold attack in the Taiyang stage is floating-tight. The Cold hurts the body Yang Qi, and the body Yang Qi cannot

body Yang has been devastated. This condition belongs to the Shaoyin stage. Such patients must have a sore throat first,[717] followed by vomiting and diarrhea.[718]

5.3 Differentiation in the Shaoyin stage

少阴病，饮食入口则吐，心中温温欲吐，复不能吐，始得之，手足寒，脉弦迟者，此胸中实，不可下也，当吐之，若膈上有寒饮，干呕者，不可吐也，当温之，宜四逆汤。

In the Shaoyin stage, a patient vomits whenever eating. After vomiting, there is still a desire to vomit, but nothing comes out. Such a situation happens for a short time, the hands and feet are cold,[719] and the pulse feels

string and slow. This condition belongs to Fullness condition (Cold-phlegm condition) in the chest.[720] Use Vomiting therapy for the treatment, not a Purging therapy. If the nausea is due to Cold water accumulation in the chest, the patient retches, Vomiting therapy should not be used. Use a Warming therapy, try the use of Si Ni Tang.

少阴病，吐利，手足逆冷，烦躁欲死者，吴茱萸汤主之。

In the Shaoyin stage, a patient vomits, has diarrhea, Jue syndrome,[721] and feels

---

seal and protect the body surface so that there is sweating. The sweat is not due to the Yang Qi floating or escaping.

[717] The Cold causes spasms in the throat so that patient feels pain in the throat.

[718] The Cold hurts the Kidney Yang Qi, which can no longer warm the Spleen-Stomach system and causes nausea and diarrhea.

Dr. Hao Wanshan: In the three Yin stages, if the disease belongs to organ deficiency, the treatment is difficult, and the outcome of the disease must be dangerous. If it is due to the pathogenic Qi overwhelming, the outcome of the disease may be promising. Here in the Shaoyin stage, if it is due to an attack of exogenous Cold, and not due to the inner Weakness of the Kidney or Heart, the outcome may be promising with proper treatment. In the previous Taiyin stage, if the disease is due to overwhelming of Dampness, the outcome is also promising with proper treatment for expelling the Dampness (or the disease can be healed naturally after a cluster of diarrhea).

Dr. Ni Haixia: This condition developed from the Taiyin stage. There was a liquid that accumulated in the middle part of the body (stomach) before the disease moved into the Shaoyin stage.

[719] Dr. Hao Wanshan: Due to the blockage of chest Yang Qi, the patient has nausea, cold hands and feet, similar to the Shaoyin stage. The cold hands and feet mean that this is Phlegm type of Jue syndrome. This is because the chest Yang Qi cannot expand to the hands and feet. The Phlegm is accumulated over the diaphragm. It should be expelled out of the body through vomit, not through Purging therapy. The Cold-water may be due to Kidney Yang deficiency,

Spleen Yang deficiency, or Stomach Yang deficiency. The treatments are different. For Kidney Yang deficiency, use Si Ni Tang; for Spleen Yang deficiency, use Lizhong Tang; and for Stomach Yang deficiency, use Wuzhuyu Tang.

[720] Dr. Hao Wanshan: Such patients also tend to have lots of salivae to spit, because body Yang Qi cannot evaporate water into warm vapor.

[721] Dr. Liu Duzhou: In the Shaoyin stage, there could be three kinds of Jue syndromes: Hotness Jue, Cold Jue (e.g., the Jue condition), and Yang-compressed Jue syndrome. Cold Jue is caused by inner Coldness, in which the body has insufficient Yang Qi to pass to the hands and feet. It is treated with Si Ni Tang, Fuzi Tang. The Hotness Jue syndrome is due to strong Hotness inside the body, which refuses and presses the Cold outwards to cause cold hands and feet. It occurs in the Yangming stage mostly, and also in the Shaoyin stage. It is treated with Baihu Tang, or Da Chengqi Tang. The third kind of Jue syndrome is Yang-compressed Jue syndrome. It means that the Yang Qi in the inner side of the body is compressed and cannot pass or expand to the hands and feet. It is treated with Si Ni San.

Dr. Hao Wanshan: The Wuzhuyu Tang condition included here in the Shaoyin stage is for distinguishment, because there is nausea, vomiting, cold hands and feet, and an annoyed feeling, all of which are similar to the Shaoyin stage. All of these symptoms in the Wuzhuyu Tang condition are caused by Cold accumulation in the stomach and Cold Qi up-rushing to cause more vomiting than diarrhea. The cold hands and feet are temporary, it happens when the vomiting is severe. It subsides after the vomiting is finished. The Cold in the stomach should belong to the Yangming Cold-attack condition. If the Cold vomit is due to Shaoyin Kidney Yang deficiency, then Si Ni Tang should be used.

extremely annoyed as wishes to die. [722] Use Wuzhuyu Tang as the primary treatment.[723]

少阴病，四逆，其人或咳，或悸，或小便不利，或腹中痛，或泄利下重者，四逆散主之。

In the Shaoyang stage, a patient has cold hands and feet (Heat-suffocated Jue syndrome). The patient may also have a cough, or palpitations, or difficulty urinating, or abdominal pain, or diarrhea with tenesmus sensation.[724] Use Si Ni Sang as the primary treatment,

少阴病得之二三日，口燥咽干者，急下之，宜大承气汤。

In the Shaoyin stage for two to three days, a patient feels dry in the mouth and throat. This case is an urgent condition. Use Da Chengqi Tang to save the patient's life (to save Kidney Water by reducing Heart Fire).[725]

少阴病，自利清水，色纯青，心下必痛，口干燥者，急下之，宜大承气汤。

---

[722] This condition is due to the accumulation of garbage water in the stomach. The water rushes up to cause vomiting and the extremely annoyed feeling. The annoyance is so great that the patient wants to die. There is also diarrhea, but mostly vomiting. Due to water in the stomach being blocked from going down to the urine, urination is difficult too.

Dr. Hao Wanshan: This condition can be seen in acute gastroenteritis.

[723] Dr. Liu Duzhou: In this condition, the vomiting and the annoyed feeling should be more severe than diarrhea. Therefore, Wuzhuyu Tang is used. If the cold hands and feet happen without the annoyed feeling, then Si Ni Tang should be used. If the cold hands and feet exist with diarrhea, and the pulse is hard to feel, use Tong Mai Si Ni Tang.

Dr. Du Yumao: This condition should not belong to the Shaoyin Coldness-transform condition. It is here for distinguishment.

[724] Dr. Hu Xishu: This condition is absolutely in the Shaoyang stage, though it is originally listed in the Shaoyin stage. The reason for the cold hands and feet is the stroke of the Yang Qi in the middle part of the body, which prevents body liquid from moving down to the hands and feet. However, such cold hands and feet are not common in the Si Ni San syndrome. The patient feels similar to the Da Chaihu Tang condition, with palpitations and tightness in the upper abdomen, and feels slightly annoyed, but has no nausea and no diarrhea.

Dr. Liu Duzhou: This condition belongs to the Shaoyin stage. It can be due to (1) the patient was given Cold medicine for the treatment of some diseases. The Cold compresses (freezes) the body inner Yang Qi. The Yang Qi cannot pass and expand to the hands and feet and causes the cold feeling; (2) extreme emotional stimulation, which also compresses the Yang Qi inside the body and causes the cold hands and feet.

Dr. Ni Haixia: Si Ni San syndrome belongs to the Shaoyin stage. It can be seen more often in gallbladder stones.

[725] Dr. Hu Xishu: This condition means that the patient initially was in the Shaoyin body surface stage for two to three days, then very quickly started to feel parched mouth and dry throat. This means the Shaoyin stage involves the Yangming inner stage. The body condition initially in the Shaoyin stage had a lack of body liquid. After the disease penetrates the Yangming stage, the Fire exhausts more body liquid, so that the body liquid will be very quickly depleted and causes a shock. The only method of treatment is to use Da Chengqi Tang to release the inner Fire in the Yangming stage, if the patient has no bowel movement. Or use Biahu Tang with Ginseng Tang if there is Fire but no firm stool in the bowel. (According to Dr. Hu Xishu, this is a Shayin-Yangming concurrent condition).

Dr. Liu Duzhou: In this case, there should be pain and bloating in the abdomen and no bowel movement, though these symptoms are not listed clearly in the original text.

Dr. Hao Wanshan: This paragraph and two other paragraphs involving the use of Da Chengqi Tang in the Shaoyin stage should be regarded as Yangming-Shaoyin successive condition. The initial Yangming inner condition develops into the Shaoyin stage too and causes depletion and exhaustion of the body Yin (liquid). To save the body liquid, use Da Chengqi Tang to remove the Fire in the bowel (Yingming stage). In olden times, it was not easy to supply body liquid quickly. Nowadays, it can be supplied easily with intravenous infusion.

This paragraph can also be understood as the Shaoyin stage changing into Yangming stage. The body Yang Qi recovers. The patient is going to get better. If the Yangming condition belongs to Cold-block condition, use Dahuang Fuzi Xixin Tang for the treatment.

124

In the Shaoyin stage, a patient has a water-like stool, the color of the stool can be blueish. The patient must also have pain in the upper stomach and have a dry mouth. This case is also an urgent condition. Use Da Chenqi Tang for urgent treatment. [726]

少阴病六七日，腹胀不大便者, 急下之，宜大承气汤。

If the Shaoyin stage for six to seven days, a patient has fullness and bloating in the abdomen, and does not have any bowel movement. This condition is urgent. Use Da Chenqi Tang for treatment.[727]

In the Shaoyin stage, patients may have a fever and an annoyed feeling (similar to inflammation in the body). Such conditions may be confused with Warm diseases.[728]

Warm diseases must be treated with Cold medicine, while Shanghan Shaoyin stages must be treated with Warm medicine. The differentiation of these two major types of diseases is very critical.

5.4 Notice of the Shaoyin stage

(1) The Shaoyin stage has the overall lowest level of metabolism. Patients feel less ambition to act, have no substantial interest in life, and feel drowsy and tired. Because of this, the pulse feels thin and faint.

(2) The Shaoyin stage is the worst phase of a disease, especially for chronic diseases. The body Yang Qi is exhausted, so the body inside becomes very cold, and there is an accumulation of water in the body.

If a patient has only Coldness but has no vomiting, no diarrhea, no constipation, no dry mouth or throat, and no sore throat, then Mahuang Fuzi Gancao Tang, or Mahuang Fuzi Xixin Tang will work well.

If there are chills and pain in the body, use Fuzi Tang.

If there is diarrhea, use Bai Tong Tang.

If there are vomiting and an annoyed feeling, use Wuzhuyu Tang.

If there is water retention syndrome, use Zhengwu Tang.

If there is diarrhea with poor sleep, use Zhuling Tang.

If there is no diarrhea, but difficulty falling asleep, use Huanglian Ajiao Tang.

If there is inside Coldness (as diarrhea), but outside Hotness (as a red face), and also cold hands and feet, use Tong Mai Si Ni Tang.

If there is a sore throat, use either Gancao Tang or Jiegen Tang. For a severe sore throat, use Ku Jiu Tang.

---

[726] Dr. Hu Xishu: This condition is not in the Shaoyin stage. It is a plague disease (an acute and very severe infectious disease characterized by acute diarrhea).

Dr. Liu Duzhou: In Yangming stage, the inner Fire has three ways to press body liquid out of the body: sweat, urine and water-like stool. Here it is the Yangming by-pass water-like bowel movement, similar to Shaoyin diarrhea so that these two stages need to be distinguished..

Dr. Martin Wang: This is a Yangming inner stage. The patient has abdominal pain, diarrhea with water-like stool and dry mouth, similar to Shaoyin diarrhea so that they need to be distinguished..

[727] Dr. Hu Xishu: This is a condition in which the Shaoyin stage develops into the Yangming stage. It is not pure Yangming stage. In a Yangming stage with such bloating in the abdomen and no bowel movement, Da Chengqi Tang is not used (it should be Xiao Chengqi Tang).

Dr. Martin Wang: This is a Shaoyin-Yangming concurrent condition. Because the background condition for the Shaoyin is insufficient body liquid, the Yangming inner stage has Fire that further exhausts the body liquid, so Da Chengqi Tang has to be used quickly to stop the Fire in the inner Yangming stage.

[728] Warm diseases: infectious diseases or epidemic diseases that are caused by an external invasion of pathogenic Qi. They are not the Shanghan diseases that are discussed in details in the book *Shanghan Lun.* For any "inflammation" diseases, pay attention to see if the background of the body constitution is the Shaoyin constitution.

Dr. Tan Jiezhong: The confusion of Warm diseases and Shanghan Shaoyin conditions are one of the major reasons why the current TCM clinic healing effects are not as sound as it was before, in ancient times. The rise of Fire-style (火神派) TCM in recent years is to correct this mistake.

If there is dryness in the mouth and throat, bloating in stomach, and no bowel movement, use Da Chengqi Tang.

(3) Annoyed feeling

The annoyed feeling needs to be differentiated with the Shaoyang stage. In the Shaoyang stage, the patient's pulse is not thin, not tiny. The patient does not look tired and doesn't tend to nap.

Here the thin-tiny pulse should be differentiated from deep-tight pulse. For the deep-tight pulse in the Shaoyang stage, the skin and muscles of the wrist, where we feel the pulse, feel tight. For the thin-tiny pulse in the Shaoyin stage, the skin and muscle of the wrist do not feel tight. The deep-tight pulse can usually be seen in those patients who have long-term stress and anxiety. The thin-tiny pulse can usually be seen in those of patients who are quiet, have no desire to act, or who do not even have the energy to get upset.

Patients in the Shaoyang stage tend to have muscle spasms (TMJ syndrome or tightness in the neck). Patients in the Shaoyin stage tend to have restless arms or legs (Huanglian Ajiao Tang condition), or shaking of the arms, hands or legs (Zheng Wu Tang condition).

(4) Sore throat or dry throat.

Dry throat occurs in Shaoyang, Yangming, Shaoyin stage, or in Warm disease. In the Shaoyang stage, the throat feels tight or as if there is a foreign mass in the throat. In the Wind-attack Yangming stage, there could be dryness and pain in the throat, which become worse with coughing.[729] If there is no coughing, the throat is not sore. A sore throat in the Shaoyin stage is continuous, regardless of coughing or not. It is usually an ulcer in the throat. In Warm disease, there would also be dryness and pain in the throat, but the pulse is floating-frequent. A patient with Warm disease likes cold environments and drinks but dislikes heat. Patients in the Shaoyin stage may prefer to drink cold water,

but drink only a little bit each time.[730] A patient in the Yangming stage or with the Warm disease also prefers to drink cold water but prefers to drink a large volume each time.

5.5 *Wrong treatment in the Shaoyin stage*

少阴病，咳而下利谵语者，被火气劫故也，小便必难，以强责少阴汗也。

In the Shaoyin stage, a patient has coughing, diarrhea, and delirious speech. This case is due to a Fire therapy used. The Fire exhausted more body Yin (Shaoyin sweat) so that urination will become difficult.[731]

少阴病，脉细沉数，病为在里，不可发汗。

In the Shaoyin stage, if the pulse is thin, deep, and fast, the disease is on the inner side of the body. Sweating therapy should not be used.[732]

---

[729] The discomfort in the throat in the Shaoyang is more a functional disorder, whereas the discomfort in the throat in the Yangming, the Shaoyin and in Warm diseases, is more of a physical disease.

[730] The dryness in the throat in the Shaoyin stage is mostly due to Yin deficiency, so the patient drinks a little bit of cold water. Those in the Yangming and the Warm disease are due to Fire, so the patient drinks lots of cold water each time.

[731] If the patient is in Shaoyin stage and has garbage water inside the body, the Fire from a Fire therapy (such as toasting the patient with fire, letting patient lie on a hot table or bed, or using Fire needle acupuncture, etc.), can stir the water and cause coughing and diarrhea. The Fire comes into the Stomach, causing delirious speech. The sweat caused by the Fire can enhance the depletion of body liquid so that urinating is difficult.

Dr. Tan Jiezhong: Frequent coughing occurring in the Shaoyin (during kidney failure, heart failure, pulmonary edema) can be treated with Zhenwu Tang. Many clinical conditions that occur after a wrong treatment of Shaoyin diseases cannot be treated simply by using the herbal formulas that are normally used for Taiyang diseases. Be careful that the Kidney function is in a damaged condition now.

[732] *Thin pulse* means weakness. *Fast pulse* means Fire. *Deep pulse* means the disease is on the inner side. The thin, fast and deep pulse means that the deficient Fire is on the inner side of the body. Typical Sweating therapy (such as the use of Mahuang Tang or Da Qinglong Tang) should not be used. More sweat will cause more depletion of body liquid in the Shaoyin stage.

少阴病，脉微，不可发汗，亡阳故也。阳已虚，尺脉弱涩者，复不可下之。

In the Shaoyin stage, if the pulse is faint (so weak that it might be difficult to detect), Sweat therapy should not be used. Such a remedy will cause Yang-devastating syndrome (亡阳). The body Yang is already in a deficient status, and if the pulse in the Chi position is weak and rough, then Purging therapy should not be used either.[733]

少阴病，但厥无汗，而强发之，必动其血，未知从何道出，或从口鼻，或从目出，是名下厥上竭，为难治。

In the Shaoyin stage, a patient has Jue syndrome and has no sweat. If a Sweating therapy were aggressively used to create heavy sweat, the blood in the body would be disturbed, and there will be bleeding from the mouth, or nose, or eyes. This condition is called lower-Jue-upper-exhausted syndrome,[734] and it is difficult to treat.[735]

Dr. Tan Jiezhong: The pulse is deep, thin and fast, suggesting that the circulation system is weak and in a compensatory status. Sweating therapy will expand the blood vessels in peripheral tissues and cause a reduction in blood pressure, resulting in shock.

[733] Dr. Ni Haixia: Before using Purging therapy, feel the pulse on the left side of the wrist. If it is weak, the Purging therapy should not be used. The left pulse (on male) represents the status of Blood in the body. Similarly, before using Sweating therapy, the pulse on the right wrist should be strong enough. The pulse on the right side (on male) represents the status of the Qi.

[734] *Patient in the Shaoyin stage has Jue syndrome* means that body blood is insufficient. In this case, heavy sweating will deplete more blood volume.

[735] *Difficult to treat*: To warm the Jue syndrome would stimulate more bleeding; to stop bleeding with Cold medicine would make the Jue syndrome worse.

Dr. Liu Duzhou: Such conditions can be seen in uremia (cold hands and feet with bleeding in the whole of the body, here and there).

Dr. Tan Jiezhong: Use Guizhi Qui Shaoyao Jia Longgu Muli Tang (救逆汤). Fire-style herbalists (火神派) may use herbal formulas containing dried ginger, Guizhi, and Fuzi. We should not use Yin herbs (e.g. the Cold herbs, such as large amounts of Shengdi, Huangbo or Huanglian).

5.6 Turnover of the Shaoyin stage

少阴病，脉紧，至七八日，自下利，脉暴微，手足反温。脉紧反去者，为欲解也。虽烦，下利必自愈。

In the Shaoyin stage, a patient has a tight pulse. After seven or eight days, the patient starts to have diarrhea and the pulse suddenly becomes faint, and the hands and feet comes however warm, the pulse feels not as much tight as before. These conditions suggest that the disease will get better. Though there is an annoyance, diarrhea will stop. [736]

少阴病，下利，若利自止，恶寒而蜷卧，手足温者，可治。

In the Shaoyin stage, a patient has diarrhea. If diarrhea stops, the patient feels an aversion to cold and lies down with body bent, the hands and feet are still warm, the disease condition can still be improved.[737]

少阴病，恶寒而蜷，时自烦，欲去衣被者可治。

In the Shaoyin stage, if a patient feels chilly and lies with a curved body, feels annoyed from time to time, and feels the willingness to remove the blanket from the body, then there is still a chance to save the life of the patient. [738]

少阴病，恶寒身蜷而利，手足逆冷者，不治。

In the Shaoyin stage, a patient feels an aversion to cold, lies down with the body

---

[736] The *disappearance of the tight pulse, warm hands and feet, and diarrhea*, all suggest that the body Yang Qi is restored, and the diarrhea is a way of expelling the pathogenic Qi. When a disease is on the inner side of the body, then diarrhea is one of the ways to remove the shrunken disease. The annoyed feeling and diarrhea here can also be regarded as a healing crisis (similar to the healing crisis in the Taiyin stage).

[737] *Diarrhea and bending the body* means that the body is very weak and cold. If the hands and feet are also very cold (Jue syndrome), the patient will die. However, if the hands and feet are warm, it means that the body Yang Qi remains, so a proper treatment may be still able to save the life of the patient.

[738] Here, the *annoyed feeling and the willingness to remove blankets on the body* can also be regarded as a healing crisis.

curved, has diarrhea and has Jue syndrome. Such a case is difficult to treat.

少阴病，吐利，躁烦，四逆者死。

In the Shaoyin stage, a patient has vomiting and diarrhea, feels annoyed and restless, and there is Jue syndrome. The patient will die.[739]

少阴病，四逆恶寒而身蜷，脉不至，不烦而躁者，死。

In the Shaoyin stage, a patient has Jue syndrome, feels an aversion to cold, bends the body when lying down, has cold hands and feet, the pulse is difficult to detect.[740] The patient does not feel annoyed but has restless arms and legs. Such a patient will die.[741]

少阴病，吐利，手足不逆冷，反发热者，不死。脉不至者，灸少阴七壮。

In the Shaoyin stage, a patient has diarrhea and vomiting, no cold hands and feet, has a fever, however.[742] In such a case, the patient will not die. If the pulse is difficult to detect, use moxibustion on the points along Shaoyin meridian for seven turns, (such as on the Taixi (KD3) point.)

少阴病，六七日，息高者，死。

In the Shaoyin stage for six to seven days, a patient has short and shallow breathing with a loud noise (has difficulty breathing). The patient will die.[743]

少阴中风，脉阳微阴浮者，为欲愈。

In Wind-attack Shaoyin stage, if the pulse feels faint in the Cun position, but floating in the Chi position, the patient is to get better.[744]

少阴病，下利止而头眩，时时自冒者死。

In the Shaoyin stage, diarrhea stops. The patient feels dizzy as drunk from time to time. Such a patient will die.[745]

少阴病，脉微细沉，但欲卧，汗出不烦，自欲吐，至五六日，自利，复烦躁，不得卧寐者，死。

In the Shaoyin stage, the pulse feels faint, thin and deep. The patient has a willingness to lie down, sweats, not annoyed, and is nauseous. On the fifth to sixth day, the patient has diarrhea, is again annoyed and has restless arms and legs, and feels difficult to fall asleep. Such a patient will die.[746]

少阴病八九日，一身手足尽热者，以热在膀胱，必便血也。

In the Shaoyin stage for eight to nine days, a patient's hands, feet, and body feel hot. This

---

[739] The Jue syndrome suggests that the body Yang Qi is exhausted.

[740] The *pulse is difficult to feel*: this means the disease involves the Jueyin stage. This is a Taiyin-Jueyin co-existing condition.

[741] The *restless arms and legs* indicate that the body liquid is exhausted, as indicated by the very weak pulse that is very difficult to feel.

   Dr. Ni Haixia: the original text should mean the dryness on lips, not restless arms and legs.

[742] Principally, in the Shaoyin stage, a patient should feel cold, no fever. Fever means that the body Yang Qi is restored.

[743] The *difficulty in breathing* indicates that the Yang Qi is escaping. Such difficulty breathing belongs to Jueyin condition, so this is a Taiyin-Jueyin co-existing condition.

   Dr. Ni Haixia: The lower part of the body (Lower Jiao) stops moving, so the inhaled air can only come in through the throat, not into the lung.

---

[744] Dr. Tan Jiezhong: Most doctors explain that the pulse here means that the pulse feels weak (mild) in the Cun position but floating in the Chi position. This might not be true in clinics. In the Shaoyin stage, the pulse in the Chi position usually is "floating" (because of Yang deficiency and the Yang tending to escape). Here it could be explained that the original deep, weak and thin pulse starts to float upon deeply pressing on the pulse.

[745] The *end of diarrhea* here is due to extreme exhaustion of body liquid. The body has nothing to change into the stool. The dizziness and drunk feeling here is the sign of escaping body Yang Qi, so the patient will die.

   Dr. Ni Haixia: The extreme diarrhea has resulted in exhaustion of blood. The brain lacks nourishment from the blood. The patient now feels as if in severe anemia or as if they have lost a heavy volume of blood.

[746] *Nauseous and diarrhea*: the Shaoyin stage also involves the Taiyin stage. There are restless arms and legs, and difficulty falling asleep because the body liquid is exhausted so that the patient will die.

   Basically in the Shaoyin stage, there should be no sweat. The sweat means that the body Yang Qi will escape.

situation means that there is Fire in the urine bladder. The patient will have bleeding in the stool. [747]

6. Jueyin stage

The Jueyin stage involves the Liver and Pericardium. In the body, the Liver meridian has an inner-surface relationship with the Gallbladder meridian (both belong to Jueyin meridian), and the Pericardium meridian has an inner-surface relationship with the Triple Jiao meridian (both belong to Shaoyang meridian). Therefore, Jueyin Liver diseases can also have similar disease locations as the Shaoyang disease. [748]

The essential nature of the Jueyin stage is also a Yin condition (e.g., lack of body blood and liquid; Coldness and Weakness), if the Jueyin stages developed from the Shaoyin stage. However, the syndrome of the Yang deficiency and Yin excess in the Yueyin stage can be worse than the syndrome in the Shaoyin and Taiyin stage.

In the Jueyin stage, the Yin aspect of the body is in its most extreme point; therefore there is a Yang development in the body too. [749] Due to the development of body Yang

Qi, diseases in this stage can have several different outcomes. First, the patient recovers (is cured). [750] This situation can happen when the Jueyin stage is caused by a direct attack of Cold and it has not developed from a disease in the Shaoyin stage. Second, the body is either in a Yang condition sometimes, but in a Yin condition at other times. Third, the Yin condition and the Yang condition co-existing in the body at the same time. [751]

The Yin condition requires Warm therapy (such as the use of Si Ni Tang), and the Yang condition requires Cold therapy for the treatment (such as the use of Baihu Tang). If the Yin condition and the Yang condition exist at the same time, then the Warm therapy and the Cold therapy are needed at the same time.

The Jueyin stage can develop from the Shaoyin stage, [752] Shaoyang stage, or from

---

[747] This is the turnover of the Shaoyin stage into the Taiyang urine bladder stage. The disease is improving from the Yin stage to the Yang stage because the Shaoyin and the Taiyang have a surface-inner relationship. The heat and bleeding can be regarded as a healing crisis.

Dr. Tan Jiezhong: The bleeding can occur in either urine or in the stool.

[748] There are lots of debates and discussions about how to understand the Jueyin stage.

Dr. Hu Xishu: The principal clinical manifestations of the Shaoyang and Jueyin are not easy to summarize because they are between the body Yang part and the Yin part. The clinical conditions are easily shared with other stages.

[749] This is a very critical concept in TCM. When the Yang goes to its strongest point, the Yang will turn to the Yin, and if the Yin goes to its strongest, the Yin will also change to the Yang. This is the Yin and Yang interrelationship. Here, the Yin is extremely strong in the Jueyin stage, and there will also be Yang starting

to develop. In the body, the disease can be Yin nature, or Yang nature, or both natures at the same time.

[750] Dr. Hao Wanshan: There is an example to explain this phenomenon. In stormy weather, the sky is full of heavy dark clouds (similar to the Yin condition in the body). Then there is big thunder (the Yang developed), followed by heavy rain (the Yin and Yang struggle), then the sky turns clear (cured). One of the functions of the Liver is to hold Minister Fire (相火) (the Heart is the Sovereign Fire, 君火). The thunder is like the exposure of the Minister Fire in the Liver, after the Minister Fire has been compressed too tightly for a while.

[751] In this case, if the developed Yang Qi located in the upper part of the body, the patient can have a sore throat, fever, and sweat. If it is in the lower part of the body, the patient will have bleeding and pus in the stool. If it is on the body surface, the patient may have abscesses under the skin.

Dr. Liao Houze: The pulse in the Jueyin stage can be big, string and tight. It can be seen more in elderly patients.

[752] Dr. Hao Wanshan: In the Shaoyin stage, the heart and kidney are already in a very weak condition. Upon passing into the Jueyin stage, the liver becomes weak too. Therefore, all of the important organs are Weakness and Coldness in the Jueyin stage. This is Organ Jue syndrome. The patient's life is in a very dangerous situation.

Dr. Du Yumao: The Jueyin stage comes more from the Taiyin stage, rarely from the Shaoyin stage.

Taiyang stage. It can also result from a direct attack of pathogenic Qi in the Jueyin stage.[753]

6.1 Four significant characteristics for the Jueyin stage

(1)   Co-existing Cold and Hot in the body

In the Jueyin stage, the body's Yin and Yang tend to be separated. The manifestation is that some part of the body has Hotness and another part has Coldness.[754]

厥阴之为病，消渴，气上撞心，心中疼热，饥而不欲食，食则吐蛔，下之利不止。

The Yueyin stage means that patients feel very thirsty,[755] feel as if hot air is rushing up to punch heart, feel pain and hot in the chest,[756] feel hungry but have no desire to eat.[757] When eat, there is vomit of roundworm. In the use of Purging therapy, there will be constant diarrhea.

- Patients feel dizzy, have poor sleep, sweat, have disorders in menstruation, have pain in the flank region, have a bloating feeling in the upper abdomen, and easily have loose bowel movements. Use Wumei Tang[758] for the treatment.

- Patients usually feel cold but have a hot sensation in the face or have lots of acne on the face, or the patients have a dry mouth and throat and like to drink cold water, but have cold hands and feet. Use Wumei Tang for the treatment.

- Patients feel hot in the upper part of the body, have chest pain and are short of breath, have a sore or dry throat, are coughing, and there is blood in the phlegm, have massive diarrhea, and have cold hands and feet. The pulse is deep and slow in the Cun position, but it cannot be felt in the Chi position. This condition is the Mahuang Shengma Tang condition. It can be understood as Liver Hotness but Spleen Coldness condition.

伤寒本自寒下，医复吐下之，寒格，更逆吐下；若食入口即吐，干姜黄连黄芩人参汤主之。

It is Taiyin –Jueyin – Shaoyin. Many diseases in the Jueyin stage can develop into the Shaoyin stage.

[753] If the Cold pathogenic Qi directly attacks the Jueyin inner organ (liver), the disease is not as dangerous as when it directly attacks the Shaoyin (heart and kidney). The treatment is relatively easier.

Dr. Zhuang Yan: The characteristic of the Jueyin disease is the insufficient reduction of the Metal Qi. The body Qi remains up-rising, but there is less falling-down. The Jueyin disease can easily occur in patients who have kidney essence deficiency. The symptoms are easily affected by weather changes. Jueyin diseases include Qi deficiency, micro-nutrition deficiency, and Weakness-Coldness conditions. It is the dislocation of Minister Fire in the body.

[754] The Hotness is true Hotness, and the Coldness is true Coldness in the Jueyin stage. In the Shaoyin stage, the Hotness is false Hotness, in which the Hotness could be floating Hotness. The floating Hotness is not true Hotness.

[755] The patient feels thirsty but has no difficulty urinating, so it is not Wu Ling San condition (i.e. not garbage water retention condition). The thirsty feeling is a sign of body Yang Qi recovery.

Dr. Liao Houze: For the thirst in the Jueyin stage, use Chaihu Guizhi Ganjiang Tang for the treatment. Do not use Nourishing herbs, such as Ginseng or Huangqi or Yin herbs such as Shengdi.

Dr. Xiao Xiangru: This paragraph is not the principle for the diagnosis of the Jueyin disease. The characteristic of Jueyin disease is the Jue syndrome.

[756] The chest cavity is weak and the abdomen cavity is cold. The Cold tends to rush up to the weakened chest to cause the up-rushing feeling.

[757] The *hungry feeling* is due to stomach Fire; the *no desire to eat* is due to spleen Coldness.

Dr. Liu Duzhou: The *hungry feeling but has no desire to eat* is due to the Coldness-Weakness of the Stomach and Spleen.

[758] Wumai Tang contains lots of Cold herbs and also many Hot herbs. The function of the herb Wumei is as an adhesive agent to combine the Yin and Yang together. To treat mixed Hotness-Coldness condition, the herbal formula usually contains both Hot and Cold herbs.

In the Shanghan disease, a patient feels weak and has Cold diarrhea initially, but the disease is treated with Purging therapy and Vomiting therapy again. This procedure results in a Cold-refusing syndrome in the stomach.[759] No Purging therapy or Vomiting therapy can be tolerated anymore. The patient vomits at once after eating.[760] As the primary treatment of such case, use Ganjiang Huangqin Huanglian Renshen Tang.[761]

In clinics, the manifestations of Coldness-Hotness mixing condition are largely variable.[762] The above conditions are just such of the examples.

(2)   Jue syndrome

凡厥者，阴阳气不相顺接，便为厥。厥者，手足逆冷是也。

The Jue syndrome means the body Yang Qi and the Yin Qi fail to connect each other, or cannot pass from Yang to Yin or from Yin to Yang.[763] It shows as a cold feeling on the hands and feet. The cold feeling can develop to as high as the elbow or knee.

Organ Jue syndrome

伤寒脉微而厥，至七八日肤冷，其人躁无暂安时，此为脏厥.

In the Shanghan disease, the pulse is faint, and the body has the Jue syndrome. Up to the seven to eight days, the skin feels cold. The patient feels restless without any cessation. Such a condition is called Organ Jue syndrome.[764]

Meridian Jue syndrome

Meridian Jue syndrome means that the Jue syndrome is a body surface condition in the Jueyin stage. There is still a chance to improve the Jue syndrome to make it move into the Shaoyang stage so that the disease can be cured.

伤寒脉促，手足厥逆者，可灸之。

With a Shanghan disease, if the pulse feels floating in the Cun position but weak and deep in the Chi position, and the patient has Jue syndrome, moxibustion can be used for treatment.[765]

手足厥寒，脉细欲绝者，当归 四逆汤主之。若其人内有久寒者，宜 当归 四逆加 吴茱萸生姜 汤主之。

---

[759] Cold-refusing condition (寒格): with a blockage in the stomach, the upper warmth cannot be conducted to the lower cold in the body, so this is an upper-Hotness and lower-Coldness condition.

[760] *Vomits after eat* suggests Fire in the stomach. If the vomiting occurs a long time after eating, it could be due to Coldness in the stomach.

[761] Dr. Du Yumao: This paragraph should be understood as the patient initially having Coldness in the lower part of the digestive system. The Coldness pushes the Yang Qi (hotness) up to cause vomiting. The doctor misunderstood this condition and used Vomiting therapy and Purging therapy. The treatments caused the Cold-blockage condition in the middle part of the body, so the patient cannot eat, and the food cannot come into the stomach at all.

[762] The Hotness-Coldness condition can be easier to see in many auto-immune disorders, such as lupus and type I diabetes.

[763] Dr. Tan Jiezhong: For Jue syndrome in the Shaoyin stage, the cold feeling in the hands or feet is evenly distributed in both hands or feet and from fingertips to the wrist (or from tips of the toes to the ankle). In the Jue condition in the Jueyin stage, however, the tips of the fingers or toes are much colder than in the wrists or ankles.

[764] Organ Jue syndrome means that there are diseases inside the body. The disease affects the function of solid organs, such as liver, spleen or kidney. The patient feels bloating in the upper abdomen, wants to vomit after eating or is nauseous, spits saliva, and has headaches, in addition to the Jue syndrome. In this case, use Wuzhuyu Tang for the treatment. If the Organ Jue syndrome includes constant restlessness in the arms and legs, then use Wumei Wan for the treatment. If the Organ Jue syndrome occurs with massive thirst, use Fuling Gancao Tang.

[765] Dr. Hu Xishu: The floating pulse in the Cun position suggests body surface condition, but the patient has Jue syndrome too, which suggests inner Weakness and Coldness condition. Therefore, the treatment should focus on warming the inner part of the body. Use Si Ni Tang.

Dr. Liu Duzhou: The original text for the pulse may be understood as a fast pulse. Because there is Jue syndrome, the fast pulse suggests Yang deficiency inside the body, so moxibustion therapy should be used.

If a patient has Jue syndrome and the pulse is very thin and faint (nearly cannot feel the pulse), use Danggui Si Ni Tang as the primary treatment. If, in this case, the patient often has Coldness condition inside the body (such as diarrhea when drinking or eating cold things), then use Danggui Si Ni Jia Wu Sheng Tang.

(3)　　　Alternating Fever-Jue condition

In the Jueyin stage, patients may feel hot some days and cold on other days (Jue syndrome). The clinical meaning is different for the number of days and the sequence of the hot and cold feelings.

伤寒先厥，后发热而利者，必自止。见厥复利。

With a Shanghan disease, if a patient has Jue syndrome first, then feel warm and have diarrhea, diarrhea will stop naturally. If the Jue syndrome occurs again, diarrhea will occur again too. [766]

伤寒始发热，六日，厥反九日而利。凡厥利者，当不能食，今反能食者，恐为除中，食以索饼，不发热者，知胃气尚在，必愈，恐暴热来出而复去也。后三日脉之，其热续在者，期之旦日夜半愈。所以然者，本发热六日，厥反九日，复发热三日，并前六日，亦为九日，与厥相应，故期之旦日夜半愈。后三日脉之而脉数，其热不罢者，此为热气有余，必发痈脓也。

With a Shanghan disease, a patient has had a fever for six days, then has Jue syndrome with diarrhea for nine days. During the Jue syndrome, the patient should not be able to eat. If indeed the patient can eat during the Jue period, be careful that this is a Middle-depletion condition (除中). [767] If the patient wants to eat and then has no fever, the disease will get improved. If the fever comes back again quickly, the condition might become worse soon (the Middle-depletion condition). After the Jue syndrome, if there is fever for an additional three days, and if the fever remains, the patient will get better in the middle of the night, because the total days of the fever is nine days (the first six days plus the later three days), which is equal to the days of the Jue syndrome (nine days). If the later fever lasts for more than three days and the pulse feels fast, it means that the body Hotness is too much and there will be abscesses in the body. [768]

伤寒先厥后发热，下利必自止，而反汗出，咽中痛者，其喉为痹。发热无汗而利必自止，若不止，必便脓血。便脓血者，其喉不痹。

With a Shanghan disease, if the Jue syndrome is followed by fever (without a sweat), diarrhea during the Jue period will stop naturally. [769] Then if the patient starts sweating and develops sores (ulcers) in the throat, [770] the throat will have long-term pain (Throat Bi syndrome). If the fever is not followed by sweat, diarrhea will stop. If diarrhea does not stop, there will be blood

---

[766] This is the alternating Jue-diarrhea and Hotness condition in the Jueyin disease, similar to alternating Hotness-Coldness in Shaoyang disease.
With Jue syndrome, the inner body is weak so there could be diarrhea. When the Yang Qi in the body is restored, the body feels hot, and diarrhea will stop. Traditional, if the inner body becomes weak again, the Jue and diarrhea will occur again.

[767] Middle-depletion condition: the exhaustion of Stomach Qi. Without Stomach Qi, the patient will die. This is also a kind of *bright-light-before-death*. It means that the patient has a desire to eat before

---

death. It is translated as a *sudden spurt of appetite before the collapse* in some books.

[768] Dr. Hao Wanshan: A long time of being hot and abscess in the body means that Yang Qi has been restored too much. The body abscess can be treated with Zhen Ren Huo Ming Yin (真人活命饮). Currently, in the clinic, it is difficult to see such diseases, which can occur as alternating Hotness and Coldness for several days in turn. This might be a disease in olden times.

[769] Dr. Hao Wanshan: The initial diarrhea is Cold diarrhea. With the restoration of the body Yang Qi, Cold diarrhea will stop. Sweat and sore throat indicate the over the restoration of body Yang Qi.

[770] The *fever with sweat and the sore throat* suggest that the Yang Qi was restored too much. The Fire (the Yang Qi) hurts the throat, causing ulcers in the throat or in the colon and causing pus and bleeding in stool. If the Fire moves down to the colon (it finds the outlet in the colon), it will not go up to hurt the throat.

Dr. Hao Wanshan: A sore throat can be treated with Gancao Tang or Jiegen Tang.

and pus in the stool. [771] If there are such blood and pus in the stool, there will not be any a long-term sore throat.

伤寒一二日，至四五日而厥者，必发热，前热者，后必厥，厥深者，热亦深，厥微者，热亦微，厥应下之，而反发汗者，必口伤烂赤。

With a Shanghan disease for one to two days, there is a Jue syndrome on the fourth or fifth day. In such a case, there will be heat/fever in the body. If the fever occurs first, the Jue syndrome will follow. The stronger the Jue condition is, the higher the Fire is. If the Jue syndrome is mild, the fever is also mild. For Hot Jue syndrome, Purging therapy should be used. [772] If a Sweating therapy is used, however, the treatment will cause severe ulcers in the mouth. Such a case is the Hotness type of Jue syndrome.

伤寒发热四日，厥反三日，复热四日，厥少热多，其病当愈。四日至七日，热不除者，其后必便脓血。

With a Shanghan disease, a patient has had a fever for four days, then had Jue syndrome for three days, and has a fever again for four days. This case means that the Jue is less than fever and that the disease will recover, (because the number of days of the fever is more than that of the Jue.) If the fever lasts for up to seven days, the patient will have pus and blood in the stool. [773]

伤寒厥四日，热反三日，复厥五日，其病为进，寒多热少，阳气退，故为进也。

With a Shanghan disease, if the Jue syndrome lasted for the first four days, the fever lasted for the following three days, then the Jue syndrome lasts again for five days. A condition as such suggests the worse of the disease. The Coldness is more than the fever; the body Yang Qi is reducing, so the disease condition becomes worse.

6.2 Treatment of Hot-cold co-existing condition

The Hotness and Coldness in the Jueyin disease is true Hotness and true Coldness. Depending on whether the patient is in the fever period or the Jue syndrome period, the treatment is different.

伤寒六七日，大下后，寸脉沉而迟，手足厥逆，下部脉不至，咽喉不利，唾脓血，泄利不止者，为难治。麻黄升麻 汤主之。

In a Shanghan disease for six to seven days, a Purging therapy was used, the pulse is deep and slow in the Cun position, there is a Jue syndrome, the pulse on the Chi position is difficult to detect, there is discomfort feeling in throat, the patient spits pus-blood, has constant diarrhea. Such a case is difficult to treat. Try Mahuang Shengma Tang. [774]

热利下重者，白头翁 汤主之。下利，欲饮水者，以有热故也，白头翁 汤主之。

With hotness diarrhea, if a patient has tenesmus sensation, use Baitouwen Tang as the primary treatment. If the patient has diarrhea and also desires to drink water, the situation indicates Heatness inside the body. Use this formula as the primary treatment too. [775]

---

[771] Dr. Hao Wanshan: The pus and bleeding in the stool are also the over restoration of body Yang Qi. It can be treated with Baitouwen Tang.

[772] This is Hotness type of Jue syndrome, not Coldness type Jue syndrome.

[773] The pus and blood in stool are due to over restoration of body Yang Qi.

[774] Dr. Hu Xishu: This condition should not be treated with this formula. There is no body surface condition, and the body is very weak and the body is seriously lacking body liquid now. Mahuang is the main ingredient of this formula, and the formula creates sweat. Sweat must absolutely not be created in this very weak condition.

[775] Dr. Hu Xishu: With hot diarrhea, there is usually also stool retention feeling. If there is blood in the stool, add herb Ajiao to the formula.

Dr. Liu Duzhou: In the Jueyin stage, diarrhea can be both Coldness diarrhea and Hotness diarrhea. This one is Hotness diarrhea. Coldness diarrhea tends to be slippery diarrhea; the Hotness diarrhea tends to have tenesmus feeling inside the anus.

Dr. Hao Wanshan: For Hotness diarrhea, there must be tenesmus, blood-pus in the stool, pain in the abdomen and thirst. The thirst is stronger than that in the Shaoyin stage, and the patient tends to drink cold water too. Such diarrhea can be seen in acute bacterial dysentery, acute and chronic amoebic dysentery or ulcerative colitis.

下利，谵语者，有燥屎也，宜小承气汤。

After diarrhea, a delirious speech[776] indicates dry stool inside the intestine. Use Xiao Chengqi Tang for treatment.

下利后更烦，按之心下濡者，为虚烦也，宜 栀子 豉汤。

After diarrhea, more annoyed feeling and soft in the upper abdomen when pressed indicates a deficient type of annoyance.[777] Use Zhizi Chi Tang for treatment.

下利，腹胀满，身体疼痛者，先温其里，乃攻其表。温里四逆汤，攻表 桂枝 汤。

After diarrhea, when there is bloating feeling in the abdomen and generalized pain in the body, use Si Ni Tang to warm up the inside of the body first, then use Guizhi Tang to cure the body surface condition later.[778]

呕而脉弱，小便复利，身有微热见厥者难治。四逆汤主之。

A patient is nauseous. The pulse is weak. Urinating becomes natural. The body is mildly hot and has Jue syndrome. Such a case is difficult to treat. Try Si Ni Tang as the primary treatment.[779]

下利清谷，里寒外热，汗出而厥者，通脉四逆汤主之。

A patient has diarrhea with undigested food in the stool. The body is Coldness on inside but Hotness outside. The patient sweats but also has Jue syndrome. Use Tong Mai Si Ni Tang as the primary treatment.[780]

下利，脉沉而迟，其人面少赤，身有微热，下利清谷者，必郁冒，汗出而解，病人必微厥。所以然者，其面戴阳，下虚故也。

A patient has diarrhea. The pulse feels deep-slow. The face looks slightly red, and the body has a slight fever. There is undigested food in the stool. In such a case, the patient will feel drunk.[781] The patient will get better after sweating. The patient will also have mild Jue syndrome. The reason is that there is a Yang-upcast syndrome, due to Weakness in the lower part of the body.

干呕，吐涎沫，头痛者，吴茱萸 汤主之。

If a patient is nauseous, spits saliva,[782] and has a headache, use Wuzhuyu Tang as the primary treatment.[783]

呕而发热者，小 柴胡 汤主之。

If a patient is nauseous and has a fever, use Xiao Chaihu Tang as the primary treatment.[784]

---

[776] Diarrhea is usually not accompanied by delirious speech. The delirious speech is a sign of the presence of firm-stool in the bowel. In such cases, if the hot feeling is strong, use Tiaowei Chengqi Tang.

Dr. Hao Wanshan: Inner Fire presses body liquid out of the body through the colon (similar to pressing liquid out of the body as sweat or urine).

[777] *Deficient annoyed* means there is no solid mass in the body to cause the annoyed feeling. This annoyed feeling is not due to excessive Fire inside the body.

[778] Such disease conditions should be listed as the Taiyin stage. This is Taiyang-Taiyin concurrent condition.

[779] In this case, the Stomach Yang Qi is very weak, so the patient feels nauseous, and the pulse feels weak. The frequent urination and the Jue syndrome are due to Weakness of the Stomach. The mild fever is a sign of the body Yang Qi trying to escape.

[780] The pulse, in this case, must be very weak, deep and even difficult to feel. The sweat is a sign of the body Yang Qi trying to escape. (Patient is near death.)

[781] The alcohol-drunken feeling suggests that body Yang Qi is restored. With sweat, the pathogenic Qi leaves the body from the body surface (Yang-upcast condition).

[782] Dr. Hao Wanshan: When a person is stressed, the person tends to feel dry mouth and tends to drink water, though the person may not admit that he or she is stressed. Here the excess amount of saliva is due to the Cold water that cannot be evaporated by Body Yang Qi. It is not due to the relaxation of the patient. Such a headache tends to locate on the top of the head and become severe in the middle night.

[783] *Spits saliva or has more water in the mouth*, are signs of cold garbage water in the stomach. The up-rushing of the garbage water causes headaches or dizziness. Such patients usually also have a hardness feeling in the stomach.

[784] This condition is the opposite of the above Wuzhuyu Tang condition. Here it is Hotness in the gallbladder.

Dr. Hao Wanshan: This paragraph is usually interpreted as the Jueyin disease moving into the Shaoyang stage to get better, similar to when Shaoyin

134

伤寒大吐大下之，极虚，复极汗出者，以其人外气怫郁，复与之水，以发其汗，因得哕。所以然者，胃中寒冷故也。

With a Shanghan disease, a strong Vomiting therapy, or a strong Purging therapy was used. The patient is very weak in body condition but has profuse sweating.[785] This situation is because the body Yang Qi is floating on the body surface, the patient was given water (to drink or to have a shower) with the aim to create sweat, but the patient starts to have a hiccup.[786] The hiccup is because the stomach is in a Coldness-Weakness condition.

伤寒，哕而腹满，视其前后，知何部不利，利之则愈。

With a Shanghan disease, if a patient has hiccups and a bloated feeling in the abdomen, check the urine and the stool to find the reason for the hiccups and give treatment accordingly.[787]

6.3 Various Jue syndromes that need differentiation

(1) Organ Jue syndrome (see page 131)

(2) Meridian Jue syndrome (see page 131)

(3) Hot Jue syndrome (see page 133)

(4) Heat-suffocated Jue syndrome (see page 124)

(5) Roundworm Jue syndrome

蛔厥者其人当吐蛔。今病者静，而复时烦，此为藏寒。蛔上入膈，故烦，须臾复止，得食而呕，又烦者，蛔闻食臭出，其人当自吐蛔。蛔厥者，乌梅丸主之。又主久利方。

A Jue syndrome can be due to roundworm inside. If the patient appears or behaves quiet, only feels annoyance from time to time, it is Organ Jue syndrome. For roundworm Jue syndrome, the uprising of the worm into the chest results in annoyance. The annoyance can stop within a short time. Upon eating, the patient feels nausea and also an annoyance. This situation is because the roundworm starts to move after it smells the odor of food. The patient would vomit the roundworm. For the roundworm Jue syndrome, use Wumei Wan as the primary treatment.[788]

(6) Phlegm Jue syndrome

病人手足厥冷，脉乍紧者，邪结在胸中。心中满而烦，饥不能食者，病在胸中，当须吐之，宜瓜蒂散。

A patient feels cold hands and feet. The pulse feels tight from time to time. This situation is due to an accumulation of pathogenic Qi inside the chest. The patient feels bloating in the upper abdomen, feels irritated, and feels hungry but cannot eat. The disease is in the chest. Use Vomiting therapy for treatment. Use Guadi San.[789]

(7) Water Jue syndrome

伤寒厥而心下悸者，宜先治水，当服茯苓甘草汤，却治其厥；不尔，水渍入胃，必作利也。

---

[785] disease move into the Taiyang stage (to urine bladder), and Taiyin disease moves into the Yangming stage.

[785] The sweat was created by giving lots of hot water to the patient to drink or allowing the patient to have a hot water bath.

[786] Dr. Hao Wanshan: For the treatment, use Wuzhuyu Tang. If the hiccups are caused by Phlegm in the stomach, use Xuanfuhua Daizheshi Tang.

[787] Dr. Hao Wanshan: If a patient has hiccups and bloating feeling in the abdomen, check urination and bowel movement. If the urination is difficult, with apparent Coldness condition in the body, use Zhenwu Tang. With apparent Hotness condition, use Zhuling Tang. If the signs for Hotness or Coldness are not clear, use Wu Ling San for the treatment. If the patient has no bowel movement, it is Hotness-fullness condition of the Yangming disease. Use Xiao Chengqi Tang for the treatment. If the patient has the hiccups, bloating in the stomach and has repeated speech (not delirious speech), it is a Weakness condition.

---

[788] For the roundworm Jue syndrome, the patient feels much pain in stomach, then has the Jue syndrome. After stop of stomach pain (the roundworm does not disturb the inside), the Jue feeling stops too. Inbetween the onset of the Jue syndrome, the patient has no discomfort.

[789] This is a Cold-entanglement condition in the chest. Such a condition is due to accumulation of Phlegm in the chest, which prevents body Yang Qi spread to the hands and feet.

In Shanghan disease, if a patient has Jue syndrome, feels palpitations in the upper stomach, the accumulated water should be treated first. Use Fuling Gancao Tang. The Jue syndrome is to be treated later. Otherwise, the retained water would move to the stomach to cause diarrhea. [790]

(8) Cold-entanglement in Lower Jiao

病者手足厥冷，言我不结胸，小腹满，按之痛者，此冷结在膀胱 关元 也。

A patient has Jue syndrome, has no discomfort feeling in the upper abdomen (The patient does not feel fullness and hardness in the upper abdomen, e.g., no evidence for Chest-bind syndrome), but feels bloating and pain in the lower abdomen upon being pressed. This condition is called Cold-entanglement condition in the lower abdomen (not inside urine bladder).

(Use moxibustion on the Guanyuan (CV4) point (in the middle of the lower stomach), or use Zhenwu Tang for the treatment. [791])

(9) Cold Jue syndrome

大汗出，热不去，内拘急，四肢疼，又下利厥逆而恶寒者，四逆汤主之。

A patient has profuse sweating, but fever continues, [792] feels muscle spasms inside the body and pain in the arms and legs, has diarrhea, has Jue syndrome and feels an aversion to cold. [793] For such case, use Si Ni Tang as the primary treatment.

大汗，若大下利而厥冷者，四逆汤主之。

A patient has profuse sweating. If the patient also has massive diarrhea and Jue syndrome, [794] use Si Ni Tang as the primary the treatment.

6.4 Turnover of Jueyin stage

厥阴中风，脉微浮，为欲愈；不浮，为未愈。

In Wind-attack Jueyin stage, [795] if the pulse feels slight floating, [796] the patient will get better. If it is not floating, then the patient is not ready to get better.

厥阴病，渴欲饮水者，少少与之，愈。

In the Jueyin stage, if a patient starts to desire to drink water, let the patient drink water little bit by little bit. Such a condition suggests that the disease is to get cured.

下利，脉数，有微热汗出，今自愈。设复紧，为未解。

If there is diarrhea, the pulse feels fast, and the patient has mild fever and sweats, allow the body to get better naturally. If the pulse turns as tight again, the disease has not cured yet. [797]

下利，有微热而渴，脉弱者，今自愈。

---

[790] In this case, the Jue syndrome is caused by water accumulation in the chest, which prevents body Yang Qi spread to the hands and feet. The tongue coating is water-like and slippery, and the pulse is slippery and strong.

[791] Dr. Hu Xishu: Use Da Wutou Jian, Da Jianzhong Tang, or Fuzi Genmi Tang (depending on further diagnosis).

Dr. Liu Duzhou and Dr. Hao Wanshan: Use Danggui Si Ni Tang or Danggui Si Ni Tang with Wuzhuyu and Shengjiang for the treatment. This disease condition can be regarded as Cold entanglement in the Liver meridian.

[792] For Baihu Tang condition (Yangming surface condition), the fever will fall after a heavy sweat.

[793] Dr. Hao Wanshan: This is Shaoyin Cold Jue syndrome. *Heavy sweat* indicates kidney Yang

deficiency and the Yang Qi cannot seal and protect the body surface. *Fever* indicates overwhelming Yin that causes the Yang Qi to float.

[794] This is also Cold Jue syndrome.

[795] Jueyin Wind-attack condition: the patient usually has a Guizhi body constitution (weak and easy to sweat).

Dr. Du Yumao: There is no introduction to the symptoms of the Jueyin Wind-attack condition. It should be a fever, mild sweating, and cold hands and feet. For the treatment, use Guizhi Tang with Chaihu and Zhishi

[796] *Float pulse* suggests that the disease is changing from the inner side to the body surface, so the patient is getting better.

[797] The mild fever, sweat, and fast pulse (tight pulse changes to the faster pulse) suggest that the body Yang Qi is restored. Yang breaks the Yin to allow the body Yang Qi to move to the body surface. This sweat is warm sweat, not cold sweat.

If a patient has a mild fever and feels thirsty, and the pulse feels weak, allow the body to recover naturally.[798]

下利，脉数而渴者，今自愈；设不差，必清脓血，以有热故也。

If the pulse is fast, and the patient feels thirsty, allow the disease to recover naturally. If not, there will be pus and blood in the stool. The reason is that there is Hotness inside the body.[799]

下利，手足厥冷无脉者，灸之不温，若脉不还，反微喘者，死。少阴负趺阳者，为顺也。

A patient has diarrhea, has the Jue syndrome, and the pulse cannot be felt. If moxibustion therapy has been used without any improvement, the pulse can still not detected, and the patient even has mild panting,[800] then the patient will die. If the pulse on the back of the foot (Yangming Stomach pulse) is stronger than the pulse on the gut position (Shaoyin Kidney pulse), the patient will not die.[801]

下利后脉绝，手足厥冷，晬时脉还，手足温者生，脉不还者死。

After diarrhea, the pulse cannot be felt; there is Jue syndrome. If the pulse can be felt again within twenty-four hours, the hands and feet become warm,[802] the patient will live. If the pulse cannot be felt within the twenty-four hours, the patient will die.

伤寒病，厥五日，热亦五日，设六日当复厥，不厥者，自愈。厥终不过五日，以热五日，故知自愈。

With a Shanghan disease, there is Jue syndrome for five days, then has a fever for another five days. If on the eleventh day, the patient does not feel the Jue syndrome, this case means that the disease will recover.[803] The reason is that the Jue syndrome lasted less than five days, and the fever is also five days. Therefore, it is known that the disease will get cured.

伤寒六七日，脉微，手足厥冷，烦躁，灸厥阴，厥不还者，死。

In Shanghan disease for six to seven days, the pulse feels faint, the patient has a Jue syndrome, feels annoyed and has restless arms and legs. Treat this condition with moxibustion.[804] If the Jue syndrome is not improved, the patient will die.[805]

伤寒发热，下利，厥逆，躁不得卧者，死。

With a Shanghan disease, if a patient has fever, diarrhea, Jue syndrome, and has restless arms and legs, the patient will die.[806]

伤寒发热，下利至甚，厥不止者，死。

With a Shanghan disease, if a patient has a fever and very massive diarrhea, and has constant Jue syndrome, the patient will die.

伤寒下利，日十余行，脉反实者死。

With a Shanghan disease, if a patient has diarrhea, which occurs more than ten times a

---

[798] The mild fever and the thirst in the Jueyin stage suggest the restoration of body Yang Qi.

    Dr. Hao Wanshan: This condition could be an attack of Cold in the Jueyin stage. The initial pulse felt tight and now it becomes mild (soft). Diarrhea can be understood as the expelling of Cold through bowel movement, so it is a self-healing process.

[799] The *pus and blood in the stool*: the over the restoration of body Yang Qi.

[800] The shortness of breath here means that the Kidney Qi is very weak and the Lung Qi will escape. The patient will die.

[801] The reason for this is that the patient still has Stomach Qi (the pulse on the back of feet is stronger).

[802] The *hands and feet feel warm*: there is still Yang Qi in the body to restore.

---

[803] On the eleventh day, if the cold hands and feet do not happen again it means that the body Yang Qi is dominated, so the body will get better after that.

[804] Do moxibustion on Taichong (LV3) points.

[805] Dr. Hu Xishu: This is the early stage of Organ Jue syndrome. On the seventh or eighth day, the skin will also feel cold, the patient feels annoyed and has restless arms and legs.

[806] When Jue syndrome is accompanied by diarrhea, it means that the Stomach Qi is exhausted. Once the restless arms and legs occur, the patient will die. The restless arms and legs are almost a bright-light-before-death. The fever means there is body surface condition. With both body surface condition and inner Taiyin and Jueyin conditions, treat the inner Taiyin and Jueyin condition urgently. Use Si Ni Tang.

day, and if the pulse felt however strong,[807] the patient will die.

伤寒六七日，不利，便发热而利，其人汗出不止者，死。有阴无阳故也。

With a Shanghan disease for six to seven days without diarrhea, and now the patient has a fever and diarrhea and constantly sweats, the patient will die.[808] The reason is that the pathogenic Qi won and the body has Yin but no Yang.

下利，脉沉弦者，下重也；脉大者，为未止；脉微弱数者，为欲自止，虽发热不死。

With diarrhea, if the pulse feels deep-string, the pulse suggests a tenesmus sensation. If the pulse feels big, the big pulse means that diarrhea does not stop yet. If the pulse feels slightly weak and fast, such a pulse means that diarrhea is to stop naturally and the patient will not die even if there is a fever.

发热而厥，七日，下利者，为难治。

If a Jue syndrome accompanies a fever for seven days, and if there is diarrhea,[809] this case is difficult to treat.

呕家有痈脓者，不可治，呕脓尽自愈。

---

[807] In such severe diarrhea, the pulse should be very weak. A strong pulse suggests the clinic manifestations and the pulse are unmatched. This is a bright-light-before-death phenomenon. Such unexpected pulse belongs to True-organ pulse (In normal conditions such pulse cannot be felt. It shows before death.).

[808] Dr. Hu Xishu: After six to seven day of the Shanghan disease, the body starts to have a fever, heavy sweating, and diarrhea. This means that the body defense energy is failing to struggle against the pathogenic Qi. The diarrhea and sweat cause the exhaustion of body liquid, so the patient will die. The body cannot hold the stool and sweat.

Dr. Liu Duzhou: The diarrhea indicates inner Coldness and the fever and the sweat are the escaping of the body Yang Qi. The sweat in the three Yin stages is a very dangerous sign of impending death.

[809] With fever and Jue syndrome, the Jue would be Hot Jue syndrome in the Yangming body surface condition. The *diarrhea on the seventh day* suggests that the disease has developed into the Taiyin stage. The disease becomes worse.

If a patient has a history of nausea and has a purulent disease in the body, do not give treatment. The disease will get better naturally after the pus is spat out entirely.[810]

6.5 *Wrong treatment in Jueyin stage*

诸四逆厥者，不可下之，虚家亦然。

With any Jue syndromes, Purging therapy should not be used. It should not be used with any weak or insufficient body condition either.[811]

伤寒脉迟，六七日，而反与 黄芩 汤彻其热。脉迟为寒，今与 黄芩 汤，复除其热，腹中应冷，当不能食；今反能食，此名除中，必死。

With a Shanghan disease and with a slow pulse for six to seven days, a patient, however, was given Huangqin Tang for the treatment (for diarrhea) to clear the Fire. The slow pulse indicates Coldness condition inside the body. The Huangqin Tang depletes Fire, so the treatment makes the body inside Colder and patient cannot eat. If the patient can indeed eat, it is Middle-depletion condition (除中), and the patient will die.

伤寒五六日，不结胸，腹濡，脉虚，复厥者，不可下，此为亡血，下之死。

With a Shanghan disease for five to six days, there is no Chest-bind condition, the abdomen is soft when pressed, the pulse feels weak, and the patient has Jue syndrome. In this case, Purging therapy should not be used. This condition suggests that the body lacks blood (Blood-exhausted), the Purging therapy

---

[810] Dr. Liu Duzhou: This case does not belong to the Jueyin stage. This is a case in which the patient has abscess inside the stomach, so the patient spits pus.

Dr. Hao Wanshan: For patients with an abscess in the stomach, the pus spitting is one of the ways by which the body expels pathogenic Qi. Therefore the vomiting should not be inhibited by aggressive treatment. This is similar to the annoyance and sudden, frequent diarrhea in the Shaoyin or Taiyin stages (a self-healing process).

[811] Dr. Liu Duzhou: If the Jue syndrome is due to a weakness condition, then Purging therapy should not be used. If it is a Hot-Jue syndrome, then Purging therapy can still be used.

(which depletes more body liquid) can cause death.[812]

下利清谷，不可攻表，汗出，必胀满。

If there is diarrhea with undigested food in the stool, Sweating therapy should not be used. Otherwise, after sweating, the patient will have bloating and fullness feeling in the abdomen.

---

[812] Dr. Hu Xishu: In such weak and Jue condition, Sweating therapy cannot be used either.

7. Six stage diagnosis: co-existing stages

In clinics, the manifestation of a disease may not be in only a single stage. Pathogenic Qi can penetrate other stages without entirely leaving the previous stage.[813] Furthermore, a patient can also have been in any of these stages before the new Cold-attack or Wind-attack comes into the Taiyang stage. Therefore, there could be two or more stages existing at the same time in the body. If the disease shows the two or more stages at the same time (the pathogenic Qi attacks the two stages at the same time), this is called *concurrent* stages/diseases (合病).[814] If the disease shows in the first stage, and then the second stage (the first stage has not finished yet), it is called *successive* stages/disease (并病).[815]

For concurrent stages, the disease in each stage needs to be treated separately. If a disease is in successive stages, treat all the stages at the same time.[22] For Taiyang-Yangming, or Taiyang-Shaoyang concurrent stages, treat Taiyang first. For Shaoyang-Yangming concurrent stages, treat the Shaoyang first. For Taiyang-Taiyin (or with Shaoyin or Jueyin), treat the Taiyin (the Yin stages) first.[816]

Here are some examples introduced in *Shanghan Lun*:

(1) 太阳与阳明合病者，必自下利，葛根汤主之。太阳与阳明合病，不下利，但呕者，葛根加半夏汤主之。

In the Taiyang-Yangming concurrent stages, if a patient has diarrhea,[817] use Gegen Tang

---

[813] Here a pathogenic Qi causes two or more previously described "diseases". Such complex disease condition is better to understand as two or more "stages", rather than two or more "diseases". The original concept of the Taiyang disease, Yangming disease, Shaoyang disease, Taiyin disease, Shaoyin disease, and Jueyin disease clearly means the "stage" of a disease. For this reason, in this chapter, I translate the co-existing "disease" as "disease stages".

[814] There is an opinion that the concurrent stages, such as Taiyang-Yangming, Taiyang-Shaoyang, and Shaoyang-Yangming are all caused by Wind-attack, not Cold-attack. The Wind pathogenic Qi belongs to Yang nature, meaning that it moves quickly inside the body and it easily causes heat and fire inside the body, attacking two or more stages of the body the same time.

[815] The "合病" was translated as "combined syndromes"; and the "并病" was translated as "complicated diseases" in some other books.

[816] Such differences in the treatment principles are very important in the Classical herbal formula system, not so much in Conventional herbal formula system. Such importance has been well documented in a book by Dr. Lu Shaokun (我的经方之路).

[817] The body health-maintaining Qi moves to the body surface, and the inner side is weak, so that there is diarrhea and/or nausea. The common cold with diarrhea and/or nausea is usually called digestive type of common cold. It may be treated with Gegen Tang, Mahuang Tang or with Guizhi Tang, depending on clinical conditions. The principle is to treat the body surface condition mostly. Do not pay too much attention to diarrhea or nausea unless they are very severe.

Dr. Hao Wanshan: The diarrhea here is caused by the disorder of Qi and Blood in the digestive system. It does not mean that the disease is in the Yangming inner stage.

Dr. Tan Jiezhong: For Taiyang-Yangming co-existing stages with panting (respiratory diseases), use Mahuang Tang. If with diarrhea (digestive system), use Gegen Tang.

Dr. Ni Haixia: In the Gegen Tang condition, the Cold pathogenic Qi seals the body surface. The body liquid from the digestive system lifts to the body surface, but cannot go out as sweat. So it returns to the intestine. The returning liquid is cold, but the small intestine is hot. The cold liquid makes the small intestine cold, to contract and cause diarrhea. The stool in such diarrhea is sticky and loose, with an awful odor. Gegen Tang lifts the liquid, so to solve the problem. Note that if the patient has had Hotness-Dampness in the middle part of the body, the tongue coating is wet and yellow, the body is obese, and the patient likes to eat oily food. After the use of Gegen Tang, the face of the patient might become red. This is because the Gegen Tang lifts the Hotness-Dampness up to the face. In this case, add Fuling to

---

as the primary treatment.[818] If the patient has no diarrhea but only nausea, use Gegen Jia Banxia Tang as the primary treatment.

(2)　太阳与少阳合病，自下利者，与黄芩汤，若呕者，黄芩加半夏生姜汤主之。

In Taiyang-Shaoyang concurrent stages, if a patient has diarrhea, use Huangqin Tang. If the patient is nauseous, use Huangqin Jia Banxia and Shengjiang Tang as the primary treatment.[819]

(3)　太阳与阳明合病，喘而胸满者，不可下，宜麻黄汤。

In Taiyang-Yangming concurrent stages, if a patient has panting and a bloated feeling in the chest,[820] try Mahuang Tang.[821] Do not use Purging therapy.

(4)　伤寒腹满谵语，寸口脉浮紧，此肝乘脾也，名曰纵，刺期门。

With a Shanghan disease, if a patient feels bloating in the abdomen and has delirious speech,[822] the pulse feels floating and tight in the Cun position, this condition means that the Liver bullies the Spleen (stomach). For treatment, use acupuncture on the Qimen (LV14) point.[823]

---

the formula to let the Hotness-Dampness be removed via urine.

[818] Taiyang-Yangming co-existing stages with diarrhea can also use Gegen Tang plus Xuejianchou. For a Warm disease with diarrhea (dysenteritis), use Mahuang Xinren Shigao Gancao Tang plus Xuejianchou.

[819] Theoretically, in the Taiyang-Shaoyang concurrent stages, the treatment should focus on the Taiyang body surface condition first. Here, however, using Huangqin Tang to treat the inner Shaoyang condition first. This is strange. Dr. Hu Xishu believed that the body Surface condition must be very mild. If the body surface condition is indeed apparent, then Gegen Qinlian Tang should be used for the treatment (as for the treatment of Taiyang-Yangming concurrent stages with diarrhea). The diarrhea condition that needs Huangqin Tang is acute dysentery. If the stool retention feeling is severe, Baitouwen Tang is needed for treatment.

Dr. Ni Haixia: Note that Hotness-diarrhea occurs not only due to wrong treatment of the common cold by a Purging therapy, but also naturally. The diarrhea that occurs after the Purging therapy in the common cold could be treated with either Gegen Qin Lian Tang (Hotness diarrhea), or Guizhi Renshen Tang (Cold-weakness diarrhea). Here the naturally developed Hotness diarrhea is treated with Huangqin Tang. The Huangqin Tang condition features pain in the abdomen. The former two formula syndromes have no apparent pain in the abdomen. There is herb Baishao in the Huagqin Tang. The Baishao works to stop the abdominal pain. There is no Baishao in the Gegen Qin Lian Tang or Guizhi Renshen Tang. Dahuang clears Fire in the Upper Jiao (including the Fire in the face and head). Huanglian clears Fire in the middle part of the body (stomach), and the Huangqin clears Fire in the small intestine and large intestine.

Dr. Du Yumao: This paragraph should not belong to Taiyang-Shaoyang co-existing stages. It should belong to Hotness in the Yangming stage.

[820] In this Taiyang-Yangming concurrent stage, the evidence for the Yangming should be no bowel movement for several days. The panting and floating feeling in the chest should belong to the Taiyang stage. Taiyang and Yangming have a surface-inner relationship. The suppressed Lung Qi affects the downwards movement of the Large intestine Qi, to cause no bowel movement for several days.

Dr. Hao Wanshan: This is the co-existing of Taiyang body surface condition and Yangming body surface condition (not the Yangming inner condition).

Dr. Ni Haixia: The Taiyang surface condition is sealed with Cold and the Yangming stage with Fire. The Fire tends to rise but is blocked in the chest by the Cold. Therefore the patient feels fullness in the chest and shortness of breath.

[821] Dr. Hu Xishu: This is not the Taiyang-Yangming concurrent stage. It is the Taiyang condition alone. To mark this as the "the co-existing of Taiyang and Yangming" is to distinguish them. Panting can occur in both Taiyang condition and Yangming condition. In the Taiyang condition, the panting is more severe than the chest fullness feeling. In the Yangming stage, the abdomen fullness is more severe than the panting. The Taiyang stage causes fullness feeling in the chest, while the Yangming stage causes fullness mostly in the abdomen.

[822] *Bloating feeling in the abdomen and delirious speech*: Yangming stage.

[823] In the original text, it is suggested to use acupuncture for the treatment.

(5) 伤寒发热，啬啬恶寒，大渴欲饮水。其腹必满，自汗出，小便利。其病欲解，此肝乘肺也，名曰横。刺期门。

With a Shanghan disease, a patient feels feverish, an aversion to cold,[824] is very thirsty and wants to drink much water. If the patient drinks much water, he will feel fullness and bloating in the abdomen. If the patient starts to sweat[825] and has regular urination, the patient will get better. This condition means that the Liver bullies the Lung (Urine bladder). For treatment, use acupuncture on the Qimen (LV14) point.[826]

(6) 二阳并病，太阳初得病时，发其汗，汗先出不彻，因转属阳明，续自微汗出，

Dr. Liu Duzhou: The floating-tight pulse means stringy pulse. So, it is the pulse of the Liver. It is the Liver bullying the Spleen to cause the bloating in the stomach. In Five-element theory, the Liver (Wood) suppresses the function of the Spleen/Stomach (the Soil). Stimulating the acupuncture point Qimen (LV14) (the point is on Liver meridian) can release the pathogenic Qi in the Liver/Gallbladder.

Dr. Ni Haixia: This is a condition with an enlarged liver, which presses on the stomach and spleen. The stomach and spleen have insufficient blood to work with. The body needs more nutrition to produce blood, so the tongue becomes thick and big. The *delirious speech* indicates Yangming stomach. The *fullness in abdomen* indicates the Taiyin Spleen condition. For the treatment, doing acupuncture on the Zhangmen (LV13) point might be better.

Dr. Martin Wang: It is hard to understand that the floating-tight pulse can be understood as the stringy pulse (the liver pulse, or the Shaoyang pulse). If the floating-tight pulse is believed to be the typical Cold-attack Shanghan pulse, the condition here should be understood as the co-existing of the Taiyang and Yangming stages. However, the acupuncture on the Qimen point does not support this understanding. Therefore, Dr. Hu Xishu feels that this paragraph is strange.

[824] *Fever and chilly feeling* indicate a disorder of Lung (the Lung dominates the body skin).
[825] Because the disease is originally in Cold-attack condition, the patient should have no sweat.
[826] In the original text, it is suggested to use acupuncture for the treatment. Dr. Hu Xishu believed that this is ridiculous to understand. In this paragraph, it is hard to find evidence indicating the involvement of the Liver system in the disease.

不恶寒。若太阳病证不罢者，不可下，下之为逆，如此可小发汗。设面色缘缘正赤者，阳气怫郁在表，当解之熏之。若发汗不彻，不足言，阳气怫郁不得越，当汗不汗，其人躁烦，不知痛处，乍在腹中，乍在四肢，按之不可得，其人短气但坐，以汗出不彻故也，更发汗则愈。何以知汗出不彻？以脉涩故知也。

In two Yang successive stages, a patient has Taiyang body surface condition and is given Sweating therapy. However, the sweat produced was insufficient, so the disease penetrates and involves the Yangming stage [827] (the Taiyang body surface condition remained). The patient later has mild sweating, but no aversion to cold. With the presence of the Taiyang body surface condition, Purging therapy should not be used. (Guizhi Tang can be used to cure this condition.) If the patient's face is pink (indicating the Yang Qi is suppressed in the body surface), use a mild Sweating therapy (Guizhi Tang), or use an Herbal-steam therapy (boil herbs such as Jingjie and A grass in water, and steam the body of the patient). If the sweat created so is not sufficient, and whenever the Yang Qi is suppressed in the body surface, the patient will feel annoyed and have restless arms and legs, feel pain here and there and cannot point clearly where the pain is. The patient feels panting and cannot lie down (wishes to sit up). These conditions are just due to insufficient sweat. Use Sweating therapy to create sufficient sweat to release the disease condition. How do we know that the sweat was not sufficient? It is known from the rough pulse. [828] (Use Da Qinglong Tang for treatment.)

(7) 太阳与少阳并病，头项强痛，或眩冒，时如结胸，心下痞鞕者，当刺大椎、第一间 (商阳穴)，肺俞、肝俞。慎不可发汗，发汗则谵语，脉弦，五、六日，谵语不止，当刺期门。

---

[827] There should be fullness feeling in the abdomen.
[828] In the original text, the pulse is "rough". Dr. Hu Xishu believed that the pulse should be "floating or floating and tight" instead. The rough pulse happens when the blood is not sufficient. It is not the case here when the Yang Qi is in a strongly suppressed condition.

In Taiyang-Shaoyang successive stages, a patient could feel intense pain in the head and nape, or dizziness as drunken, or feels a hardness and pain in the upper stomach from time to time (similar to a Chest-bind syndrome). [829] Use acupuncture on the Dazhui (GV14), Shangyang (LI1), Feishu (BL13), and Ganshu (BL18) points. Do not use Sweating therapy. Otherwise, the patient will become delirious, and the pulse will feel like string. [830] If the delirious speech has continued for five to six days without stop, use acupuncture on the Qimen (LV14) point.

(8)　太阳少阳并病，心下硬，颈项强而眩者，当刺大椎、肺俞、肝俞，慎勿下之。

In Taiyang-Shaoyang successive stages, a patient could feel the hardness in the upper abdomen, feels tightness on the nape, and feels dizzy. Use acupuncture on the Dazhu (GV14), Feishu (BL13) and Ganshu (BL18) points. Do not use Purging therapy. (Or use Xiao Chaihu Tang for the treatment.)

(9)　太阳少阳并病，而反下之，成结胸，心下硬，下利不止，水浆不下，其人心烦。

In Taiyang-Shaoyang successive stages, a patient was treated with Purging therapy by mistake. The patient has the Chest-bind syndrome, feels the hardness in the upper abdomen, have constant diarrhea,[831] cannot drink or eat anything, and feels annoyed.

(10)　太阳中风，下利呕逆，(表解者，乃可攻之)。其人蛰蛰汗出，发作有时，头痛，心下痞硬满，引胁下痛，干呕短气，汗出不恶寒者，(此表里未和也)，十枣汤主之。

In Wind-attack Taiyang stage, a patient has diarrhea, retch, nausea, [832] (Only after the body surface conditions are released, then Purging therapy can be used). The patient lightly sweats at fixed times, has headaches, a hardness feeling in the upper abdomen which creates pain in the flank region, belches and pants, and sweats but no aversion to cold. [833] (Such a condition suggests that the body surface and inner side is not harmonized). Use Shi Zao Tang as the primary treatment. [834]

---

[829] *Strong headache:* Taiyang stage. *Dizziness, hardness, and pain in the upper stomach from time to time*: the (atypical) Shaoyang stage. For the atypical Shaoyang condition, use acupuncture for the treatment.

This co-existing condition needs to be distinguished from Fire-water entanglement condition.

Dr. Hu Xishu: For such conditions, Xiao Chaihu Tang can also be used.

Dr. Ni Haixia: For such conditions, Xiao Chaihu Tang is not recommended. The patient with such conditions has had a deficiency of stomach water. The patient feels thirsty and drinks lots of water. The drink cannot solve the thirst. The use of Xiao Chaihu Tang can exhaust more body water by creating lots of sweat, to make the deficiency worse.

[830] *Delirious speech*: Yangming stage. *Stringy pulse*: Shaoyang stage. Sweating therapy can take the disease deeper into the Shaoyang and Yangming stages.

[831] Purging therapy not only makes the pathogenic Qi shrink into the Shaoyang to cause Chest-bind syndrome but also make it shrink to the Yangming to cause Hot diarrhea.

[832] In the Wind-attack disease condition, the patient also feels nausea and diarrhea. Use Gegen Tang first to cure the body surface condition. Then treat the remaining Shaoyang condition.

[833] From *the slightly sweating...* to the *no aversion to cold*, all of these symptoms indicate the presence of water accumulation inside. It is similar to water in the chest cavity or pericarditis.

[834] Shi Zao Tang condition can be seen in pleural effusion, tuberculous effusion pleurisy, cirrhotic ascites, pneumonia and pulmonary edema, hydrothorax and ascites caused by nephrotic syndrome.

Dr. Hao Wanshan: In clinics, if there is clear Hotness-water entanglement, it is Da Xianxiong Tang condition. If it is without apparent Fire, it is Shi Zao Tang condition. The clinical manifestations of these two conditions are very similar. Shi Zao Tang condition is a Water-Dampness accumulation syndrome.

Dr. Ni Haixia: Normally, after sweating, the water that has been activated from stomach to skin now will return to the stomach. If the water did not return to the stomach, but to the diaphragm, the diaphragm becomes heavy. If there isn't much water, and the patient feels dizzy, this is Ling Gui Zhu Gan Tang condition. If there is much water, it is Shi Zao Tang

(This is Taiyang-Shaoyang concurrent stages.)

(11)　　阳明病，脉迟，汗出多，(发热)，微恶寒者，表未解也，可发汗，宜桂枝汤。

In the Yangming stage, the pulse is slow, sweat is profuse, the patient (has a fever), and has a slight aversion to cold. Such a case means that the body surface condition still exists. Sweating therapy can still be used. Use Guizhi Tang. [835]

(12)　　阳明病，脉浮，无汗而喘者，发汗则愈，宜麻黄汤。

In the Yangming stage, the pulse feels floating, the patient does not sweat but has panting. Sweating therapy can release the condition. Use Mahuang Tang. [836]

---

condition. Shi Zao Tang can be used for the treatment of water accumulation in the lung, the heart, the liver and in the abdominal cavity.

[835] Dr. Hu Xishu: This is Yangming condition with Taiyang body surface condition. Therefore, treat the Taiyang body surface condition first. The pulse is slow and there is sweat, so use Guizhi Tang.

　　Dr. Liu Duzhou: The *slow pulse, aversion to cold, and sweat* all are from Yangming body surface condition. The treatment for Yangming body surface condition is the same as Taiyang body surface condition.

　　Dr. Du Yumao: The Yangming stage here only means that the patient has had bloating in the abdomen and no bowel movement for several days. It is a reminder, not a diagnosis that such conditions are the Yangming stage.

　　Dr. Martin Wang: This should be Taiyang-Yangming concurrent condition, both of which involve body surface condition. If it belongs to Taiyang-Yangming successive condition, the herbal formula needed might be Guizhi Jia Gegen Tang.

[836] Dr. Hu Xishu: This is also Yangming condition with Taiyang (cold-attack) condition. Therefore treat the Taiyang body surface condition first. For the lack of sweat, use Mahuang Tang.

　　Dr. Liu Duzhou: The floating pulse, no sweat and panting, all indicate Yangming body surface condition, not Taiyang body surface condition, though the treatment for the Yangming body surface condition and the Taiyang body surface condition are the same.

　　Dr. Du Yumao: Similar to the above paragraph, the Yangming stage here only means that the patient has had bloating in the abdomen and no bowel

(13)　　阳明中风，口苦咽干，腹满微喘，发热恶寒，脉浮而紧，若下之，则腹满小便难也。本证中，发热恶寒，脉浮而紧为太阳表证; 口苦咽干为少阳证; 腹满微喘为阳明证. 三阳合病, 不可单用下法, 否则表邪更陷, 加重阳明证. 若表证重, 用桂枝加大黄汤. 若少阳阳明证重, 用大柴胡汤治之.

In Wind-attack Yangming stage, a patient has a bitter taste in the mouth, has a dry throat, bloating in the stomach, has slight panting, has a fever with an aversion to cold, and the pulse is floating and tight. If Purging therapy is used, the patient will feel bloating in the abdomen and difficulty urinating. In this case, the fever with aversion to cold and floating-tight pulse suggest the Taiyang stage. The bitter taste in the mouth and dry throat suggest the Shaoyang stage. Bloated stomach and slightly pants suggest the Yangming stage. Such three Yang concurrent stages should not be treated with Purging therapy alone. Otherwise, the body surface pathogenic Qi would sink deeper to make the Yangming stage worse. If the body surface condition is severe, use Guizhi Jia Dahuang Tang for treatment. If the disease conditions in both the Shaoyang stage and Yangming stage are severe, use Da Chaihu Tang for the treatment. [837]

(14)　　三阳合病，腹满身重，难以转侧，口不仁，面垢，谵语，遗尿，发汗则谵语(甚)，下之则额上生汗，手足逆冷，若自汗出者，白虎汤主之。

With three Yang concurrent stages, [838] a patient feels bloating and fullness in the abdomen, heavy in the body, has difficulty turning over the body, discomfort in the

---

movent for several days. It is a reminder, not a diagnosis. It is not the Yangming stage, it is the Taiyang stage, but the patient has abdominal bloating and has had no bowel movement for several days.

[837] The three Yang co-existing condition described here is indicated in the original text as "concurrent" condition. However, it might belong to "successive" condition, because the herbal formula recommended is to treat all the three condition the same time (with relative focus on one or two stages). For concurrent condition, the treatment should focus on one stage each time.

[838] Dr. Liao Houze: The three Yang co-existing conditions can be seen more in Warm diseases.

144

mouth, [839] a dirty tint on the face, [840] delirious speech, and leak urine. [841] If Sweating therapy is used as the primary treatment, the patient would have severer delirious speech. If Purging therapy is used, the patient would have Jue syndrome with sweat on the front of the head. [842] If there is spontaneous sweat, use Baihu Tang as the primary treatment (Fire-clearing therapy). [843]

(15) 三阳合病，脉浮大，上关上，但欲眠睡，目合则汗。

In three Yang concurrent stages, the pulse feels floating and big in the Guan position.[844] The patient wants to sleep and sweats after falling asleep.[845]

(16) 阳明病，脉浮而紧，咽燥口苦，腹满而喘，发热汗出，不恶寒反恶热，身重。若发汗则躁，心愦愦反谵语。若加温针，必怵惕烦躁不得眠。若下之，则胃中空虚，客气动膈，心中懊浓，舌上胎者，栀子豉汤主之。

In the Yangming stage, a patient has a floating-tight pulse, has a dry mouth and throat, a bitter taste in mouth, [846] bloating and fullness in the abdomen with panting, is

---

[839] *Discomfort feeling in mouth*: some doctors have thought that this means that the patient cannot taste food. It includes numbness in the mouth lips and in the tongue.

[840] Dr. Cai Changfu: This should be understood as an oily face. It also means some chloasma, swab spots, or dark spots on the face. (蔡长福。蔡长福老师济南经方会议讲课. 李鹏 整理。
http://blog.sina.com.cn/s/blog_a208215e0101k4iu.html)

[841] This condition belongs to Dampness-Wind disease. A heavy feeling in the body means that there is Dampness in the body surface, which is due to inner Fire that pushes Dampness from inside to the body surface and the Dampness has not become sweat yet. If sweating occurs, there will be no heavy feeling in the body. The *Dampness* belongs to body surface Taiyang. *Fullness-bloating feeling in the abdomen, delirious speech, leaking urine* belong to Yangming and the *discomfort in the mouth, dirty face* belong to Shaoyang. With Taiyang condition, Purging therapy should not be used. With Shaoyang condition, Sweating therapy and Purging therapy should not be used. With Dampness condition, Purging therapy cannot be used. So, use Baihu Tang to clear the inner Fire, because it is the inner Fire that makes the inner water move to the body surface to cause the body surface condition and causes inner dryness condition in the bowel. Although there is delirious speech indicating the use of Purging therapy, the Dampness on the body surface suggests that the stool in the bowel has not become solid yet. Therefore, the delirious speech is not an absolute indication for the use of Purging therapy.

[842] Dr. Hao Wanshan: Sweat here is an indication that body Yang Qi is escaping. Such sweat is sticky as an oil (not as pure water that flows). Such sweat is called escaping sweat (脱汗, sweating from exhaustion).

Dr. Du Yumao: In this paragraph, there is no sign of Taiyang or Shaoyang. It is entirely the Yangming stage, so use Baihu Tang for the treatment. This paragraph is just like the Huangqin Tang condition, which is not the three Yang co-existing conditions. It is entirely Hotness in the Yangming stage.

[843] Fire is severe in the three Yang stages but more so in the Yangming stage, so use Baihu Tang first.

Dr. Hao Wanshan: This is not three Yang co-existing condition. The Taiyang condition and the Shaoyang condition either were not written or these two stages aren't there. It is mostly the Yangming stage.

[844] *Floating pulse*: Taiyang stage. *Big pulse*: Yangming stage. The *pulse feels floating and big in the Guan position of the wrist*: the Shaoyang stage.

[845] In this three Yang stages, the body has Fire inside and on the body surface too. The Fire rushes up to make the mind cloudy (slow and retarded reaction to the surrounding environment, a condition similar to mild coma).

Dr. Liu Duzhou: Here, *night-sweat* belongs to Shaoyang stage.

Dr. Tan Jiezhong: Patients with Gallbladder Hotness can also desire to fall asleep and sweat after falling asleep. Patients with Shaoyin disease also desire to fall asleep, but may not really fall asleep. Patients with Shaoyin diseases may just want to lie down and have no desire to act for life or work.

[846] Dr. Hao Wanshan: The condition here is not three Yang co-existing condition. The bitter taste can be due to the Shaoyang stage, but can also be due to Stomach Fire. If it is due to Shaoyang, the bitter taste and dry mouth occur usually in the early morning. If it is due to Stomach Fire, it can occur in the afternoon, or after a nap after lunch. The floating pulse indicates Fire, and the tight pulse indicates that the pathogenic Qi is strong.

feverish and sweats, has no aversion to cold but has an aversion to hot, and feels heavy in the body. [847] Such a complex condition should not be treated with a Sweating therapy. Otherwise, the patient would have a restless body, feel frighted, scared and irritated feeling in the heart and have delirious speech. If Warm-needle acupuncture is used as the primary treatment, the patient would have scared feeling, annoyed feeling, and feel difficulty falling into sleep. If Purging therapy is used, the stomach will become empty; pathogenic Qi would pouch the diaphragm, which makes the patient feel annoyance. If there is white and thick tongue coating, use Zhizi Chi Tang as the primary treatment. [848]

(If the patient feels very thirsty, has dry mouth and throat, use Baihu Jia Renshen Tang as the primary treatment. If the patient has a fever, are thirsty with the desire to drink water, has difficulty urinating, and floating pulse, use Zhuling Tang as the primary treatment. Zhuling Tang should not be used if the sweating is heavy.)

(17)　阳明中风，脉弦浮大而短气，腹都满，胁下及心痛，久按之气不通，鼻干不得汗，嗜卧，一身及面目悉黄，小便难，有潮热，时时哕，耳前后肿，刺之小差。外不解，病过十日，脉续浮者，与小柴胡汤。脉但浮，无余证者，与麻黄汤；若不尿，腹满加哕者，不治。

In Wind-attack Yangming stage, the pulse feels string, floating and big. The patient feels bloating and fullness in the whole abdomen and has pain in the upper abdomen and the flank region. If the abdomen is pressed for a long time, the patient will have difficulty breathing. The patient has a dry nose, does not sweat, and has the desire to lie down. There is a yellow color in the face, eyes, and whole body (jaundice). The patient has difficulty urinating, has a tidal fever from time to time, hiccups from time to time, and has swelling in the front and back of the ears. Acupuncture can only release little symptoms. The body conditions remain for more than ten days, and the pulse still feels floating. In such case, use Xiao Chaihu Tang for treatment. If the pulse is floating but no any other symptoms, use Mahuang Tang for treatment. If there is no urination, there is bloating and fullness in the abdomen, and hiccup, the disease is difficulty in treating. [849]

(This is Taiyang, Yangming and Shaoyang three Yang concurrent stages. [850])

---

[847] The heavy feeling in the body suggests Dampness. It is not so severe as to cause difficulty in turning the body.

Dr. Hu Xishu: This is a concurrent co-existing condition of Taiyang, Yangming, and Shaoyang. Floating-tight pulse indicates the Taiyang stage. Dry mouth and bitter taste are from the Shaoyang stage. Bloating and fullness in the abdomen and asthma, fever with sweat, and heavy body suggest the Yangming stage.

Dr. Liu Duzhou: All of the symptoms belong to Yangming body surface Fire condition, including the floating-tight pulse, bitter taste, and dryness in the throat. Zhizi Chi Tang is used to clear the Fire from the Yangming body surface stage.

[848] This paragraph should belong to three Yang concurrent conditions, though in the original text it says that this is a Yangming stage. The floating-tight pulse is the Taiyang stage; the bitter taste in mouth and dryness in the throat is the Shaoyang stage; the other symptoms belong to Yangming stage. With three Yang concurrent conditions, treat the Shaoyang first.

[849] Dr. Hu Xishu: *Floating pulse and no sweat* indicate the Taiyang. *Stringy pulse, fullness and pain in the upper-abdomen and in the flank region, pain in front and back of ears*, all belong to Shaoyang. *Dry nose, fullness in abdomen, tidal fever, and hiccups* belong to Yangming. This is three Yang concurrent conditions with jaundice, so use Xiao Chaihu Tang to cure the Shaoyang condition first. It is hard to understand the use of Mahuang Tang here.

Dr. Liu Duzhou: The *floating-big pulse and no sweat* belong to Yangming (not the Taiyang). This is Shaoyang (Hotness-Dampness) plus Yangming body surface plus jaundice condition. The use of Xiao Chaihu Tang here needs some modification. In such conditions, if the pulse feels floating only, use Mahuang Tang. The Mahuang Tang is used to release the Yangming body surface condition. If the pulse is not stringy (no Shaoyang), and there is no fullness in the abdomen (no Yangming), then Mahuang Tang can be used to treat the Jaundice.

[850] In this case, *floating pulse* indicates the Taiyang. The *bloating and fullness feeling in the flank region,*

(18)　脉浮而大, 心下反硬，有热. 此为太阳阳明证. 脉浮为太阳病, 脉大为阳明病. 心下硬却未到腹满地步, 故此时该汗, 该下, 颇为难定. 论中提示: 若临床表现主要为阳明腑证 (即大便难), 不可发汗; 若临床表现主要为阳明经证 (即发热汗出, 不恶寒, 反恶热), 不可用利小便法. 利小便法 (如用猪苓汤) 会致病陷阳明腑证.

The pulse is floating and big, the stomach feels hardness, and the body has a fever. This is Taiyang-Yangming co-existing stages. The floating pulse indicates the Taiyang stage. The big pulse and hardness feeling in stomach area indicate Yangming stage. There is hardness feeling in the upper abdomen, but it has not developed into fullness in abdomen yet. At this movement, it is difficult to decide if a Sweating therapy or a Purging therapy should be used. According to *Shanghan Lun*, if the clinical condition shows more on Yangming inner stage (difficulty in bowel movement), Sweating therapy should not be used; if there are more apparent conditions indicating Yangming body surface condition (e.g., fever, sweat, no aversion to cold but to hot), Diuretic therapy should not be used. The Diuretic therapy, such as use Zhuling Tang can bring the disease more in-depth into the Yangming inner stage.

(19)　伤寒四、五日，身热恶风，颈项强，胁下满，手足温而渴者，小柴胡汤主之。

With a Shanghan disease for four to five days, a patient feels feverish, has an aversion to wind, feels intensive tightness on the neck

tends to lie down, swelling in front and back of the ears, and string pulse belong to the Shaoyang. The *fullness and bloating in the whole abdomen, shortness of breath, hiccups, tidal fever, dry nose, and big pulse* belong to the Yangming stage. The difficulty in urination suggests there is an accumulation of garbage water inside the body. Because there is no sweat, and there is difficulty urinating, jaundice has formed. For the treatment, try Xiao Chaihu Tang. This is a difficult condition to treat, which can be seen in acute hepatic jaundice.

Dr. Martin Wang: The jaundice is due to Hotness-Dampness in both Shaoyang and Yangming stages, not only from the Shaoyang stage. Because of the *no sweating and difficulty urinating*, the Hotness and Dampness became jaundice.

and nape, feels fullness in the flank region, has warm hands and feet, and is thirsty. For such a case, use Xiao Chaihu Tang as the primary treatment. [851]

(20)　伤寒六、七日，发热微恶寒，支节烦疼，微呕，心下支结，外证未去者，柴胡桂枝汤主之.

With a Shanghan disease for six or seven days, a patient feels feverish and has a slight aversion to cold, has an annoying pain in joints, [852] slight nausea, obstruction feeling in the upper abdomen. If the body condition remains, use Chaihu Guizhi Tang as the primary treatment. [853]

(This is a Taiyang-Shaoyang successive stages.)

(21)　伤寒五、六日，头汗出，微恶寒，手足冷，心下满，口不欲食，大便硬，脉沉细, 为阳微结. 阳气结于表. 小柴胡汤治之.

With a Shanghan disease for five to six days, a patient sweats only on the head, has a slight aversion to cold, has cold hands and feet, fullness in the upper stomach, has no desire to eat, has a firm stool, and the pulse is deep-

---

[851] In this case, *the aversion to wind and tight neck and nape* suggest Taiyang stage. *Bloating in the flank region* is the Shaoyang stage. *Fever and thirst* suggest the Yangming stage. This is three Yang concurrent conditions. Use Xiao Chaihu Tang to treat the Shaoyang first.

[852] Dr. Hao Wanshan: The annoying pain should belong to the Taiyin stage. Therefore this is a Taiyang, Shaoyang and Taiyin co-existing stages. The annoying joint pain is never described in the Taiyang stage.

[853] Here, the *fever, aversion to cold, joint pain, slight nausea* suggest the Wind-attack Taiyang stage. The obstruction feeling in the upper stomach suggests the Shaoyang stage. The *slight nausea* can be both of the stages.

Dr. Hu Xishu: We can also use Xiao Chaihu Tang with herbs such as mint, yam or Juhua to increase sweating. It is not proper to only use Xiao Chaihu Tang or to use Sweating therapy alone. Chaihu Guizhi Tang can be used in (1) various fever diseases with joint pain (similar to Xiao Chaihu Tang); (2) digestive diseases with joint pain; (3) mental diseases or nervous diseases with joint pain. It is used also in seniors with movement pain in the muscles.

147

thin. [854] This condition is called Yang mild-bind syndrome (阳微结), meaning that body Yang Qi is bound in the body surface. Use Xiao Chaihu Tang for treatment. [855]

(22)　　脉浮发热口干鼻燥，能食者衄。

The pulse feels floating. The patient has a fever and has a dry mouth and nose. In such a case, if the patient can still eat, the patient would have nosebleeding.

(This condition is the three-Yang co-existing stages. [856])

(23)　　阳明病，脉迟，汗出多，微恶寒者，表未解也，可发汗，宜 桂枝 汤。

In the Yangming stage, if the pulse feels slow, the patient has profuse sweating and has a slight aversion to cold, such a case means that the body surface condition remains. Use Sweating therapy for treatment. Use Guizhi Tang. [857]

(24)　　阳明病，脉浮，无汗而喘者，发汗则愈，宜 麻黄 汤。

In the Yangming stage, the pulse is floating; the patient has no sweat but has panting. For such a case, use Sweating therapy (Mahuang Tang) to cure the body surface condition first. [858] Use Mahuang Tang.

---

[854] The syndrome can be understood as a Taiyang-Shaoyang-Yangming concurrent condition. *Slight aversion to cold*: Taiyang stage. *Fullness in the stomach and has no desire to eat:* Shaoyang stage. *Cold hands and feet, firm stool, thin (or deep and thin)* pulse: Yangming Cold-attack stage. Use Xiao Chaihu Tang for the treatment.

[855] If this syndrome is understood as the three Yang successive conditions, then Chaihu Guizhi Ganjiang Tang can be used (as suggested by Dr. Hu Xishu).

[856] In this case, the *fever and floating pulse* indicate body surface Taiyang. The *dry mouth and nose* indicate Shaoyang. The *ability to eat* suggests inner Fire, a Yangming stage.

[857] The Taiyang condition here is a Wind-attack condition. This is Taiyang-Yangming concurrent condition (both are in body surface conditions)

[858] The Taiyang condition is a Cold-attack condition. Here is Taiyang-Yangming concurrent condition (both are in body surface condition).

8. Diagnosis and treatment of Cholera

Cholera (here it means sudden turmoil) is different from Shanghan diseases. It is a group of diseases characterized by sudden vomiting and diarrhea. It includes cholera, acute gastroenteritis, and others. There are Dry type cholera disorder and Dampness type of cholera. In the former, a patient feels nauseous but cannot vomit, and wants to have a bowel movement but cannot pass any stool. In the latter, the patient vomits and has diarrhea. Usually, this disorder refers to Dampness type of cholera. There is some similarity between cholera and the Shanghan diseases, so the differentiation diagnosis is essential.

问曰：病发热，头痛，身疼，恶寒，吐利者，此属何病？答曰：此名霍乱。自吐下，又利止，复更发热也。

Asked: A patient has a fever, headaches, generalized pain, an aversion to cold, and has vomiting and diarrhea (from the beginning days of the disease). What disease is it?

Answered: This is cholera disease. Such a patient has vomit and diarrhea. If diarrhea stops, there would be a fever again.[859]

伤寒，其脉微涩者，本是霍乱，今是伤寒，却四五日，至阴经上，转入阴必利，本呕下利者，不可治也。欲似大便而反矢气，仍不利者，属阳明也，便必硬，十三日愈，所以然者，经尽故也。

In the Shanghan disease. The pulse feels slightly rough. The disease condition is initially cholera; now it is Shanghan disease. The disease lasted for four to five days and penetrated and located in Yin meridians, so there would be diarrhea. If the vomit happens before diarrhea, the treatment is difficult. If the patient wants to have a bowel movement, but there is only farting and no stool, then it is the Yangming stage of the Shanghan disease. The stool will become firm. The

disease will be over on the thirteenth day. The reason is that, after thirteen days, the disease has moved and finished all meridian.

下利后，当便硬，硬则能食者愈；今反不能食，到后经中，颇能食，复过一经能食，过之一日，当愈。不愈者，不属阳明也。

After diarrhea, the stool should become firm. If the stool is indeed firm and the patient can eat, the disease will be over. If the patient cannot eat, and if the disease lasts to the later time of the meridian course, and starts to eat. After over one meridian course and then can eat, after one day, the disease will get recovered.[860] If the disease is not over, the disease does not belong to the Yangming stage of the Shanghan disease.[861]

恶寒脉微，而复利，利止，亡血也，四逆加人参汤主之。

A patient has an aversion to cold; the pulse is faint; the patient has diarrhea again. If diarrhea stops, the stop means blood collapse (亡血) condition. Use Si Ni Jia Renshen Tang as the primary treatment.[862]

霍乱，头痛，发热，身疼痛，热多欲饮水者，五苓散主之；寒多不用水者，理中丸主之。

With the cholera disease, a patient has a headache, fever, generalized pain. If the fever is intense and the patient desires to drink water, use Wu Ling San as the primary treatment.[863] If there are relatively more chills (cold) and the patient has no desire to drink water, use Lizhong Wan as the primary treatment.

---

[859] Because of the fever, headache, pain, and aversion to cold, the sudden turmoil disorder is very similar to the Shanghan disease. But in the former, the vomiting and diarrhea occur in the first or second day of the disease, while that in the Shanghan disease, if any, happens after several days.

[860] The original Chinese texts "到后经中，颇能食，复过一经能食，过之一日，当愈" are difficult to translate.

[861] This paragraph is very difficult to understand and to translate. It seems not consistent with the text of the whole text of the book *Shanghan Lun*. It mentioned lots of meridian concepts.

[862] Dr. Liu Duzhou: The herb Ginseng here is used to save body liquid (the body Yin). Fuzi is used to save body Yang (body warm energy).

[863] Dr. Liu Duzhou: *Wu Ling San syndrome*: the body has Dampness. *Lizhong Tang condition*: the body has Coldness-Weakness condition. The dosage of Lizhong Wan needs to be increased until the body feels warm (either on the head, or back, on the stomach, or on the whole body).

吐利止而身痛不休者，当消息和解其外，
宜 桂枝 汤小和之。

If the vomiting and diarrhea stop, but there is
still a generalized pain in the body, the
disease condition is better to be treated with
Guizhi Tang to calm the body condition.

吐利汗出，发热恶寒，四肢拘急，手足厥
冷者，四逆汤主之。

If there is vomiting, diarrhea and sweating,
fever and an aversion to cold, muscle spasms
in the arms and legs, and Jue syndrome, use
Si Ni Tang as the primary treatment.

既吐且利，小便复利而大汗出，下利清谷，
内寒外热，脉微欲绝者，四逆汤主之。

With vomiting and diarrhea, the urination
becomes regular, but the patient has profuse
sweat, has undigested food in the stool. This
case is an inner Coldness and outside Hotness
condition. If the pulse is difficulty in feeling,
use Si Ni Tan as the primary treatment.[864]

吐已下断，汗出而厥，四肢拘急不解，脉
微欲绝者，通脉四逆加猪胆汁汤主之。

Vomiting and diarrhea stopped. The patient
sweats and has Jue syndrome; there are
muscle spasms in the arms and legs, and the
pulse is faint and difficulty in feeling. Use
Tong Mai Si Ni Tang Jia pig gallbladder
juice as the primary treatment.

吐利发汗，脉平，小烦者，以新虚不胜谷
气故也。

After vomiting and diarrhea, Sweating
therapy was used. The pulse feels calm; the
patient feels slightly annoyed. This condition
means that the body condition is in a weak
condition and there is not enough energy for
digesting food.

---

[864] The sweat here means that Yang Qi will float.
    Dr. Liu Duzhou: The herbal formula used here
should be Tongmai Si Ni Tang.

9. New conditions after recovery from Shanghan disease

After recovering from Shanghan disease, the body condition is weak. The body needs time to get back to its original health. During this recovery period, if the patient does not pay attention to proper diet and physical activity, the patient may have new symptoms, though this time they may not indicate Shanghan disease.

伤寒，阴阳易之为病，其人身体重，少气，少腹里急，或引阴中拘挛，热上冲胸，头重不欲举，眼中生花，膝胫拘急者，烧裈散主之。

In the recovery period following a Shanghan disease, a patient may get Yin-Yang transmission syndrome. The patient feels heaviness in the body and is short of breath. There are spasms in the lower abdomen, or the spasm pain contracts and causes pain in the sexual organ. The patient feels hot up-rushing feeling, feels that the head is so heavy to lift it, has a blurring vision, and spasms in the knees and calves. Use Shaokun San as the primary treatment.[865]

大病差后，劳复者，枳实栀子汤主之。若有宿食者，加大黄如博棋子大五六枚。

After recovery from a severe disease, if a patient feels discomfort,[866] which is caused by a substantial physical work or labor (劳复),[867] use Zhishi Zhizi Tang as the primary treatment. If such a condition is due to retained food (宿食) in the bowel, add Dahuang[868] to the formula.

伤寒差已后，更发热者，小柴胡汤主之。脉浮者，以汗解之；脉沉实者，以下解之。

If the patient has a fever again after getting recovered from a severe disease, use Xiao Chaihu Tang as the primary treatment. In such a case, if the pulse feels floating, use Sweating therapy as the primary treatment. If the pulse feels deep but not weak, use Purging therapy.[869]

大病差后，从腰以下有水气者，牡蛎泽泻散主之。

After recovering from a severe disease, a patient has a heavy feeling from the lower back to the legs,[870] use Muli Zexie Tang as the primary treatment.[871]

大病差后，喜唾，久不了了者，胃上有寒，当以丸药温之，宜理中丸。

After recovering from a severe disease, a patient likes to spit for a long time without cessation. This condition suggests the presence of Coldness and retained water in

---

[865] This is a disease condition, which occurs in the later recovery period of the Shanghan disease, due to the sexual activity between the male and female. It is called Yin-Yang transmission syndrome.

Dr. Du Yumao: For the treatment of this syndrome, we can also use formula Danggui Si Ni Tang. If there is Jue syndrome, add Fuzi; if there is Cold, add Wuzhuyu and dried ginger.

[866] The discomfort here means annoying fever and a bloating feeling in the abdomen.

[867] The reasons also include over-eating, or eating undigestable food; over-work; has long baths; physical exercise, etc.

[868] Dahuang is added if the stool is dry and firm.

[869] Dr. Hu Xishu and Dr. Hao Wanshan: Purging therapy here means, in most cases, Da Chaihu Tang. There's a small chance to use Chengqi Tang. If the new condition is hard to diagnose as either body surface condition or inner condition, use Chaihu-containing formulas.

[870] This means that there is swelling from the lower back down to the legs.

[871] If the swelling is mostly in the lower part of the body, use Diuretic therapy. Muli Zexie San is one such herbal formula. Another herbal formula that can be used is Fangji Fuling Yin (防己茯苓饮). These are just some of the examples.

Dr. Hu Xishu: If the patient feels thirsty, use Gualu Muli San (瓜蒌牡蛎散), or Wu Ling San.

Dr. Liu Duzhou: Muli Zexie San is used in Excess condition, in which the body has water accumulation and Hotness, the pulse feels deep and strong, there is difficulty urinating, bloating in the abdomen, and swelling in the legs, which feel hard when pressed. If the over-accumulation of water is due to a weakness condition, this formula should not be used. In the weakness condition, if the swelling in the legs and the lower abdomen is soft when pressed, then the herbal formula used should be Shi Pi Wan (实脾丸) or Shen Qi Wan (肾气丸).

the stomach. Use Warm therapy, such as Lizhong Wan. [872]

伤寒解后，虚赢少气，气逆欲吐者，竹叶石膏 汤主之。

After recovering from Shanghan disease, a patient feels weak, short of breath, and is nauseous. In such case, use Zhuye Shigao Tang as the primary treatment. [873]

病人脉已解，而日暮微烦，以病新差，人强与谷，脾胃气尚弱，不能消谷，故令微烦，损谷则愈。

It is known from the pulse that the patient has recovered, but the patient feels mildly annoyed in the later afternoon. The reason is that the stomach is weak after the recovery, but the patient overate food or had undigested food. The food stays in the stomach, causes the annoying sensation. Let the patient reduce the amount of food to eat and have a break.

---

[872] Dr. Hu Xishu: Wuzhuyu Tang can also work for such Cold conditions in the stomach. In the Wuzhuyu Tang condition, the patient feels nauseous, dizziness, or has headaches. It is more a severe condition than Lizhong Tang condition.

Dr. Liu Duzhou: If the frequent water-spitting is due to Coldness-Weakness condition in the lung, use Gancao Ganjiang Tang (甘草干姜汤).

[873] Dr. Hu Xishu: This is a condition in which the stomach is lacking liquid (Yin), and there is Fire in the stomach.

10. The time in which a patient recovers

It is possible to predict when a patient will get better. For example, for a disease in the Shaoyang stage, the patient can get better between 3 am and 9 am. The usefulness of the getting-better time zone is that, if we allow the patient to drink herbal tea before that time, the herbal tea will start working during the time zone, the healing effect and the body energy status will match each other, and the healing effect of the herbal tea will be much stronger. [874] However, with modern lifestyles, people go to bed very late and get up late, drink alcohol, have too much stress, or use improper treatment, and so on. Therefore, the getting-better time pattern may not be apparent. [875]

In *Shanghan Lun*, different disease stages have different getting-better time zones. [23]

太阳病，欲解时，从巳至未上。

For the Taiyang stage, the getting-better time is from 9 am to 3 pm.

少阳病，欲解时，从寅至辰上。

For the Shaoyin stage, the getting-better time is from 3 am to 9 am.

阳明病，欲解时，从申至戌上。

For the Yangming stage, the getting-better time is from 3 pm to 9 pm.

太阴病，欲解时，从亥至丑上。

For the Taiyin stage, the getting-better time is from 9 pm to 3 am.

少阴病，欲解时，从子至寅上。

For the Shaoyin stage, the getting-better time is from 11 pm to 5 am.

厥阴病，欲解时，从寅至卯上。

For the Jueyin stage, the getting-better time is from 1 am to 7 am.

There are different explanations for how a disease could have such getting-better time zones. One explanation is the Yang Qi status in the body, which can affect the disease status in the body because the status of the six-stage of a disease is the overall result between the intensity of the pathogenic Qi and the Yang Qi (the health-maintaining Qi) inside the body.

In the morning, the intensity of Yang Qi is increasing in nature, the body Yang Qi is also rising, which increases the intensity of the Yang Qi in the Shaoyang stage (the Shaoyang is the rising movement of Yang Qi in the body). A disease in the Shaoyang stage has an increased chance to counteract the pathogenic Qi and get better.

Around noon (between 9 am and 3 pm), Yang Qi in nature is at its highest, and the Yang Qi is on the surface of the earth. So is the Yang Qi in the body. With Taiyang stage diseases, pathogenic Qi seals and compresses the body Yang Qi on the body surface. Now with the highest Yang Qi in nature, the body Yang Qi also comes to its peak intensity. On the body surface, the body has more Yang Qi to counteract the disease. Therefore, the Taiyang stage gets better.

In the afternoon, the Yang Qi in nature is falling, and so is the Yang Qi in the body. A Yangming stage disease results because of the difficulty of the Yang Qi in the digestive system to reduce. Now with the help of the downwards-falling Yang Qi in the body, the Yangming stage diseases can get better.

---

[874] Dr. Du Yumao: The getting-better time zones match the reality of clinical observations.

[875] Dr. Hu Xishu: The getting-better time zone theory may not be true.

Dr. Liu Duzhou, Ni Haixia, Tan Jiezhong, and Li Keshao believe in this getting-better time zone theory.

There is an opinion that the time-course of the Zi Wu Liu Zhu (子午流注, the time zone for energy flow in the body meridians, or the midnight-noon ebb-flow) may not work and may not be useful in acupuncture.

Dr. Gong Shicheng: The getting-better time zone may only work for the body surface conditions of the Taiyang, Yangming (non-wave fever phase), Shaoyang, Taiyin, Shaoyin, and Jueyin stages, not for the Yangming body surface condition (tidal fever in the Qi phase). Also, the overall rule of the severity of a disease described in the book *Huangdi Nei Jing*, that a disease can be quiet and calm in the morning and noon, worse in the afternoon, and severe at night, only applies to exogenous diseases, not to miscellaneous diseases.

The getting-better zones for the three Yin stages are at night with much overlap amongst them, because, in nature, the Yang Qi shrinks deep into the Earth (is not floating like during daytime). Likewise, the Yang Qi in the body shrinks deeply into the body. The characteristics of the three Yin stages are the lack of body Yang Qi with different extents. Now with the returning of body Yang Qi deep within the body at night, the body has more Yang Qi at night to counteract the pathogenic Qi, so the three Yin stage diseases get better mostly at night.

In recent times, there is opinion[13,24] that there should also be a getting-worse time zone for each of the stages, and that the getting-worse time pattern is also the same for a disease as the getting-better time zone. For example, the getting-better time zone for Taiyang stage is from 9 am to 3 pm, so the getting-worse time zone for the Taiyang disease is also from 9 am to 3 pm.

Some others[25] believe that the getting-worse time zone should be the opposite time zone to the getting-better time zone. For example, the getting-better time zone for Shaoyang stage diseases is from 3 am to 9 am, so the getting-worse time zone for the Shaoyang diseases should be from 3 pm to 9 pm.

The belief that the getting-worse time zones for the six-stage diseases are opposite to, or the same as, their getting-better time zones, seem to be theoretical speculation. Some doctors[26] totally do not believe this is true. We believe that the getting-worse time zone can be the opposite of the getter-better time zone for the Taiyang, Shaoyang and the Yangming stages, but they are the same time zones for the three Yin stages. For example, the getting-worse zone of the Shaoyang stage is in the afternoon, and that for the Yangming stage is in the morning. For the Taiyang stage, the getting-worse time zone is at night. We know that the symptoms of a common cold or flu are worse at night, at which time the patient can have a stronger stuffy nose and fever, but the symptoms are less around lunch time. However, for the three Yin stages, the getting-worse time is also at night, the same as their getting-better time zones. This is true when there are Yang-floating signs in the patient because of excess Yin in the body. At night the excess of the Yin Qi in the body becomes strongest due to the excess of Yin Qi in nature. The increase in the Yin Qi inside the body makes the disease worse. This phenomenon matches clinical reality.

It should be pointed out that the getting-better time zones in the book *Shanghan Lun* are not the same as the time zones of energy flow in the meridians (the midnight-noon ebb-flow theory). The classification of diseases in the *Shanghan Lun* six stages are not the same as those of the meridian theory that is used in acupuncture treatment.

Expert opinions:[27]

Dr. Gu Zhishan (顾植山) believed that the getting-better time for the six-stage diseases comes from the idea or switch-pivot theory. The function of the switch-pivot effect of the three Yang regions and the three Yin regions can be verified in clinics.

Dr. Zhang Zhicong (张志聪) said that the six diseases usually get better when the disease's nature matches the daytime zone (for example, the Yangming disease gets better during the Yangming time zone of the day). Dr. Chen Xiuyuan (陈修园) had the same idea.

Dr. Gu said that the Jueyin is the end of the Yin regions. It is the time of the Yin moving into the Yang region (Shaoyang region). The Jueyin region is extraordinary. If the daytime zone helps the Jueyin disease (e.g., the Jueyin disease is in the Jueyin time zone, the 1 am to 3 am zone), the pathogenic Qi returns, and the body Health-maintaining Qi becomes stronger. The patient will get better or even be cured. Otherwise, if the Jueyin disease does not get help from the time zone, the Jueyin disease will get worse, and return to the Shaoyin disease to die. For any stubborn diseases and severe diseases, if the symptoms occur or become worse during 1 am to 3 am, all can be treated with Wumei Wan, the leading herbal formula for the treatment of Jueyin diseases.

Supplementary readings

1 Background for *Shanghan Lun* and its spread

Dr. Hao Wanshan (郝万山): 4

The *Shanghan Zabing Lun* was written by Dr. Zhang Zhongjing (AD 150-219) in about AD 200. There are 16 volumes in total. Before this book was published, a few other TCM books in medical theory and herbal formulas had already been produced. These medical theory books discussed body physiology and pathology. They include the following: *Huangdi Nei Jing* (黄帝内经), *Huangdi Wai Jing* (黄帝外经), *Bianque Nei Jing* (扁鹊内经), *Bianque Wai Jing* (扁鹊外经), *Baishi Nei Jing* (白氏内经), *Baishi Wai Jing* (白氏外经), and *Baishi Pang Jing* ((白氏) 旁经).

Formula books are a summary of clinical experience. There are eleven such books, including *Tang Ye Jing* (汤液经). Dr. Zhang Zhongjing combined the two kinds of the books, creating a new kind of book that talks about medical theory, principles of treatment, the content of herbal formulas, application of herbal formulas, and methods for diagnosing diseases. Therefore, it sets up a foundation for TCM diagnosis and treatment.

Theoretical books include basic theory about medicine. They are not used for clinical practice. Classical herbal formulas (Jing Fang), formula books, are collections of clinical experiences without a theoretical explanation. Only after the appearance of *Shanghan Zabing Lun*, was there a medical book that combined medical theory and clinical practice. From this point of view, Dr. Zhang Zhongjing is the founder of TCM clinical medicine. He is also the founder of individual treatment (treatment based on the disease status of an individual patient) and treatment according to syndrome differentiation (e.g., not adding up the herbs according to the number of symptoms present). He served a significant role in TCM history by linking medical theory with actual clinical practice so that clinical practice came under the guidance of medical theory.

Shanghan Zabing Lun has sixteen volumes. Due to various reasons, it was challenging to preserve and protect the book during its long history. During the Western Jin dynasty of China, Dr. Wang Shuhe (王叔和) summarized and edited the book and could only find ten volumes. The ten volumes mostly talk about differentiation diagnosis, so he gave the book a new name *Shanghan Lun* (ten volumes and 22 chapters).

Dr. Wang Shuhe had his book too. It is called *Mai Jing* (脉经) (about the pulse). In his book, he included many things from *Shanghan Lun*, but not the formulas.

During the Tang dynasty, Dr. Sun Simiao (孙思邈) wrote *Qian Jin Yao Fang* (千金要方). In the book, he included some contents from *Shanghan Lun*. In his other book, *Qian Jin Yi Fang* (千金翼方), he included all the contents of *Shanghan Lun*.

During the Tang dynasty, there was an exam for doctors. The content from the *Shanghan Lun* was worth many marks, so the spread of *Shanghan Lun* during the Tang dynasty was vast. However, the books were hand copied. The version of *Shanghan Lun* (Kang version) we see now in Japan has hand-copying citations from the Tang period (65 paragraphs).

During the Tang dynasty, there was another doctor named Wang Tao (王焘). He wrote *Wai Tai Mi Yao* (外台秘要). In this book, he also used some content from *Shanghan Lun*. However, besides the contents from *Shanghan Lun*, there are also many items that can be seen in the later book, *Jin Kui Yao Luo* (金匮要略). Therefore, it is believed that the contents from *Shanghan Lun* in his book did not come from Dr. Wang Shuhe, but from somewhere else. It might be some other version of *Shanghan Lun*.

From the Tang dynasty, there are two books: *Qian Jin Yao Fang* by Dr. Sun Simiao and *Wai Tai Mi Yao* by Dr. Wang Tao. Both books are essential reference sources for today's doctors when editing the *Shanghan Lun*.

The first time that *Shanghan Lun* was fixed and printed (rather than hand copied), occurred in the Song dynasty. Dr. Lin Yi (林亿), Dr. Sun Qi (孙奇) and Dr. Gao Baoheng

(高保衡) in the Song National Medical Press edited and printed a version of *Shanghan Lun* in Song Zhiping second year (1065 AD). The Song version of the *Shanghan Lun* is also called the Zhiping version, which can no longer be found nowadays. What we can find is the reprinted version of the Song version, by Dr. Zhao Kaimei (赵开美) from the Ming dynasty (Wangli 27th year, e.g., 1599 AD). He gave the reprinted version a new name, *Fanke Song Ban Shanghan Lun* (翻刻宋版伤寒论). He also reprinted the books *Zhujie Shanghan Lun* (注解《伤寒论》) by Dr. Cheng Wuji (成无己, 1044 AD), *Shanghan Lei Zheng* (伤寒类证) by Dr. Song Yinggong (宋英公), and *Jin Kui Yao Luo* (金匮要略). He called these four books the *Zhongjing Quanshu* (仲景全书).

The book *Shanghan Ming Li Lun* (伤寒明理论) by Dr. Cheng Wuji from the Jin dynasty mostly explains the words and terms used in the book *Shanghan Lun*.

Only because the book *Fanke Song Ban Shanghan Lun* was reprinted by Dr. Zhao Kaimei, can *Shanghan Lun* be passed on to today, allowing us to see the original texts of *Shanghan Lun*. For this reason, Dr. Zhao Kaimei was indispensable in preserving *Shanghan Lun*.

In 1982, Dr. Liu Duzhou (刘渡舟), Qian Chaochen (钱超尘) and I (郝万山) edited the book *Fanke Song Ban Shanghan Lun* (翻刻宋版伤寒论) and, in 1991, published *Shanghan Lun Jiaozhu* (伤寒论校注).

If we say that the first, second, third, fourth and fifth editions of the TCM textbook for *Shanghan Lun* are based on the book *Fanke Song Ban Shanghan Lun* (翻刻宋版伤寒论), then the sixth edition was edited from the book *Shanghan Lun Jiaozhu* (伤寒论校注).

The Song dynasty's National Medical Book Edition Press also printed *Jin Kui Yu Han Jing* (金匮玉函经) with eight volumes in total. By glancing at the name of the book, it is easy to misunderstand that it includes content from *Jin Kui Yao Luo* (金匮要略). However, its content is from *Shanghan Lun*. It is the same book with a different name.

The Song dynasty's National Medical Book Edition Press also found another book called *Jin Kui Yu Han Yao Luo Fang Lun San Juan* (金匮玉函要略方论三卷). They found that the first volume of this book includes citations for *Shanghan Lun*. They inferred that the second and the third volumes of the book should have citations of texts for the treatment of miscellaneous diseases and female diseases from *Shanghan Zabing Lun*. They omitted the first volume of *Jin Kui Yu Han Yao Luo Fang Lun San Juan* (金匮玉函要略方论三卷), reorganized the second and third volumes of the book into another three volumes (including the formulas), but still used the same title, *Jin Kui Yu Han Yao Luo Fang Lun San Juan* (金匮玉函要略方论), which goes by the short name of *Jin Kui Yao Luo* (金匮要略). Because of the works printed by the Song dynasty's National Medical Book Edition Press, the book *Shanghan Zabing Lun* was separated into the current *Shanghan Lun* (ten volumes, 22 chapters) and *Jin Kui Yao Luo* (three volumes).

Dr. Hu Xishu (胡希恕): 2

Dr. Huang Fumi (皇甫谧) in the Jin dynasty said in his book, *Zhenjiu Jiayi Jing* (针灸甲乙经), that Dr. Zhaong Zhongjing "Lun guang *Tang Ye Jing* several ten volumes". What he meant is that Dr. Zhang Zhongjing wrote the book *Shanghan Lun* from the basis of book *Tang Ye Jing* (汤液经). Dr. Huang Fumi was not only good at medicine, but he was also a historian. His book *Zhenjiu Jiayi Jing* included the contents of *Shanghan Lun* but not the preface in the book by Dr. Wang Shuhe. In the preface of the book by Dr. Wang Shuhe, it says that Dr. Zhang Zhongjing's book *Shanghan Lun* was based on the chapters *Su Wen* (素问), *Jiu Juan* (九卷), *Bashiyi Nan* (八十一难), *Yin Yang Da Lun* (阴阳大论) in the book *Huangdi Nei Jing*.

If indeed there was a preface in the original *Shanghan Lun*, it is impossible that Dr. Huang Fumi would not have respected Dr. Zhong Zhongjing's preface by saying that *Shanghan Lun* was developed from somewhere else. Dr. Huang Fumi says that *Shanghan Lun* was developed from *Tang Ye Jing*, suggesting that there was no such preface in his time. Therefore, we believe that this preface is not real, that it is false. Dr. Wang Shuhe himself composed the preface.

This preface affected doctors very much. Many doctors believed that *Shanghan Lun* followed the book *Huangdi Nei Jing*, just because of what it said in this preface. To me, there is no relationship between *Shanghan Lun* and *Huangdi Nei Jing*.

Dr. Lin Zhiman (林之满):[28]

It is generally believed that the chapters of Bian Mai Fa (辩脉法), Ping Mai Fa (平脉法), Shanghan Li (伤寒例), and the later eight chapters in the book *Zhujie Shanghan Lun* (注解伤寒论) by Dr. Wang Shuhe were written by himself (not by Dr. Zhang Zhongjing). When comparing these chapters with his book, *Mai Jing*, we can see that this believing is correct.

Other versions：

The book *Shanghan Zabing Lun Guilin Guoben* (伤寒杂病论桂林古本) is said to be the 12th version of *Shanghan Zabing Lun* by Dr. Zhang Zhongjing. This version of the book was never seen in history. In the late Qing dynasty, Zhang Shaozu (张绍祖), who is the 64th descendant of Dr. Zhang Zhongjing, passed this book on to his student Dr. Zuo Shengde (左盛德). Dr. Zuo again passed this book on to his student Dr. Luo Zhechu (罗哲初). In 1934, Luo Zhechu lent the book to Dr. Huang Zhuzhai (黄竹斋). The last hand copied the book and named it *Bai Yun Ge Cangben* (白云阁藏本). In 1939, this version was edited by Zhang Boying (张伯英) and published to the public. Because this version of *Shanghan Lun* was never seen before the late Qing dynasty, the truth of this version is highly questioned by other doctors.

Kangzhi version of *Shanghan Lun*. This version of the *Shanghan Lun* was hand copied by people in the Tang dynasty. It is a short-cited version of *Shanghan Lun*, consisting of only 65 paragraphs and 50 formulas. On the back of the book, there are texts of "written in the Tang dynasty, Zhenyuan Yiyou year (唐贞元乙酉岁写之)." Traditional, in the year 1143, the book was hand copied again by Japanese Shamen Lechun (沙门了纯). It was found again in the middle of 1800. It was published in the year 1858 by Kyoto Shulin Publishing. In the year 1982, it was photocopied and published by Traditional Chinese Medicine Publishing House in China.

Kangping version of *Shanghan Lun*. The Kangping version was hand copied by Japanese Dan Bo Ya Zhong (丹波雅忠) in the year 1060 according to the copy of *Shanghan Lun* kept in his family. In the year 1346, Japanese TCM doctor He Qi Chao Chen (和气朝臣) hand copied this book. This copy is also called Heqi version of Shanghan Lun. In 1936, Japanese TCM doctor Da Zhong Jing Jie (大冢敬节) acquired this copy from the Shangfang family. He referred to his own family's copy of Kangping, as well as the book *Heqishi Guben Shanghan Lun* (和气氏古本伤寒论), and he published a new version in the year 1937. Later, he presented this book to Chinese TCM doctor Dr. Ye Juquan (叶橘泉). The latter published it in the year 1947 in China.

There are two characteristics of the Kangping version:[29] First, it is written with some lines having fifteen words, some lines with fourteen words and some other lines with thirteen words. Scholars regarded the 15-word lines as the original text of the *Shanghan Lun*, the 14-word lines as close-to-original text, and the 13-word lines as a new text. This characteristic was not seen in any other versions. Second, among these texts, there are many inserted words and parallel words. Such inserted and parallel words are included in other versions of *Shanghan Lun*.

2 The relationship between the Six stages in the Six Stage diagnosis system and the Six Jing in *Huangdi Nei Jing*:

There has been a long-standing argument about the relationship between the books *Shanghan Lun* and *Huangdi Nei Jing*. The issue of this debate is whether we should understand and explain the content in the book *Shanghan Lun* from the viewpoint of *Huangdi Nei Jing*. In recent times, those doctors who believe that the theoretical basis of the *Shanghan Lun* comes from *Huangdi Nei Jing* include Dr. Liu Duzhou (刘渡舟) and Hao Wanshan (郝万山). Whereas those doctors who do not think so, but believe that the theoretical basis of *Shanghan Lun* comes from another book, such as *Tang Ye Jing Fa* (汤液经法), include Dr. Hu Xishu (胡希恕), Dr. Cao Yingfu (曹颖甫), and others.

The reason for such different beliefs is because the commonly used Song version of *Shanghan Lun* has a preface. In the preface, it is clearly written that the book *Shanghan Lun* was written by Dr. Zhang Zhongjing after he referred to the chapters in the book *Huangdi Nei Jing*, including *Su Wen* (素问), *Jiu Juan* (九卷), *Ba Shi Yi Nan* (八十一难), *Yin Yang Da Lun* (阴阳大论), *Tai Lu* (胎胪), and *Yao Lu* (药录). Of course, another reason is that in *Shanghan Lun*, there is also acupuncture treatment, and the content of the acupuncture matches the acupuncture ideas from *Huangdi Nei Jing* too.

On the other hand, the opposite argument is that these chapters were inserted by Dr. Wang Shuhe (王叔和) and other doctors, not originally written by Dr. Zhang Zhongjing. They are not the original texts from *Shanghan Lun*. In *Shanghan Lun*, the sequence of disease transference and development is different from that described in *Huangdi Nei Jing*. The treatment principles for the three Yang diseases (Sweating therapy for Taiyang disease, Conciliating therapy for Shaoyang disease, and Purging therapy for Yangming disease) are distinctly different from those in *Huangdi Nei Jing* (in which Sweating therapy can be used for all three Yang diseases). In *Shanghan Lun*, the Purging therapy should not be used for diseases in all three Yin stages, but in *Huangdi Nei Jing,* this therapy

can. In *Shanghan Lun*, the Taiyang diseases involve the Taiyang Urine bladder, Taiyin Lung; and Taiyin diseases only involve Taiyin Spleen, not Taiyin Lung. Therefore, some doctors say that *Huangdi Nei Jing* mostly deals with physiology and that *Shanghan Lun* deals with pathology.

It might be understood that, in the *Huangdi Nei Jing*, after broadly describing human body physiology, the book mostly introduces acupuncture treatment. Acupuncture works more for meridian-related diseases. Meridian-related diseases are relatively simple. For complex diseases, it does not work satisfactorily. *Shanghan Lun* focuses on herbal treatment. It pays much attention to the whole body's reactions when attacked by exogenous disease-causing factors (pathogenic Qi). Such reactions involve the whole body, and many body systems and organs at the same time, not only one or two meridians. Please note that in Chinese history, the treatments of several kinds of severe infectious disease were treated with herbal therapy, not acupuncture. Even now, acupuncture is used mostly as a symptom-reducing therapy. This is why, in *Shanghan Lun*, there is content for acupuncture, but mostly it talks about herbal therapy. Acupuncture is used as a complementary therapy to the herbal therapy.

Whether or not *Shanghan Lun* borrowed from *Huangdi Nei Jing*, we have to admit that the manifestations of diseases, the regular patterns of diseases, are the objective description in the book *Shanghan Lun*. The question is how we can use *Huangdi Nei Jing* to explain such objective clinical phenomenon.

In addition, beside the book *Huangdi Nei Jing*, there are other medical theory books that were produced at the same or near the same time as *Huangdi Nei Jing* was, such as *Huangdi Wai Jing* (黄帝外经), *Bianque Nei Jing* (扁鹊内经), *Bianque Wai Jing* (扁鹊外经), *Baishi Nei Jing* (白氏内经), *Baishi Wai Jing* (白氏外经), and *Baishi Pang Jing* ((白氏) 旁经). What do these books talk about? Before we know the contents of these books, we have to ask a question: are the contents in the book *Huangdi Nei Jing* the only, and the whole, acceptable theory about human body physiology, the relationship between the health and disease, and the relationship between the human and nature, understood by ancient Chinese?

Dr. Liu Duzhou (刘渡舟): 3

Dr. Zhang Zhongjing clearly said that he "referred to the chapters *Su Wen* (素问), *Jiu Juan* (九卷), *Ba Shi Yi Nan* (八十一难), *Yin Yang Da Lun* (阴阳大论), *Tai Lu* (胎胪), *Yao Lu* (药录), [from *Huangdi Nei Jing*]." How can we deny the medications in the six meridian differentiations in *Su Wen-Re Lun* (素问·热论) (from book *Huangdi Nei Jing*)?

In *Shanghan Lun*, the first title is "Taiyang disease, floating pulse, headache, stiff neck and aversion to cold." It is the response to the content in *Su Wen-Re Lun* (素问·热论) that "Great Yang belongs to Yang meridian; its meridian connects to the Fengfu point." They are the same pathologic reaction of the body. At the same time, there are many sections in *Shanghan Lun* talking about meridians and the passage of disease through the meridians. For example, for the treatment of Taiyang disease, "If the Taiyang stage has lasted for seven days and it subsides by itself, this means that the disease will not progress into another stage(s). If there are signs of it progressing into the next stage, perform acupuncture on points on the foot Yangming meridian to prevent its development." If there is no meridian, there would be no way to use acupuncture to stimulate the Yangming. Another example says, "In Taiyang disease, after Sweating therapy, the patient feels more annoyed. Use acupuncture on Fengchi and Fengfu points. Then use Guizhi Tang again." Without a meridian, how can we perform acupuncture?

The Six-stage diagnosis in *Shanghan Lun* is used to verify the objective reaction of body organs and meridians during a disease course. It is ridiculous to talk about distinguishing of the six meridians without knowing this.

Dr. Hao Wanshan (郝万山): 4

Ancient Chinese believed that Yin and Yang theory is the natural source of life. But they also felt that Yin and Yang separation is not sufficient to determine the quantity changes in the Yin and Yang. They can only show us the quality change, from Yin to Yang, or if they are either Yin or Yang. So, they separate the Yin and the Yang into three parts. These are the three Yin phases and three Yang phases. The aim is to use these new concepts to tell the amount of either Yin or Yang. Among the three Yang phases, the Taiyang phase is triple the amount of Yang, the Yangming is double, and the Shaoyang is one Yang. Among the three Yin phases, Taiyin is triple the amount of Yin, Shayin is double, and Jueyin is one Yin.

In nature, there is s change from Yin to Yang, and from Yang to Yin. Such changes can be gradually changed with the change in quantity. Doctors used the three Yin and the three Yang to describe and to mark the quantity of the Yin and Yang in meridians and organs. Therefore, in the book *Huangdi Nei Jing*, there are the names of organs and meridians.

In *Huangdi Nei Jing*, the Stomach meridian and Stomach organ are Yangming, and the Urine bladder meridian and Urine bladder are Taiyang, based on the physiology function, the amount of Yang Qi in the meridians and organs, and also on the amount of sunshine received on the body surface. They used the names Taiyang, Shaoyang, Yangming, Taiyin, Shaoyin, and Jueyin to tell the amount of Yang or Yin in these organs and meridians.

We should say that the three Yin and three Yang, in *Shanghan Lun*, is not physiology, but pathology.

If in the *Huangdi Nei Jing*, we mention the feet Yangming Stomach meridian, and feet Yangming Stomach, they are physiological concepts. In *Shanghan Lun*, when we mention Yangming, we mean the Yangming disease. If we mention Taiyang, we mean the Taiyang disease. They are pathological concepts. Since they are pathological concepts, the name of the Yin or Yang is related to the location of a disease, the nature of a disease, and the tendencies of a disease's development.

As for Taiyang disease, is the disease location, as described in *Huangdi Nei Jing*, related to feet Taiyang urine bladder meridian, Urine bladder organ, hands Small intestine meridian, or hand Small intestine organ? No, not at all.

In his time, Dr. Zhang Zhongjing collected many cases of diseases. He wrote about these cases on bamboo plates. At that time, there was no differentiation thought of yet. He said, "How can I separate these diseases into groups?" In one group, he put diseases which occurred in the feet Taiyang Urine bladder, feet Taiyang Urine bladder, on the body surface, and occurred due to Cold pathogenic Qi attack on the body surface. He called this group of diseases Taiyang diseases because the body surface contains the most amount of body Yang Qi. He thought that the source of the body Yang Qi is the Urine bladder and the Kidney in the lower cavity. The nature of the disease is a disease in the Yang phase. The tendency of the disease is the early stage of a disease. We say that Taiyang contains the most amount of body Yang Qi, but from the development of a disease in the body, it is the early, lower level of the disease's extent. [876]

The Six-stage diagnosis by Dr. Zhang Zhongjing follows the actual situation of a disease. It does not follow the subjective separation of the amount of Yang or Yin in the body. The six stages in the Six-stage diagnosis system represent the comprehensive results between pathogenic Qi and the health-maintaining Qi of the body. The terminology of the six kinds of diseases, share the same names used in *Huangdi Nei Jing* but have entirely different meanings in *Shanghan Lun*. The names of the diseases in the Six Stage diagnosis system in the book *Shanghan Lun* tell the location, the nature, and the tendency of a disease's development. The name of the disease is a summary of a disease condition.

Dr. Cai Changfu (蔡长福): **30**

Six Stage was not proposed by Dr. Zhang Zhongjing, but rather by the book *Huangdi Nei Jing*. The Six meridians (in *Huangdi Nei Jing*) and the Six stages (in *Shanghan Lun*) are the same things. Without Six meridians, there would be no six stages. Even the Six diseases have been described in *Huangdi Nei*

Jing. They are from the dialog between Huangdi (黄帝) and Qibo (岐伯). Dr. Zhang Zhongjing simplified the six stages (six diseases) from *Huangdi Nei Jing*. He is great.

Dr. Hu Xishu (胡希恕): **2**

Taiyang diseases not only pass into the Half-surface-half-inner of the body but also into the inner side of the body. They can pass directly into the Yangming phase to cause Yangming disease. What does this mean? It means that the Taiyang disease can pass deep into the body, into either the Shaoyang or Yangming phase. This concept is different from what is said in *Huangdi Nei Jing*. In *Shanghan Lun*, Dr. Zhang Zhongjing cited words from *Huangdi Nei Jing,* but very few. We can see that Shaoyang disease can pass to Yangming, but not from Yangming to Shaoyang.

Before Dr. Zhang Zhongjing's writings, there was a book named *Tang Ye Jing* (汤液经). In that book, such basic concepts are readily present, such as the names of the six diseases. During the writing of *Shanghan Lun*, Dr. Zhang Zhongjing referred to and based his thoughts on *Tang Ye Jing*. Dr. Huang Fumi (皇甫谧) was good at medicine, and he was also a historian. He said that Dr. Zhang Zhongjing learned medicine from Dr. Zhang Bozhu (张伯祖). Dr. Huang Fumi lived in the Jin dynasty. The time during which Dr. Huang Fumi lived was similar and closer to the time during which Dr. Zhang Zhongjing lived. If indeed there was a preface in the book *Shanghan Lun*, which said that *Shanghan Lun* referred to the contents of *Huangdi Nei Jing*, it would be impossible that Dr. Huang Fumi did not respect Dr. Zhang Zhongjing's preface, and to say that *Shanghan Lun* came from *Tang Ye Jing*. Most probably there was no preface in the book *Shanghan Lun*. The preface was most likely added by other doctors, such as Dr. Wang Shuhe (王叔和). This preface has affected us a lot. Many scholars and doctors believed that *Shanghan Lun* was based on *Huangdi Nei Jing*, just because of the preface. I believe that they have no relationship.

The six meridians (diseases) in *Shanghan Lun* and the six meridians (diseases) in *Huangdi Nei Jing* are not the same. In the latter, it said that the Taiyang, Shaoyang, and

---

[876] Dr. Martin Wang: The name Taiyang here no longer represents the amount of Yang Qi, but the intensity of the disease. The term Taiyang here no longer means to tell the amount of body Yang Qi.

Yangming are all in the body surface and that Sweating therapy can be used for all three diseases. After three to four days, the disease passes into the inner organs, which are Yin diseases, and that all Yin diseases can be treated with Depleting therapy (such as Purging therapy). This concept is different from the concepts in *Shanghan Lun*. Especially for the sequence of disease passing, it is not first the Taiyang, then Yangming, then Shaoyang. The sequence is funny. It says that on the fourth day, the disease is in Taiyin, on the fifth day, in Shaoyin and on the sixth day, in Jueyin. After the Jueyin, the disease returns to the Taiyang. Who saw such a disease? Is this a strange disease? There is no such disease. Therefore, in *Huangdi Nei Jing*, it tells of the disease passing with such a fixed path. The disease passes from Taiyang to Yangming, Yangming to Shaoyang. We never see such a disease in clinics. Neither is there a disease going from Jueyin back to Taiyang.

Shanghan Lun tells that a disease can pass from the body surface to the inner side, either to Shaoyang, or directly to Yangming, or Shaoyin, etc. The progression pattern is not fixed. Besides, *Huangdi Nei Jing* says that the Taiyang, Yangming, and Shaoyang all dominate the body surface, and diseases in all three phases can be treated with Sweating therapy. But in *Shanghan Lun*, the Yangming disease and Shaoyang disease should not be treated with Sweating therapy.

Shanghan Lun does not tell that diseases pass along meridians. It does not say that the Taiyang meridian is sick or the Yangming meridian is sick, ever.

Ancient people found the patterns of diseases, and their development, via clinical practice. It is an objective presence. It is there. The six diseases are six types of diseases. Why are diseases in just these six big groups? He wanted to explain the reasons. He remembered the six meridians in acupuncture. So, he used the names of the six meridians. However, this affected us a lot (caused difficulty in understanding).

Dr. Feng Shilun (冯世纶): [31]

It is very common in *Huangdi Nei Jing* to use Five-element theory and Four Qi theory to explain body physiology and pathology. Such theories have been developed in China (especially in the middle part of China) even further.

It is known that the main formulas in *Shanghan Lun* come from another book, *Tang Ye Jing Fa* (汤液经法). The latter also uses the Five-element theory for five-organ diagnoses. However, Dr. Zhang Zhongjing used only 39 formulas from it and refused to use the names of the herbal formulas. The formulas named in *Tang Ye Jing Fa* suggest whether the function of the formula is to deplete or to nourish. Instead, Zhongjing used eight-principle diagnosis. The whole book talks about the Six-stage diagnosis and formula-syndrome diagnosis. *Six-stage* means the Taiyang, Yangming, Shaoyang, Taiyin, Shaoyin, and Jueyin. Throughout the book, the original word "病" is called "disease", but actually, it means a "disease stage, disease condition, or disease situation". *Shanghan Lun* is used to diagnose the six stages, then give the herbal formula indications. There is no need to use the Five elements. … Here we should know that in *Shanghan Lun*, the chapters *Ping Mai Pian* (平脉篇) and the first chapter of the book *Jin Kui Yao Luo* (金匮要略) were inserted by Dr. Wang Shuhe (王叔和). For this, it is further known that *Shanghan Lun* does not use Five-element theory or Six Qi theory.

Huangdi Nei Jing uses the Five organs, Five-elements, and Qi circulation in meridians as physiological bases. Its characteristic is to emphasize Five Xing (五行) and Six Qi (六气), to try to match the Five organs to the Five Xing and so on. The treatment of an organ can start from the sick organ, or from other organs. Therefore, its differentiation treatment is Five factor, or the Five-element theory (every treatment consideration includes the Five organs).

Shanghan Lun uses Six Stage diagnosis, then formula syndrome diagnosis. For any disease, first, verify which stage the disease condition belongs to. For the treatment, further, identify which formula syndrome the body condition belongs to. With the verification of the syndrome, use the corresponding herbal formula. Therefore, *Shanghan Lun* is a one-factor theory.

161

Huangdi Nei Jing pays more attention to the diagnosis of the nature of the pathogenic Qi, such as if the disease is caused by Fire, Dampness, Wind, Cold or others, and on the mechanism (reason) for the disease. For the treatment, it tends to deduce the body condition, the Deficiency or Excessiveness, Coldness or Hotness, body Exterior or Interior side, the Yin or the Yang nature, and if it is in the meridians or the organs. The treatment plan is modified according to the nature of the pathogenic Qi, the weather, and the season, during which the disease occurs.

Shanghan Lun makes its diagnosis based on the disease manifestations in the body. It uses the body manifestation to deduce the nature of the disease. The treatment targets Coldness or Hotness, Deficiency or Excessiveness, body surface or inner side, the Yin or the Yang nature, of the body condition (the indication). It does not deduce the exact name of the pathogenic Qi, or the status of Qi circulation in meridians.

More importantly, the two books use the same name for a disease, but the treatment principle is different. *Huangdi Nei Jing* says that all three Yang diseases, the Taiyang, Shaoyang and Yangming diseases can be treated with Sweating therapy. In *Shanghan Lun*, the Shaoyang stage (diseases) should be treated with Conciliating therapy, not Sweating therapy. Yangming stage (diseases) should be treated with Purging therapy, not Sweating therapy. For the treatment of Yin stages (diseases), the difference between the two books is even more apparent. *Huangdi Nei Jing* says that, if a disease has existed for more than three days, use Depleting therapy. In *Shanghan Lun*, only the Shaoyin body surface condition can be treated with Sweating therapy. For Taiyin and Jueyin stages (diseases), it is forbidden to use Sweating therapy and Depleting therapy.

Huangdi Nei Jing separates diseases into Deficiency or Excessiveness conditions, the inner damage disease or exogenous diseases. The treatment is either Weakness-nourishing therapy or Excess-depleting therapy. The treatment principle is different.

Shanghan Lun does not separate a disease into clearly inner deficient disease or exogenous disease. For the treatment,

Depleting therapy and Nourishing therapy are most often used at the same time. This is to nourish the body Health-maintaining Qi first and let the body Health-maintaining Qi works to struggle against the disease.

Dr. Zhai Wangchao (寨王潮): [32]

Always trying to understand *Shanghan Lun* from the meridian theory and meridian-association theory is the primary source of misunderstandings about *Shanghan Lun*. When the three Yin stages (diseases) and three Yang stages (diseases) are summarized into six meridians, the original meanings of the six-stage (disease) concepts in *Shanghan Lun* was simplified into nearly meaningless "disease location". ... Such simplification of the three Yin and three Yang stages (diseases) in *Shanghan Lun* is in fact to narrow the application of *Shanghan Lun*.

Dr. Fang Guoqiang (方国强): [33]

The "treatment" mentioned in *Huangdi Nei Jing* is only suitable for acupuncture, not for herbal therapy. In this book, there are only 13 formulas, and the herbal therapy did not form a systematic theory. So, for the herbal therapy, this book can only supply "diagnosis", not "treatment" by herbal therapy.

There are also differences between the book *Shanghan Zabing Lun* and its predecessor, *Tang Ye Jing Fa*. ... Therefore, Dr. Zhang Zhongjing is not only the direct successor of *Tang Ye Jing Fa* but he also further developed and expanded the application of the herbal therapy in the original book. He actually has jumped out of the region of *Yiyin Tang Ye Jing*, but established his own Shanghan style of TCM.

3 The relationship between the Six-stage diagnosis and meridians

Is the six stages (diseases) in the book *Shanghan Lun* the same as the six meridians in the book *Huangdi Nei Jing*? This issue has also divided many doctors since there is also acupuncture treatment in *Shanghan Lun* too. For example, Dr. Liu Duzhou (刘渡舟) believed that the six "diseases" in *Shanghan Lun* reflect the disease in the meridians and their associated inner organs. It is a summary of the meridians and the organs. For example, the Taiyang disease is actually a disease in the hand Taiyang urine bladder meridian and feet Taiyang small intestine meridian. Also, the Yangming disease in *Shanghan Lun* is the disease in feet Yangming stomach and hand Yangming large intestine meridians as in *Huangdi Nei Jing*.

However, the six meridians, such as Taiyang, Shaoyang, Yangming, Taiyin, Shaoyin, and Jueyin, and the Taiyang, Shaoyang, Yangmin, Taiyin, Shaoyin, and Jueyin stages (diseases) in the book *Shanghan Lun* are different meanings, though their names are the same.

The concept of them in the two books may have overlaps in concept, but they are not at all the same. For example, the Taiyang stage (disease) in *Shanghan Lun* involves the Urine bladder and Lung but rarely involves Small intestine.[877] (The disease in the Taiyang Small intestine in *Shanghan Lun* is reflected more in the Taiyin disease in *Shanghan Lun*.) While for diseases in the foot Taiyang Urine bladder, there are minimal symptoms for the urine bladder.[878] During an exogenous disease, if manifestations of meridian

---

[877] The diseases in the hand Taiyang Small Intestine meridian and organ small intestine are: deafness, yellow color in eyes, swelling in the jaw, sore and swelling in throat, stiffness on neck, pulling feeling in shoulders, fracture feeling in hip, bloating and pain in small abdomen, frequent urination, diarrhea or constipation.
[878] Diseases in the foot Taiyang Urine bladder meridian are: fever, dislike wind and cold, nose stuff, running nose, headache, stiffness on neck, eye bulging, shoulder and pulling, hip as fracture, Popliteal as with knob, ankle as broken; epilepsy, madness, malaria, hernia; pain on the back of leg.

diseases occur, then of course acupuncture can be used for the treatment. This is how we work in clinics; the clinical condition is treated according to its indications. If there is an indication for the use of herbal therapy, we use herbal therapy. If there are indications for using acupuncture, we use acupuncture. If there are indications for both herbal therapy and acupuncture, then we use both. However, we cannot say that the six stages (diseases) in *Shanghan Lun* are the same as the meridians in the book *Huangdi Nei Jing*. At least, the six stages (diseases) in *Shanghan Lun* cannot include the diseases in the eight extra meridians in the Meridian diagnosis system (as in *Huangdi Nei Jing*).

Dr. Ma Wenhui (马文辉): [34]

The diagnosis frame of *Shanghan Lun* is the Six Disease diagnosis and followed formula indication diagnosis. The Six Disease diagnosis is used to verify the disease location and its nature. The disease location in the Six Disease diagnosis is not the meridians or organs. It is the three layers of the body: the body surface, the inner side, and the phase between the surface and the inner side. In *Huangdi Nei Jing* there are only the body surface and the inner side layers. The three layers in *Shanghan Lun* are the layers of disease intensity, and they have physical structures to support the existence of the location.

The three Yin and three Yang in *Shanghan Lun* only summarize the body symptoms and signs. The concept is different from that in the book *Huangdi Nei Jing*. It is similar to the Wei, Qi, Ying Yue diagnosis system developed by Dr. Ye Tianshi (叶天士). Though the disease names are the same as in *Huangdi Nei Jing*, the meanings are entirely different. The six disease concept in *Shanghan Lun* includes the disease nature (Yin or Yang, Coldness or Hotness), the location (body surface, inner side, or between the surface and the inner side), and the body condition (Weakness or Excessiveness).

The Six Meridians and the Six Diseases are two groups of entirely different concepts. The Six Meridians talk about body physiology. The circulation of the meridians has a fixed path. Even if there is no disease, they still exist. The Six Diseases is the pathological concept. It is made of manually separated groups of diseases. If there is no disease, there are no Six Diseases. Meridians, no matter if they are on the body surface or inside the body, they are a line, and the disease occurs only along the path it distributes and along the organs or body tissues it associates with. The Six Diseases manifest in the whole body. The Yin or Yang nature of the meridian tells us the Yin or Yang association of the body tissue and structure, which is decided by the association of its associated organ and the part on the body it passes through. While the Yin or Yang nature of the Six Diseases tells the disease association, it is determined by the disease intensity, the disease location, and the diseased body status.

Dr. Du Yumao (杜雨茂): [35]

The six meridians in *Shanghan Lun* are not the same six meridians that are in *Huangdi Nei Jing*. For example, the chapter *Su Wen – Re Lun* (素问-热论) in *Huangdi Nei Jing*, talks about body surface symptoms, and Hotness symptom. For the treatment, it only mentions Sweating therapy and Purging therapy. Based on this, can we say that *Shanghan Lun* has only body surface symptoms and Hotness symptoms and that there are only Sweating therapy and Purging therapy in *Shanghan Lun*? Of course, we cannot.

Then, is there a hand meridian disease in *Shanghan Lun*? From the contents of the six meridian diseases in the *Shanghan Lun*, … previously, it generally included "no bowel movement, diarrhea, nausea" in the Taiyang meridian (disease) as a disease in the stomach and large intestine. But it is also related to the small intestine. …. All together, there are hand Taiyang small intestine diseases in the Taiyang diseases.

The diseases of the hand Taiyin Lung meridian (disease) is a Taiyang disease. In the chapter of Taiyang diseases, 13 paragraphs talk about coughs or asthma. … They all belong to the Lung meridian (disease).

In the Song version of *Shanghan Lun*, eleven chapters that include *Bian Mai Fa* (辨脉法), *Ping Mai Fa* (平脉法), *Shanghan Li* (伤寒例), *Bian Buke Fahan Bing Mai Zheng Bingzhi*

(辨不可发汗病脉证并治), *Bian Ke Fahan Bing Mai Bingzhi* (辨发汗后病脉证并治), *Bian Buke Tu* (辨不可吐), *Bian Ke Tu* (辨可吐), *Bian Buke Xia Bing Mai Ping Zhi* (辨可下病脉证并治), *Bian Ke Fahan Bing Mai Zheng Bingzhi* (辨可发汗病脉证并治), *Bian Fahan Tu Xia Hou Bing Mai Bingzhi* (辨发汗吐下后病脉证并治), are all edited and inserted by later doctors, and are not the original text of Dr. Zhang Zhongjing.

Dr. Zhu Liangchun (朱良春): [36]

The theory in *Shanghan Lun* was developed and expanded from *Huangdi Nei Jing*. As for the six meridians in the former, they were developed from the chapter *Su Wen-Re Lun* (素问·热论) of the latter. However, Dr. Zhang Zhongjing inputted new contents and made the six meridians in the *Huangdi Nei Jing* more complete so that they can guide clinical diagnosis and treatment.

I believe that the Six Meridians and the Six Diseases are different concepts. The term "six meridians" was shown in *Huangdi Nei Jing* earlier than in *Shanghan Lun*. In the former, they mean meridians. In the latter (*Shanghan Lun*), the Taiyang, Shaoyang, Yangming, Taiyin, Shaoyin and Jueyin, all contain many more meanings. They no longer only mean the meridians but include the results of the body structure and functional status. "Six Meridians" in *Shanghan Lun* summarized the six physiological units. When diseases invade, the "Six Meridians" are the disease locations. Six Diseases is no longer a physiological concept but a pathological concept. They are the principles of diagnosis and the targets of treatment.

With this understanding, the "Six Meridian (diseases)" in *Shanghan Lun* include the location of disease (meridian and organ); disease nature (Coldness or Hotness, Deficiency or Excess, Body surface or inner side, Yin or Yang); and the principle of treatment. These three aspects are the basic contents of indication diagnosis. The "Six Disease Indication treatment" has a broad meaning in clinics. Is there any disease that is not a disease of an organ, meridian, Qi, blood, or body liquid? No any. Is there any disease that cannot be included in the Yin or Yang, body surface or inner side, Coldness or Hotness, Deficiency or Excessiveness? No any. Just because the six diseases focus on herbal formula indications, different diseases, if they have the same indications for a particular herbal formula, can also be treated with the same formula. Similarly, if the same diseases have indications for different formulas, then different herbal formula should be used for the treatment. After understanding that this is the real meaning of the "Six Disease diagnosis", the formulas in *Shanghan Lun* can be used for the treatment of Shanghan diseases, Warm diseases, as well as miscellaneous diseases too.

4   The relationship between Six Jing (six stages, or six diseases) diagnosis and other diagnosis systems

Dr. Hao Wanshan (郝万山): 4

Several diagnosis systems have been developed through the history of TCM, such as Eight Gang diagnosis, Organ and meridian diagnosis, Qi Blood Jingye diagnosis, Disease-causing factor diagnosis, Wei Qi Ying Xue diagnosis, Triple Jiao diagnosis and more. Then what is the relationship between the Six Jing diagnosis (in book *Shanghan Lun*) and these other diagnosis systems? It should be said that the Eight Gang diagnosis system was developed from the Six Jing diagnosis system.

Within the Six Jing diagnoses, the Taiyang diseases are more often body surface diseases, Yangming disease and Shaoyang disease are more often inner-body diseases. This way, we can separate a disease into either body surface or inside. The three Yang diseases are more often Yang nature diseases, and the three Yin diseases are more often Yin nature diseases. So we can separate the Yin and Yang nature diseases. The diseases in three Yang disease stages are more often in Excess condition, and the diseases in the three Yin diseases are more often in Deficiency condition. So, we can separate the Deficiency or Excess conditions of the body, and separate Coldness and Hotness. Therefore, the Eight Gang diagnosis system is extracted from the Six Jing diagnosis system. [879]

The weakness of the Eight Gang diagnosis is that it cannot guide the clinical use of herbal formulas. If you diagnose a disease as body surface or an inner side disease, is it body surface Coldness or Hotness? Is it a Wind-attack or a Cold-attack disease? We cannot tell. Therefore, the Eight Gang diagnosis system cannot be used directly for deciding the herbal formula to be used. Dr. Liu Duzhou (刘渡舟) has an interesting example of this. He says the diagnosis is like sending a letter. The Eight Gang diagnosis allows you to know the name of the street, but not the

number of the apartment. Without knowing the number of the apartment, you do not know which room you should deliver the letter to. However, the Six Jiang diagnosis system allows you to know the number of the apartment and the number of the room. If the Six Jing diagnosis system tells that the disease is Taiyang body surface Excessiveness condition, we know that we need to use Mahuang Tang. If a disease belongs to Yangming inner condition, the Hotness dominates, and the organ Qi is sluggish, then we know that we need to use Tiaowei Chengqi Tang. Therefore, the Eight Gang diagnosis tells us broad information, whereas the Six Jing diagnosis tells more detailed information.

The Organ and Meridian diagnosis system was summarized by more modern doctors. They listed the possible diseases in each organ and each meridian, as Coldness or Hotness, Deficiency or Excess. Therefore, in the Meridian diagnosis system, some contents come from the meridians in *Shanghan Lun*. For example, if the Taiyang meridian is sick, and the patient has headaches and stiffness in the nape, then such symptoms are included in the later Meridian diagnoses as a disease in the Taiyang meridian. In *Shanghan Lun*, it mentions that the Yangming diseases can have a frontal headache, redness in the face, sore eyes and dry nose, and difficulty to falling asleep. Such manifestations are also included in later Meridian diagnosis as the Yangming meridian diseases.

Similarly, using the Organ diagnosis system, later doctors listed the possible disease manifestations in the organs. Some contents were also collected from *Shanghan Lun*. … Therefore, the Six Jing diagnosis supplied disease manifestations allowing later doctors to use in the Organ diagnosis. However, the two diagnosis systems cannot replace each other.

The clinical manifestations found in Six Jing diagnosis (*Shanghan Lun*) are a summary of the real clinical phenomenon. All of the symptoms and body signs can be seen in actual clinical practice. The symptoms and the body signs in the Organ and Meridian diagnosis system are, however, imaged and deduced from a doctor's mind. After doctors

---

[879] Dr. Martin Wang: The Eight Gang diagnosis system is a way of looking at the Six Jing system at a different angle.

analyzed the present data in front of them, they supplied the missing data by logical deduction.

Nowadays, along with the change of disease pattern (spectrum), there are more Warm diseases in clinics. So, after the Ming dynasty and Qing dynasty, doctors found that some herbal formulas used in *Shanghan Lun* worked unsatisfactorily for the treatment of some exogenous diseases. So they developed Wei Qi Ying Xue diagnosis and Three Jao diagnosis. As we know now, the former is mostly used for the diagnosis of Warm diseases and febrile diseases, whereas the latter is used for the diagnosis of Dampness-Hotness diseases. The Six Jing diagnosis, as everyone knows, is for the diagnosis of Wind-Cold attack to the body. With the use of all the three diagnoses systems, the diagnosis for all the exogenous diseases can be completed.

Dr. Xu Jiadong (许家栋): [37]

The aim of Six Jing diagnosis (Taiyang disease, Yangming disease, Shaoyang disease, Taiyin disease, Shaoyin disease, and Jueyin disease) is to separate the body's reactions to a disease invasion into six main domains, e.g., six significant syndromes. Every Jing (disease) has its own unique disease location, disease nature and status. Such a diagnosis system allows doctors to verify the nature of disease quickly from complex clinical manifestations.

Dr. Liu Zhijie (刘志杰): [38]

The critical theory of the diagnosis in *Shanghan Za Bing Lun* is Six Jing diagnosis (Six principle diagnosis).

The Eight Gang diagnosis is an incomplete Yin and Yang diagnosis system. It is not a complete theory. It does not solve the problem of diagnosing a "Half condition". The Six Gang diagnosis system (in book *Shanghan Lun*) included the Yin and Yang into three Yang diseases and three Yin diseases. It allows the diagnosis of "Half conditions" of a disease and puts the three Yin and three Yang diseases into a dynamic flowing phase. It is a complete theory. The Eight Gang diagnosis was proposed by doctors in the Qing dynasty only. It does not represent ancient TCM truth.

Six Gang diagnosis in *Shanghan Lun* and the later Eight Gang diagnosis are the principal methods of diagnosis. The Eight Gang should not be called Eight Jing, and the Six Gang should not be called Six Jing. The term Six Jing is the term used for meridians. It was named by Dr. Zhu Gong (朱肱) in the Song dynasty. The term should not be used without care. The theory should not be mixed up.

Traditional doctors use the "Jing" in meridian theory to explain *Shanghan Lun*, and believe that Six Gang as the same as Six Jing. Some other doctors use Five-element organ theory to understand Six Gang or use Six Qi theory to understand it. All come into the wrong region, making things a mess and reducing the healing effect.

Some doctors say that, if we are not using the Five-elements, the Organ and Meridian theory, how can we make a diagnosis? Such an opinion is a preconceived idea. It is very superficial. Let us examine the book *Zhou Yi* (周易). Is there any Gang Branch and Five-element theory in it? However, the book *Zhou Yi* explains the change and exchange of every movement on the Earth and in the universe in a much simplest way. The Six Gang diagnosis in the book *Shanghan Lun* is also the simplest way to separate diseases. [880]

---

[880] Dr. Martin Wang: In *Shanghan Lun*, the exogenous diseases are separated into six "diseases" in the Chinese word. The diseases are not separated into six "Jing", "meridians", "Gangs", or "principles". The "six meridians", "six Gangs", "six principles" are terms used by modern doctors based on their own understanding of the meaning of the six "diseases". My own interpretation is this: if the diagnosis system in *Shanghan Lun* is used for the diagnosis of exogenous disease, the diagnosis can be regarded as the "six stages diagnosis system (or six phases diagnosis". If it is used for diagnosis of a miscellaneous disease, it can be regarded as "six diseases" diagnosis system.

5 Difference between Classical formulas and Conventional formulas

TCM, through its long development, started from using a single herb, to using herbal groups, and gradually formed a systematic theory system. Nowadays, the most commonly used herbal formula systems are the Classical formulas (经方) and the Conventional formulas (时方). The Classical formulas here means the herbal formulas introduced in the book *Shanghan Zabing Lun*, whereas the Conventional herbal formulas mean the formulas that are organized according to the theory in book *Huangdi Nei Jing* (黄帝内经) and later book Bencao Gangmu (本草纲目).

The most critical point in the Classical herbal formula system is the match between the disease manifestation and the herbal formula. The book *Shanghan Lun* uses Six Stages (Diseases) as the target of the diagnosis, describing the development path and the corresponding treatment of all the exogenous diseases. *Jin Kui Yao Luo* (金匮要略) targets the diagnosis of miscellaneous diseases. Both books emphasize the exact match between the disease manifestations and the herbal formulas, in order to verify and to find the indications in a disease condition for the use of an herbal formula. The indication diagnosis does not pay much attention to verifying if the Qi is sluggish or if there is blood stagnation, Liver stagnation or Kidney deficiency and so on. The "reason and mechanism" of the disease situation or status is very rarely talked about. This does not mean that there is no pathological basis for a disease condition, but it bears in the herbs used.

The critical point of the Conventional herbal formula system based on the Yin-Yang, Five-element, meridian, and Yunqi (Five Yun and Six Qi theory). The impact of this TCM style is powerful and broad. It is the mainstream of TCM from ancient history to nowadays. The books published from the Han, Tang, Ming and Qing Dynasties in China mostly belong to this style of TCM, such as the books *Huatuo Shenqi Mizhuan* (华佗神医秘传), *Xiaoer Yaozheng Zhijue* (小儿药证直诀) by Dr. Qian Yi (钱乙), *Yixue Qiyuan* (医学启源) by Dr. Zhang Yuansu (张元素), *Jingyue Quanshu* (景岳全书) by Dr. Zhang Jingyue (张景岳), and *Bianzheng Lu* (辨证录) by Dr. Chen Shiduo (陈士铎) and so on. The characteristic of this style of TCM is to find out the weakness or excessiveness status of body Qi and Blood, and those of the organs, to find out the reasons for the disease conditions, and then to set up the principle treatment. The herbal formulas, such as Xiebai Sang (泻白散), Zuo Jin Wan (左金丸), Dao Chi San (导赤散), and Long Dan Xie Gan Tang (龙胆泻肝汤), have already shown such thought patterns. The Conventional formula system emphasizes the recognition of disease mechanism (reason for the disease status).

There are many differences between the two herbal formula systems and the understanding of the functions of an herb or an herbal formula. Especially after the Jin and Yuan Dynasties, the recognition for herbs in the Conventional herbal system became much complex and led to the development of the "Eighteen clash herb groups" (十八反) and "Nineteen incompatibility herb groups" (十九畏). Such warnings seemingly do not apply to the Classical herbal formula system. For example, in this Conventional herbal system, the herbs Banxia and Fuzi should not be used at the same time. However, in the Classical herbal formula system, in formula Fuzi Genmi Tang, the herb Banxia is used together with the herb Fuzi.

In the Conventional herbal formula system, the formula takes care of every aspect of the disease conditions. The formula contains a large number of herbs, and the herb category is highly variable. The diagnosis is relatively broad. On the contrary, the Classical herbal formula system contains a small number of herbs. The formula works straight forwards to target the disease. The diagnosis is relatively more precise.

Although Dr. Zhang Zhongjing is known as a "holy doctor", and the healing effect of the Classical formula is commonly described as "marvelous", how come the spread of the Classical formula system is not as broad and not as popular as the Conventional herbal formula system? We believe the reason is that because *Shanghan Lun* was explained from the *Huangdi Nei Jing* point of view by

Dr. Cheng Wuji (成无己) (Jing dynasty), and that the real meaning of *Shanghan Lun* has been mostly twisted. It severely impacted the understanding of *Shanghan Lun* for later doctors. From recent and current history, Dr. Cao Yingfu (曹颖甫), Wu Peiheng (吴佩衡), Hu Xishu (胡希恕) and Fan Zhonglin (范中林), are real Classical formula experts.

Dr. Tan Jiezhong (谭杰中): 6

Chinese medicine is separated into the Classical formula system (style) and Conventional formula system (style). Not only do the Chinese know this, but the Japanese know this also. The Classical formula system is called "Ancient style", and the Conventional formula system is the "Traditional style". Both in China or in Japan, TCM doctors know that the separation of the two systems was done by the "Jin Yuan (dynasty) Four experts". It refers to the four TCM experts in the Jin and Yuan Dynasties of China. Another doctor who lived much earlier than them is Dr. Zhang Yuansu (张元素). He did a terrible thing in TCM history, which caused TCM to separate into these two major systems. The "bad thing" is that he introduced the "meridian association theory" – some herbs go to such and such meridian(s), or such and such organs in the body.

Is this theory completely wrong? In most of the times, it is right. Such a theory is also applied mainly in clinics. It allows doctors to know where an herb targets the body, to quickly understand and remember its function. For beginner TCM students, yes, it is useful. However, is it entirely correct? Not really, because it mostly "narrowed" the functioning regions of an herb.

Both formula systems use herbs for treatment. If the herbs are chosen and used according to the books *Shennong Bencao Jing* (神农本草经) or *Tang Ye Jing Fa* (汤液经法), then the formula is called a Classical herbal formula. The herbal formulas used in the Tang dynasty, and up to the Song dynasty, still belong to the Classical formula system. If the herbs are chosen and organized according to the "Meridian association" theory, this is called the Conventional formula system. In the Conventional formula system, the understanding of the herb function is different from that of the Classical formula system. In the earliest book, *Shennong Bencao Jing* (神农本草经), it only tells about the nature and taste of herbs, such as the herb's name are if they are cold, hot, cool or warm. Later, many books written up to the Tang dynasty were mostly about finding new functions but did not explain more in theory about the book *Shennong Bencao Jing* (神农本草经).

It was Dr. Zhang Yuansu who edited the ancient formulas…and classified each herb into one or two meridians. Is this classification wrong? Not really. The herbs are indeed working in specific regions or parts of the body, such as Guizhi in Taiyang meridian, Gegen in Yangming, and Chaihu in Shaoyang… and so on. However, the problem is that herbs do not only work this way. Such a classification is too careless. It makes it easier to remember where in the body each herb targets, but this is "only seeing the tree, not the forest". It omits the real nature of the herbs and the real function of the herbs.

However, such a way to learn herb nature and function is easy to remember and to use. Also, Dr. Zhang Yuansu was indeed a high-level TCM doctor. So, the "Jin Yuan four experts" were naturally his followers and also had good reputations in clinical work. For example, the formula Buzhong Yiqi Tang (补中益气汤) by Dr. Li Dongyuan (李东垣), which was created by himself or which he modified from the formula Longdan Xie Gan Tang (龙胆泻肝汤), is a famous formula.

However, the "Meridian association theory" only reflects part of the truth, not the whole of the truth. The above five doctors were educated from *Huangdi Nei Jing*. They did not divert TCM too much yet. After them, more and more herbal formulas were created but the healing effects were less and less marvelous. In the time *Shanghan Lun* was written, an herb effect was "one dose allowing the patient to feel effective and two doses cure the disease". Whereas in later times, doctors asked patients to "drink the herbal tea for half a month, then come back to see if it works or not and see if other herbal formulas need to be tried". Of course, some doctors felt that something might be wrong in Chinese medicine and they wanted to end such "useless" herbal therapy. They tried to re-edit the book *Shennong Bencao Jing* and attempted to find the reason for the source of the herbal therapy. Though they achieved a little, the overall results were not so satisfactory.

In the Ming dynasty, Dr. Li Shizhen (李时珍) collected all the theory and herbal nature and function records. He wrote the book *Bencao Gangmu* (本草纲目). His book was criticized terribly by Dr. Ni Haixia (倪海厦). However, the *Bencao Gangmu* is not the source of corrupt herbal theory. The real source is Dr. Zhang Yuansu. When he said that "Gegen brings pathogenic Qi into Yangming", "Chaihu brings pathogenic Qi into Shaoyang" and "Shigao is strong Cold and should not be used in large doses", he entombed the three primary herbs in the Classical formula system for eight hundred years. There are no such things at all! (He is completely wrong!)

In the early stage of Taiyang disease, and if the patient has indications for the use of Gegen Tang, we should use Gegen Tang. Dr. Fu Qingzhu (傅青主) used Xiao Chaihu Tang to treat Wind-attack in the early stage of common colds. It worked very well, and the Chaihu did not bring the pathogenic Qi deep into the Shaoyang region. The Shigao is only cool, not very Cold. Without using up to eight *qian*, four *liang* or one *jin*, it is hard to see its healing effect. But after Dr. Zhuang Yuansu, everyone said the same thing, and most TCM doctors feel nervous in the use of Shigao in large doses, and tried not to use the Classical formulas described in *Shanghan Lun* and *Jin Kui Yao Luo*.

Until Qing dynasty, things started to change a little. Theory in the book *Shennong Bencao Jing* became re-emphasized. This result is not due to the book *Shengnong Bencao Jing Du* (神农本草经读) by Dr. Chen Xiuyuan (陈修园) or the book *Shennong Bencao Jing Bai Zhong Lu* (神农本草经百种录), by Dr. Xu Lintai (徐灵胎), but due to the contributions by Confucians in the Qing dynasty. Some Confucians were also TCM doctors. The important books are *Ben Jing Shu Zheng* (本经疏证) by Dr. Zou Shu (邹澍), and *Bencao Si Bian Lu* (本草思辨录) by Dr. Zhou Yan (周岩). They tested the herbal functions in *Shanghan Lun* by "deduction".

For example, if there are two formulas, then one formula contains only one additional herb. With the addition of the "extra" herb, the two formulas work for very different disease conditions. So, they deduced the effects of this "extra" herb. They then tested this prediction in more other herbal formulas to confirm. For example, if there are two formulas: one contains an additional herb, Baishao, and all other ingredients are the same between the two formulas. The formula that contains the Baishao works for more clinical conditions. So, they deduced that the function of the herb Baishao is responsible for that "extra function". They checked this prediction for the function of Baishao in other formulas (also considering the different dosage ranges). Similarly, there are two formulas, and the difference between them is that one formula contains the herb Shigao, and another one does not. They checked to see what function had been lost without the Shigao, so that they could deduce the function of the herb Shigao in that formula.

This way, they gradually found the functions of each herb at the same or different doses. It is very exciting that the findings of the herbal functions by this method are the same as the herbal functions that have been indicated in the book *Shennong Bencao Jing* (神农本草经). The herbal functions listed in this book had been as difficult to understand before as to understand the book of God. So, the riddles of this book and the riddles in the book *Shanghan Lun* were solved at the same time.

If some herbs did not allow sufficient time for such deductions, Dr. Zou Shu (邹澍) would try secondary authorized books, such as *Qian Jin Fang* (千金方) and *Qian Jin Yi Fang* (千金翼方) by Dr. Sun Simiao (孙思邈). They continued such "deductions", analysis, conclusions, and comparisons with the books *Shennong Bencao Jing* and *Shanghan Lun*. Such a work sounds so difficult but they fulfilled it! This is really the spirit of scholarship. Ordinary TCM doctors have no time and no interest in doing such "research".

Another doctor, who did something similar several years after Dr. Zou Shu (邹澍) is Dr. Tang Ron Chuan Shi (唐容川氏). His theory was introduced in detail in his book *Bencao Wenda* (本草问答), which is included in the book *Zhongxi Huitong Yishu Wu Zhong* (中西医汇通医书五种). His book is of the same important as another book, *Ben Jing Shu Zheng* (本经疏证) by Dr. Zou Shu (邹澍). His theory is that the herbal nature of Metal herbs and that of Wood herbs are opposite and that the herbal nature of Water herbs and Fire herbs are opposite. This is similar to the book *Fu Xing Jue* (辅行诀), which was unearthed from Dunhuang (敦煌). The great secret of "Chinese Ancient Herbalism" was finally opened to the public at the end of Qing dynasty. We, who live in the time of the Republic of China and learn TCM at this time, should feel lucky and happy.

But, is Conventional herbalism really wrong and dangerous? Sometimes, I feel it is difficult to tell. There is a Conventional herbalist of expert level who created an herbal formula, the healing effect of which was as significant as the formulas created by Dr. Zhang Zhongjing. His name is Fu Qingzhu (傅青主). He is a great medical doctor as well as a writer. His book *Fu Qingshu Nan Nu Ke* (傅青主男女科) is a handbook at home. Especially for the treatment of female diseases, his formulas work much better than the herbal formulas prescribed by other doctors in the market.

Dr. Fu Qingzhu based his theory on Conventional herbalism, with Five-element theory, to set up his herbalism and reached the top of TCM. Some other doctors did not follow the *Shanghan Lun* style of TCM but were also famous for their clinical skills. For example, Dr. Yun Ziyu (恽子愉) "gave herbal prescriptions by seeing the reports of lab tests and X-rays". Dr. Peng Yijun (彭弈竣) "did not use Classical herbal formulas". Dr. Pi Shashi (皮沙士) used ordinary, mild, and calm herbal formulas. However, the clinical healing effects by them are also marvelous. It seems hard to tell how, without following the Classical herbal formula system, Conventional doctors can also be pretty good in their clinical practice. Does it really depend on personal skill?

Dr. Ruan Jinping (阮劲平): [39]

Clinical observation shows that most diseases can be treated, improved, or cured by Classical formulas and can also be treated by Conventional formulas. For small kinds of diseases, Classical formulas work better, but in most cases, diseases are better treated with Conventional formulas. Even if a disease can be treated with both types of formula systems, Conventional formulas are safer.

I have thought that the reason might be due to the body constitution and disease spectrum in modern times. The body constitutions of modern people have more Yin deficiency, Dampness-Hotness, and less Yang deficiency. Modern people have a higher life level, have a more ensured life in every aspect, have longer average ages, but they also have some problems. The diet contains more quantity of heat, and people have more incoming heat but less physical activity. The energy absorbed into the body is not entirely consumed; nutrition is not fully metabolized, so there is more metabolic garbage accumulation in the body. This situation is Dampness and Hotness. Also, due to stress in work, the pressure in emotion, shorter sleep times, the body Yin gets hurt. Besides, overeating spicy food also hurts the body Yin and stimulates Dampness.

TCM believes that sleeping is a way to nourish the body Yin. At night, the Yang moves into the Yin, so that a person can fall asleep. However, nowadays, people usually go to bed after midnight. The middle of the night is the time when the body Yin is in its excessiveness status. If a person does not fall asleep at this time, there could be more damage to the body Yin. Also, as mentioned in *Huangdi Nei Jing,* after 40 years of age, the body Yin Qi reduces half. Nowadays in clinics, middle-aged people and the elderly are the most common patients. Among these groups of patients, most of them suffer from Liver-Kidney Yin deficiency. Therefore, overall the body constitution of current people is: excess Fire or Dampness-Hotness in children and youth, Yin deficiency and Liver Hotness in middle-aged or older, or Yin deficiency and Dampness-Hotness in middle-aged or older. Therefore, in the treatment, we must pay more attention to clearing Fire, to dissolve the Dampness and nourish Yin, so the healing effect can dramatically increase. This is the advantage of the Conventional formula system. The herbal formulas in the Classical formula system are relatively more Warm and Dryness. Though these formulas work very well if the body indication and the herbal formula match well, they could also create some discomfort to patients who also have inner Hotness, or insufficient Yin in the body, as well as the formulas intended to impair body Yin. This is the reason that people say that old formulas do not work for current diseases.

My father, Dr. Kong Bohua (孔伯华) has rich experience in the treatment of Warm diseases and miscellaneous diseases. I learned from him and felt that the body constitution for children or young adults is more often Fire or Dampness-Hotness, and for middle-aged or older people it is more often Yin deficiency and Liver Hotness, or Yin deficiency and Dampness-Hotness.

For exogenous diseases, fewer kinds of diseases belong to Shanghan diseases, and more belong to Warm diseases. Among Warm diseases, most are hidden pathogenic Qi syndrome. The nature of the latter is Yin deficiency with inner Fire or Yin deficiency with Dampness.

Because the body with Yin deficiency and inner Fire usually has Dampness, after being attacked by exogenous pathogenic Qi, the disease tends to have Hotness transform faster in the body. In the treatment, we need to clear Fire, as well as to nourish the Yin and to disperse Dampness at the same time.

In the treatment of miscellaneous diseases, keep to the same principle: pay more attention to nourishing Yin and to dispersing Dampness. Many diseases can be cure with such treatment bases.

Exogenous diseases

Nowadays the exogenous diseases are more often Wind-Warm type. Modern people more often have inner Hotness body constitution. During a common cold or flu, the disease easily transforms into Fire inside the body. In my way of treatment, I use spicy cooling herbs, the calm formula, mild formula, and heavy formula together. For example, I use the formulas Sang Ju Yin (桑菊饮), Yinqiao San (银翘散), and Baihu Tang (白虎汤) at the same time. The body surface condition and inner Fire condition are treated at the same time. The most common results are the disappearance of symptoms after drinking the herbal tea. During the treatment, some Dampness-dispersing and Yin-nourishing herbs are also added, such as Shihu, Chao Zhimu, Chao Huangbo, Huashi, etc.

Miscellaneous diseases

Currently, there are not many patients who have Spleen Yang deficiency or Spleen Qi deficiency, but many patients who have disharmony between the Liver and Spleen, a Dampness block in the stomach-bowel, so that the body Qi up-down movement is in disorder. The treatment should be to nourish Spleen, disperse Dampness, calm the stomach, and conduct Qi up-down movement, by using Er Chen Tang (二陈汤), with the addition of some Liver-dredging herbs. In Er Chen Tang, Jupi (橘皮) is replaced by Juzi He (橘子核, orange kernel), and Juluo (橘络, orange kernel and tangerine pith) to increase the function of conducting Qi and meridians. Add Xuanfuhua and Daizheshi to bring down reversed Qi, and use Chao Zhike (炒枳壳), whole Gualou (全瓜蒌), Laifuzi (莱菔子), and Dafupi (大腹皮) to bring down Qi and conduct the bowel. Add Liu Shen Qu (六神曲) and Baidouku (白豆蔻) to conciliate stomach and improving digestion. Chaihu (柴胡) is not used for fear of its possible impairing Liver Yin. Use Xiangfu (香附) to replace Chaihu. Add Shihu (石斛) to nourish Stomach Yin.

The Yin deficiency, Liver Hotness, and Spleen Dampness in inner impaired diseases

For the treatment of current Yin deficiency, Liver Hotness, and Spleen Dampness, the focus of the treatment is in the Middle Jiao and Lower Jiao. An example of the formula is:

Muli 15g (cook first), Shijueming 30g (cook first), Daizheshi 12g, Xuanfuhua 12g (fold with cotton cloth), Sangjisheng 30g, Fried Zhimu 10g, Fried Huangbo 10g, Chuanniuxi 15g, Huashi 5g, Juhe (orange kernel) 15g, Juluo (tangerine pith) 15g, Banxia 10g, Fuling 30g, Shihu 30g, Hubo 5g.

This formula is used very often. It is used for various diseases with some modification for each kind of disease and each patient, such as high blood pressure, stroke, diabetes, gynecological diseases, menopause syndrome, various tumors, and so on.

Half of my clients were treated with this formula with more or less modification.

Dr. Feng Xuegong (冯学功):[40]

At present, Chinese medicine practitioners are almost all trained in TCM colleges and universities. What the school teaches is mainly based on the syndrome differentiation of the viscera (Organ diagnosis), plus the diagnosis and treatment pattern of the syndrome differentiation of Qi and blood and body fluid. The formulas used are mostly the formulas that were developed from and after the Song dynasty, based on Classical formulas with some modifications, or formulas created by the practitioner, i.e., Conventional formulas. To base mostly on the Organ diagnosis, and to use Conventional formulas, are the main ways of currently practicing TCM. Schools teach this way, and doctors practice this way too, after graduation.

There was an article in the Journal Yixue and Zhexue (医学与哲学) in the year 2003, saying that the TCM education system in China did not educate a sufficient number of TCM doctors of high quality. The author surveyed in the year 2000 students who graduated from Henan TCM University in the year 1999, about the jobs the graduated students participated in. They found that 40% of the graduates worked in a medical area, 20% in TCM related job and only 2% worked in TCM clinics and used TCM as the primary means of the treatment. How embarrassing these figures are! I heard from a friend that in his school, there had been two TCM classes, totaling 100 students. Ten years after graduation, when they re-gathered, they found that there were only several students who continued to practice TCM.

Why is there such a situation for TCM in China? Where is the spring (of TCM)? How do we find our way back to the spring? After many years of study and practice, I believe that by following Classical formulas, we may be able to return to the spring of TCM.

I initially practiced TCM for many years. I felt that TCM did not bring me more or less confidence, not to speak of dignity. The experience of applying Classical formulas in disaster areas has completely changed my feelings. I now feel that TCM is indeed good.

I can still solve a large number of clinical problems, many of which cannot be solved by Western medicine. So I sum up my feelings in four points: Jing Fang (Classical formulas) gave me self-confidence, Jing Fang gave me self-esteem, Jing Fang gave me happiness, and Jing Fang gave me a future. I also realized that every industry has its core technology. The core technology of TCM is the theory of *Shanghan Lun*, and the core technology of the theory of Classical formulae is the core technology of *Shanghan Lun*. As long as we are good at the prescriptions of the Classical formulas, then we have mastered the core technologies of TCM. We can be in an invincible position.

After I learned to use the Classical formulas, I gained a lot. Most of the experts in our current team (Zhongjing theory, professional committee of the Beijing Institute of TCM) are young, some of them being only 30 years old, but they are already famous experts in various hospitals. They have a large group of patients.

We often go out for meetings to exchange experience and see many young doctors working hard for many years but who still feel challenged to practice TCM effectively. After they begin using the Classical formula system, the curative effects of their treatments are greatly increased, and their confidence becomes increased. They are deeply grateful for the Classical formulas and Dr. Zhang Zhongjing.

Why do some doctors look down the Classical formulas and believe that the Classical formula system that emphasizes the Indication diagnosis, is too childish? Why do some other doctors like Classical formulas very much and feel that Classical formula system brings them hope and future? How come there are entirely different clinical experiences and views about Classical formulas? To be able to answer these questions, we have to clarify the Classical formulas, to see what the Classical formula system is.

The Classical formula system emphasizes the match of formula indications (symptoms and body signs) and the herbal formula to be used. This is Indication diagnosis (verification). It omits the process of the diagnosis but pays more attention to verifying the primary indication, which can be symptoms or body signs. To choose an herbal formula, let the function of the herbal formula match the disease conditions (indications). It works as if using a key to open a lock. The disease condition is the lock, and the formula is the key. The doctor has many keys in hand. We need to decide which key is needed to open that lock.

The prominent characteristic of Indication diagnosis is that the diagnosis and the treatment are one unit. Diagnosis is the treatment. For example, if the diagnosis is Guizhi Tang condition, use Guizhi Tang. Once the diagnosis is set up, the formula is ready to use. If a patient has Huangqi body constitution, consider the use of Huangqi-containing herbal formulas. Whichever the body constitution is, that is which herb is to be used. The herb and the patient's body constitution are the same units. The "indication" is the relatively fixed symptoms and body signs, which correspond to a given herbal formula. The "indication" bears relative objectiveness and certainty.

On the other hand, the "Mechanism diagnosis", which is more popularly used in the Conventional formula system, is used to find out the reason for the current disease manifestation. One diagnosis can be treated with various formulas. It is subjective and uncertain. It focuses on the "reason" of the disease's current manifestation, such as Spleen Qi deficiency, or Heart Yin deficiency, and so on. The "mechanism" of the current manifestation is the target of the treatment.

Such differences between the two herbal systems are reflected in the clinic as if ten doctors are treating the same patient. If all of these doctors use the Organ diagnosis (the Mechanism diagnosis), there could be eight to nine different formulas prescribed. If those doctors have a consulting meeting, there would be entirely different opinions. However, if ten doctors in the Classical formula system see the same patient and use Indication diagnosis, eight to nine herbal prescriptions could be pretty much the same. Discussions among doctors using this system can be held and treatment agreed upon. This is because the indication for an herbal formula is relatively fixed and entirely.

Because the Mechanism diagnosis in the Conventional herbal formula system is not difficult to master, the theory and the diagnosis seem easy and is known, but the treatment is also easy to get wrong. So, the strange results are that many students studied very hard in school. They had outstanding marks, and they each feel that they would be an excellent TCM doctor. After graduating, they use the Organ diagnosis or the Mechanism diagnosis, and they feel that their diagnosis is correct. Their prescription seems perfect, but the results make them collapse again and again.[881] However, if they use the Indication diagnosis system, it follows the Classical formula system, and the success rate would be much higher.

Clinical situations are complex. Especially nowadays, disease conditions for many patients are complicated. Many patients have developed disappointment with conventional medicine because their diseases are hardly improved. Only after failure in various departments in Western medicine, does the patient finally come to Chinese medicine.

In the face of such complex cases, if using Classical formula system, we commonly use several formulas at the same time (formula co-use). We use two or more formulas at the same time in one prescription. Such co-use of herbal formulas has also been well introduced and demonstrated in the book *Shanghan Lun*. It is not a new way to follow. To use two formulas together is because there are indications for both the herbal formulas to be used.

In the Conventional formula system, the treatment of complex diseases is achieved by modification of herbal formula, by adding more herbs for each symptom. Such a way of clinical practice results in the big-prescription phenomenon. There are many kinds of herbs and large amounts of herbs in one prescription.

---

[881] Dr. Martin Wang: They may feel there is "something" missing between their knowledge and the disease.

We should know that, in the Classical formula system, the treatment path is clear. The use of a formula has an apparent reason. This is true even with co-used formulas. While for Conventional formulas, the treatment is easy to get wrong in the last step. The last step means during the prescription. The diagnosis only points out the direction (such as Heart Yin deficiency), but the herbal formulas or herbs that are used for the treatment of the diagnosed disease condition are not the only ones. There can be many. It does not mean that any of these similar available formulas or herbs would be able to solve the disease condition with the same level of efficiency. It is not easy for the doctor to control this step. [882]

Theoretically, the Classical formula system was created a long time ago, say, at least 1800 years. For a long time after that, the herbal formulas and herbs must have gone through much development. Deduced from this, it can be expected that there would be limitations for the Classical herbal formulas and herbs used. However, as I know, many Classical formula experts have cured so many complex and stubborn diseases just by the use of simple Classical formulas. If we really want to find a weakness of the Classical formula system, it might be that the indications for some formulas are not so clear yet, and the maximum dosage of some herbs for the best healing results is not set up yet.

---

[882] Dr. Martin Wang: The prescription, therefore, becomes a subjective "guess".

6 If the Classical formula system is good, why is it not the majority in TCM?

Dr. Feng Xuegong (冯学功):

This is an unavoidable question. I think there are three reasons: First, the Classical formula is relatively cheap. It is hard to have a good income by practicing this style of herbal therapy. This problem is more severe in the big background of the market economy. Second, many Classical formulas are spicy and Dryness in herbal nature. Many doctors worry that it may cause side effects if the herbs do not match the disease condition. So they quit using Classical formulas. Third, doctors want to use it but do not know how to master it. I think that this might be the most possible reason.

No TCM doctor wants to waste effective and cheap ways for treatment. But in school, teachers did not teach them how to use it. After graduation, they had no chance to study Classical formulas. So, after a while, they forget the Classical formulas. All TCM graduates had studied, more or less, the books *Shanghan Lun* and *Jin Kui Yao Luo* when they were in school. Some of them have a good memory of the paragraphs of the books and their marks for that lesson were also very good. Why do they routinely not use the Classical formulas in clinics? The most important reason is that they did not really learn the Classical formula system. They studied, and studied very hard, but still do not know how to use it. When seeing a Classical formula, they only feel familiar. Why? The most possible reason for not really mastering the Classical formulas is because the way they learned was wrong. Here we have to point out that there are different ways of studying Classical formulas.

I have summarized four styles of studying Classical formulas: the style of Six Jing Eight Gang –indication style; the Body constitution-indication style; the Indication style; and the Six Jine Organ Meridian style.

The Indication style is the classical style. It is what Dr. Zhang Zhongjing asked students to do. I just follow, such as Dr. Huang Shipai (黄仕沛) does in Guangdong province.

Body constitution-indicating style emphasizes the indication and also pays more attention to the body constitution. One practitioner is Dr. Huang Huang (黄煌) in Nanjing TCM University, who emphasizes Guizhi constitution, Mahuang constitution, Banxia constitution, and so on. The body constitution can point out the main direction for the indication diagnosis, so this style is a unique style.

Six Jing Organ Meridian style is used to explain *Shanghan Lun* using theory in *Huangdi Nei Jing*. This style is relatively sophisticated. This is the way that *Shanghan Lun* is taught when we are in TCM schools. It is still the primary way used in TCM schools nowadays. To learn *Shanghan Lun* this way is tough to know *Shanghan Lun* really and to master the ways of using the Classical formulas. This conclusion is supported by the fact that good marks in school do not ensure being good at using the knowledge learned in school.

Another style is one used by Dr. Hu Xishu (胡希恕) and Dr. Feng Shilun (冯世纶). They believe that *Shanghan Lun* and *Huangdi Nei Jing* do not share the same theoretical basis. The Classical formula is developed from a single herb in each herbal formula, a system developed from the books *Shennong Bencao Jing* (神经本草经), *Tang Ye Jing Fa* (汤液经法), and then used in *Shanghan Zabing Lun* (伤寒杂病论). The theoretical basis for this group is Six Jing Eight Gang and Indication diagnosis. The diagnosis system has no strong relationship with organs and meridian.

I feel that among these styles, Dr. Hu Xishu's style is the fastest way to learn *Shanghan Lun*. In clinics, make the Six Jing (disease) diagnosis first, then use Eight Gang (principle), then the herbal indication. The diagnosis process is simple and clear. It is easy to learn and to understand. Many Classical formula followers, whom I know, get to know the Classical formulas and have improved their clinic healing effect by following this way. Following this way, they feel hope for TCM. Therefore, this is a promising way to follow. [883]

---

[883] Dr. Martin: There is no need to emphasize the Eight Gang diagnosis. Once the Indication diagnosis is

A TCM expert once said that TCM doctors could come through the TCM gate only after being 60 years old. When I heard this, I felt uneasy in the heart. What does it mean? It means that it is tough to become a TCM expert. The time length is too long. If we graduate from a TCM school in our 20's, it will take decades to reach 60. During those years, if we did not become good at clinical work, from where comes our confidence and dignity and how can we manage our daily income in the clinic? Just because many graduates cannot tolerate a miserable life and loneliness, (and failure in the clinic), many of them change jobs. If we tell this story and truth to high school students, can we expect that there are still students wanting to go to TCM universities?

Is there any fast and short way to learn Chinese medicine? Yes, there is. It is the Classical formula system. To learn from masters, and to get trained along with the master with real patients, is the best way to learn Chinese medicine. Undoubtedly during this course, we need to get trained in clinical experience and the morals of being a doctor. However, most of all, the most critical point is to learn how to identify the formula indications and how to modify the formulas.

Why are some old TCM doctors somehow conservative and hesitate to pass along their experience to young doctors? It is because it was not easy for the doctor to learn their skills in the clinic. The doctor has spent so many years in the clinic and found the tricks (indications) for the use of each herbal formula. Such a clinic work might be the learning course for the Conventional formula style.

What is the Classical formula system? It is the summary of the clinical experience of so many previous generations of doctors in clinics. It is a mature and reproducible herbal system. The experience is in front of us to share. Because they changed to the Classical formula, many doctors around me, and doctors I know have become famous while they are still young. I feel that, if we still use the Conventional formula system only, the

chance of becoming an expert at so young an age is minimal. Many clinical experiences that could once only be felt and summarized by the age of 60, due to following the Classical formulas system, can now be mastered within a shorter time and such a way of study can shorten the years needed to become an expert.

Dr. Xiao Peng (肖鹏): [41]

Dr. Lu Jiuzhi (陆九芝) in the Qing dynasty said that from his point of view, the best way is to follow the *Shanghan Lun* system. It is hard in the beginning, but it is easy in later practice. If we start from the Conventional system, it is easy in the beginning but it is difficult later in clinical practice. I recommend the books by Dr. Huang Huang (黄煌). At the same time, refer to other books in the Classical formula system. Try to know "what it is" first, not "why it is". Get familiar with the experience of ancient doctors, learn from their experience as if following an operations manual, and try to use these experiences in your clinic, to feel if it works. Do not jump into "theory trap". Do not become eager to know too much from the beginning.

---

achieved, the Eight Gang diagnosis has been finished at the same time.

Dr. Gao Jianzhong (高建忠): [42]

No matter whether we are using the Classical formula or Conventional formula, or even a single herb, the basis of healing efficiency is set matching herbs and disease conditions. In a book, there could be many indications listed, and many formulas can be chosen, but we often feel challenged to use the knowledge or information in the books. The indication match does not mean such a disease pattern can be treated with such and such formula, as shown and demonstrated in textbooks. It means the matching of the formula and the disease's real condition.

In textbooks, they separate the disease conditions into several syndromes and tell us which syndrome it is recommended to be treated with such and such formula. Such a way, no matter how many kinds of syndromes the doctor knows, and some doctors are good at talking blah, blah, does not ensure that he would become an expert. However, some experts only use several formulas or use only a single herb or only several herbs, and the healing effect is pretty good. How and why? The point is that the herbs match the disease conditions. As Dr. Feng Shilun (冯世纶) said, whether using the Classical formula system or the Conventional formula system, the final point is to let the herb or herbal formula match the disease conditions. In other words, the match between the herbal formula and the disease condition is the top requirement of TCM.

Dr. Huang Huang (黄煌):

The textbook works like a tourist map. The pictures on the paper are not the same as the vivid view on the spot. Therefore, to believe that the knowledge and information in the textbook is the whole of TCM is wrong. Especially some textbooks are edited in very low quality, like a low-quality tourist map, with mistakes for the locations and names of a feature spot. If we follow it, we will miss our way. To learn Chinese medicine is like going on a trip. A correct and proper tourist map is useful, but we still need to go by ourselves to enjoy the spot.

7   College TCM and folk TCM

Dr. Qiu Yue (邱岳): [43]

Some college-educated doctors, who graduated from formal medical school, look down on folk doctors, saying that they did not go to university for a formal education in TCM. What the folk doctors know is personal skill, using folk therapy, or secret formulas. On the other hand, some folk doctors do not respect the college-educated doctors either, believing that they are good at talking theory and have no satisfactory healing effect. I feel that either way is not a proper way.

For the treatment of some diseases, the folk doctors indeed are better at giving treatment. They are good at a technical level, but cannot tell why. They can cure some kinds of diseases with marvelous results. The trick for the treatment is what they depend on for earning a living. We should be patient and modest to learn from them.

Dr. Xiong Jibai (熊继柏): [44]

It is very important to learn TCM from an expert. We can learn many experiences. But medical theory is also very important. TCM is the science that needs both clinical experience and theory.

For example, in the countryside, there are many TCM doctors. They have a clinic and have had rich experiences. They can treat and cure many kinds of diseases. However, for some complex diseases, they can feel challenged. The reason is that they have no theoretical basis, so the level of clinical work is difficult to be improved further.

In our clinic, we have met some extraordinary cases. We cannot cure the disease condition 100%, but we can treat many. What we depend on is TCM theory.

For example, I had a female patient. She complained of frequent urination, but the urine color was not yellow. She had to pass the urine once she felt bloating in the urine duct. If she tried not to go, she would feel bloating pain in the hands between the palm and the wrist. After passing urine, the bloating and painful feeling disappeared too. For such a strange disease, how do you think about it? It needs to come up to the theory level. The palm is the region where the hand Shaoyin Heart meridian and hand Jueyin Pericardium meridian pass. The passage of urine is controlled by the urine bladder. The Kidney is associated with the Urine bladder. The Kidney belongs to Water, and the Heart belongs to Fire. The Water inhibits the Fire. In other words, it is the assaulting of the Heart by the Kidney. I used the formula Wu Ling San plus Danshen. The disease condition came under control.

The formula looks simple but if there is no theoretical guidance, how can you think of the solution? We need to think that the urine is controlled by the urine bladder, of the relationship between the urine bladder and the kidney, of the passing zones of the Heart meridian, of the relationship between Heart and Kidney, and finally think of the formula Wu Ling San, and with the addition of herb Danshen to conduct Heart blood circulation. Within several minutes of think as such, there had been so many theories floating in mind.

179

8 The Relationship between the TCM classic books and TCM textbooks

Dr. Huang Huang (黄煌): [45]

Though our TCM theory involves secrets of the universe, from the beginning, we still have to start from one disease, one formula, one herb, and one acupuncture point. So, we cannot avoid Classical books. The books *Shanghan Lun* (伤寒论) and *Jin Kui Yao Luo* (金匮要略) are the basis of TCM learning. Without this basis, it is useless to talk about other theories. In the beginning, when I studied *Yi Jing* (易经), I also tried to launch more research topics on other aspects. I invited mathematicians to analyze the Five-element relationship and invited astronomers to study the connection between TCM and astronomy. On the surface, it sounds fascinating, but the conclusion cannot solve real problems in the clinic. Finally, we stop such trying and start something related to the clinic. Because I am a clinical doctor, I have to study the books above, similar to an acupuncturist needing to study *Lingshu* (灵枢) in the book *Huangdi Nei Jing* (黄帝内经). I have surveyed 330 TCM experts and found that they all believed that the three books above are the basis of TCM and that they are the basis of the basis.

How about the current TCM textbook? It is fine. However, it is only a manuscript for beginners. It is a step for us to learn Classical books.

I mean that the textbook is a book for first-year students. On top of them, there are high school students, university students, graduated students and Ph. D. students. They still have a lot to learn. The contents of TCM are extensive. Its essence is in Classical literature. Its essence is in clinical practice. *Shanghan Lun*, *Jin Kui Yao Luo* and *Huangdi Nei Jing* are from clinics. Do not think that they are out-of-date. They have very practical usefulness.

TCM must be learned from Classical literature. To learn Classical literature, we can then go on the normal path. Why do so many people become confused and puzzled when learning TCM? The reason is that they did not learn the Classical literature of TCM, they only tried to recite the textbook. The contents in the textbook look very organized and easy to remember, but these are words on paper and on blackboards. You cannot find them in clinics.

Therefore, many students can only tell Yin deficiency, Yang deficiency, Qi deficiency, or Blood deficiency. They cannot even identify a Kidney deficiency. If a patient complains of being sore and weak in the lower back and legs, they would say that it is Kidney deficiency. Actually, many patients with neurosis are sore and weak in the lower back and legs.

If a patient fears cold, they would say that it is Yang deficiency. For example, some patients feel cold hands and feet, but actually, they do not have Yang deficiency at all. Their Yang is extensive. They only need to dress in a thin layer of clothes. Why do they feel cold hands and feet? They have Yang stagnation! Their body Yang Qi is blocked on the inside. It is not at all Yang deficiency. Therefore we say that to learn TCM, we need the textbook, but the textbook is not at all the whole of TCM. We should go beyond the textbook and go into Classical literature. By this way, you could feel that you open a new window in front of you. You can see the whole vivid world of TCM through this window. That is where we should live.

Why should we learn Classical literature? In short, it is to train a perspective, an ability to identify truth. TCM is too difficult to learn. TCM has a long history. There are essential things and useless things in it too. If our way of thinking is wrong, we will fall into that trap during our study. Many students had clear minds, knowing how to learn and how to question when they just started studying TCM. Gradually, they become numb, become persons with religious faith. They no longer have the ability to doubt. No doubt means there would be no practice. They dare not propose different opinions. They only believe that they cannot practice in the clinic with high healing effect because "My heart is not sincere." What is the reason? The reason is that they have no science spirit. They cannot separate what is truth and good from what is bad and false.

To learn TCM is like going to a buffet. You need to choose for yourself. Do you see any old TCM doctors learning ready-to-use TCM? Everyone has to try to start by himself, to practice in a clinic. Therefore we say that TCM is not easy to learn and that you cannot become good at TCM without differentiation spirit. If a person has no such differentiation of mind, do not come to learn TCM. Otherwise, you cannot become good at TCM, and you would feel that there are too many falsehoods in TCM. It's not strange that TCM is the result of lifestyle, ways of thinking, and choosing life values by people who lived in different times. It includes folk culture, religion spirit--all in one. It is not as simple and well organized a knowledge system as current science. It is not as easy as current science to understand. We need to learn literature because we need to know our history. Classical literature gives you a stomach, allowing you to digest knowledge, to have a standard way of thinking. This is the goodness that Classical literature can offer us.

Nowadays there is the argument of whether we should continue to use the textbook or change to Classical literature. I insist we turn back to Classical literature. The TCM textbook has shifted direction. The original textbook was edited by old experts. They have clinical experience. The textbooks are of good quality. Conventional textbooks became less and less valuable, and far, far away from the clinical experience. The more people try to target perfect cures, the farther away the textbook becomes from the essence of TCM. TCM is not as good as described by the textbook. The TCM is very sincere and honest. It has actual herbs, actual acupuncture points. Some of them are in books, some in folk medicine, and some others in the minds of experienced doctors. Therefore we say that TCM is difficult to learn. Without a background in Classical literature, without clinical experience, and without a scientific mind, you cannot become good at TCM practice.

I have practiced TCM for many years. In the first ten years, I was puzzled and confused. I read many books, especially many books about various doctors' clinical experiences. After comparison, I eventually found that the books are just that much. You do not need to be confused by too many books. In fact, start from *Shanghan Lun*, from Classical literature.

I always say that the Chinese have contributed to the world too. The Classical formula system is one of the ways we have. Such mixtures of natural herbs can only have come from the land of China. As a big country with so many herbal samples, people tried these herbs and those herbs; people shared their experience and findings. The experience became set (into a fixed arrangement of herbs). If this were a small country, there would be no significant amount of plants, together with frequent wars in history, the Classical formula could not be developed in a small country.

Chinese people have tried and used herbs for thousands of years. They tested the function of each herb with their mouth! Their experiences had terrible costs: many poisoning cases and death! Therefore we should respect what they learned. We should revere our ancient ancestors and Classical literature. We should know the difficulties the old time people had. Many doctors like to add random herbs to a formula. It seems that if they do not do so, there is no way to show their ability. This is the problem caused by the textbook. The textbook emphasizes to organize prescription according to clinical manifestations (the mechanism and reasons of the disease manifestations). It seems that this principle is to add more herbs. In fact, this is unnecessary. If you do not have a high level of experience, do not add herbs at will. I suggest that my students try fixed formulas first. To use a fixed formula does not mean that you are a doctor of low level. Quite the opposite, it means that you know TCM. The structure of Classical formulas is very exact. There are many herb combinations in a formula, which we call the "formula root". They were formed during a long time of practice.

Classical TCM emphasizes the whole body. We believe that a disease condition (status) is related to a person's mind, emotional status, psychological nature, even to a person's social position.

The herbal formula Huangqi Guizhi Wu Wu Tang (黄芪桂枝五物汤) treats Blood Bi syndrome. What kind of people does this

181

formula work for? It works for people of dignity and honor, e.g., the people who have proper nutrition and no need to work hard. Therefore, in the eyes of Dr. Zhang Zhongjing, a disease is not only a disease status but a person of sickness. This way of practice is the real "holistic view".

The current textbooks talk about a disease that is termed by Western medicine. They separate the "disease" into different "patterns". By talking this and that, the book still talks about a disease, not a human being. Why is body constitution theory emphasized nowadays again? Classical literature talks about the body constitution. The only thing is that *Shanghan Lun* tells about the diagnosis and treatment of acute diseases, the course of which emphasizes disease indications. In the book *Jin Kui Yao Luo*, various body constitutions come into a discussion: persons of dignity and honesty, persons with loss of essence, persons of Dampness, persons of a strong body, persons of withered body and so on. We should pay attention to such a way of thinking.

Dr. Lu Jiuzhi (陆九芝) said that to learn *Shanghan Lun*, in the beginning, it seems difficult. However, later it becomes easier. If we start from Conventional disease patterns, it is easy in the beginning, but difficult later. To become a famous TCM doctor, you need to learn Classical literature. The books are *Shanghan Lun*, *Jin Kui Yao Luo* and *Huangdi Nei Jing*.

Dr. Feng Xuegong (冯学功):

The current model of TCM education graduates a large number of students from TCM universities. The textbook is a very important thing in our minds. It is the yardstick. It is the standard. The textbook is right. However, is the textbook right? Not necessarily. I will tell you why not with examples from our authorized textbook for TCM.

For example, the patterns of the stroke, in the textbook, are separated into Liver Yang excessiveness and Wind-Fire up-rushing. The clinical manifestations are paralysis, whole body numbness, stiff tongue, difficulty speaking, or inability to speak, skew of tongue and eye, and so on. TCM diagnosis has two aspects. First is the diagnosis. Based on paralysis and several other main indications, you can diagnose the disease condition as stroke, not any other diseases.

However, can you treat it with the diagnosis alone? Can you start a prescription? Can you start to use herbs? No, you cannot. But Western medicine can. If the diagnosis is ischemic cerebrovascular disease, then Western medicine can start to improve blood circulation, to dissolve blood clots, to protect the nerve system, and so on. TCM cannot. TCM must find more information from the main symptoms. TCM needs to know the Deficiency or Excess, Yin or Yang, body surface or inner side, Coldness or Hotness, before any treatment.

Using Eight Gang diagnosis system, you need to at least know the nature of the disease and the location of the disease, before the start of the herbal therapy. Therefore, after the Liver Yang Excessiveness, and Wind-Fire up-rushing, we note dizziness, headaches, red face and eyes, bitter taste in the mouth, dry mouth, annoyance, easily gets upset, red urine and dry stool, red-purple tongue, and string-strong pulse. All of these manifestations are the indications for TCM treatment.

The textbook tells us that the treatment principle is to suppress Liver, to deplete Fire, and to conduct meridians. The formula recommended is Tianma Gouteng Yin (天麻钩藤饮). This formula is well known. Many TCM doctors have excellent knowledge of Western medicine. They even paid much more attention in the study of Western medicine than to TCM.

If you mention high blood pressure, they can remember Liver Yang up-rushing. If you mention Liver Yang Up-rushing, they can remember Tianma Gouteng Yin. It becomes a chain reaction. Western medicine is good. But if you use the mind and ways of Western medicine to guide the practices of TCM, you become "poisoned". You have a severe and deep "toxin" in your body.

Can all the manifestations be summarized as Liver Yang Excessiveness, and Wind-Fire Up-rushing? Can the use of Tianma Gouteng Yin solve the disease condition?

TCM emphasizes the co-relation among the five organs. Do all the above manifestations belong to Liver Fire Up-rushing? I think that it is not complete. Of course, as a textbook, it tells of typical conditions, to make the learning easier. But among the above manifestations, is there Heart Fire? Stomach Fire? Or Gallbladder Fire too? It is not enough to conclude the disease condition as Liver Fire alone. The five organs are connected, and the solid organs and hollow organs are connected. The Fire is so intense now, how can you only deal with Fire in the Liver alone?

Is the use of Tianma Gouteng Yin complete? Why use Tianma Gouteng Yin? This formula contains Duzhong (杜仲), Niuxi (牛膝), and Sangjisheng (桑寄生). The Fire is so intense, how can you still use Duzhong and Sangjisheng to nourish Kidney with Warm herbs? This formula is not a new one. It was used in the 1950's TCM textbook edited by Dr. Hu Guangci (胡光慈).

Why add Duzhong and Sangjisheng? It is because pharmacological studies show that these herbs reduce blood pressure. They are added to the formula by combining current scientific research data into the TCM herbal system. Now, the body Fire is so strong, and I do not think that it is proper to add them in the formula. They are Warm in herbal nature. It is not proper to use Warm herbs in such high Fire condition.

In fact, many problems in TCM are due to formula modification. With the addition or deletion of an herbal ingredient, the formula loses its original purpose. Why the big prescription, expensive prescription, or prescription consisting of more than 40 ingredients?

What is the proper way of treatment for the above stroke condition? From the view of the Six Jing diagnosis system (e.g., the diagnosis system in the book *Shanghan Lun*), clearly, the disease is Shaoyang-Yangming co-existing condition. Use Da Chaihu Tang with Shigao. The formula also contains Dahuang. The whole formula works to clear Fire out and to conduct the Fire via the bowel at the same time. It might be better than Tianma Gouteng Yin.

Can the healing effect be good if the herbal formula does not match the disease condition? We have many rules for the treatment of stroke. How are they followed in the clinic? It is not clear, though I admit that the separation of disease conditions into several patterns is very scientific, a separation done after analyzing a lot of clinical case data. People spend a lot of effort and energy to summarize such patterns. They have contributed to the regulation of TCM. But its application is not satisfactory in clinical practice. What is the problem?

I believe that the problem is that they finished the pattern separation, but they did not match each pattern with the herbal formula needed for the treatment. The critical problem is that the textbook way did not finish the match between the disease condition and the formula. Therefore the results in the treatment of stroke using TCM are not satisfactory. We have to find another way to improve it.

Furthermore, from the Six Jing diagnosis point of view, we need to know which pattern of stroke is more popular. We have had a look. The Shaoyang-Yangming co-existing condition occupied about 35.7%. Among 300 cases of stroke, 107 cases belong to this co-existing condition. Such a distribution is a commonly seen pattern from the Six Jing diagnosis system. Here, the co-existing condition includes both successive and the concurrent conditions. It is hard to separate them sometimes. The separation is not very significant. The next most popular patterns are Shaoyang disease, then Shaoyang-Yangming-Taiyang co-existing condition. Many patterns are around the Shaoyang.

The formulas to use are in *Shanghan Lun*. The most commonly used formulas are Da Chaihu Tang and Si Ni San. Among the 300 above cases, 89 cases have indications for Da Chaihu Tang.

Another finding is that in the acute stage, there is more co-existing condition than a single condition. Among the 300 above cases, 198 cases belong to co-existing conditions, suggesting that the disease condition for stroke is complicated and hard to treat. In the treatment of the co-existing condition, there is a treatment sequence for the emphasis. For example, if a patient has Shaoyang-Yangming co-existing condition, and it is more Shaoyang condition and less Yangming condition, then we use the formula for the treatment of Shaoyang mostly and firstly. What about the treatment of Yangming? Should we use Baihu Tang? Not really. We may use Si Ni San. If the patient only has a bitter taste in the mouth, only add Shigao, there is no need to use the whole Baihu Tang.

As you can see, the clinical condition of stroke is very complex, how can you use only a single herbal formula learned from textbook to cure it?

9 More about Shaoyang diseases

Expert opinion: [46]

We talk a lot about Shaoyang diseases because, in clinics, Shaoyang diseases are relatively more common. Historically, *Shanghan Lun* is interpreted by Organ (Five-element) and Meridian theory. Even the TCM expert Lui Duzhou (刘渡舟) said clearly that without Organ Meridian theory, *Shanghan Lun* is tough to understand.

However, in recent years, along with the spread of formula-indication match theory, emphasized by Dr. Feng Shilun (冯世纶), public interest in his supervisor, Dr. Hu Xishu (胡希恕), became stronger. Dr. Hu Xishu separates the disease location in the body into body surface, inner side, and half-surface half-inner phase. His opinion has had a powerful impact on TCM society. Though such influence has not reached everyone, it can be believed that there will be a day when people discover its vast energy and hidden power. Of course, what I am saying here does not deny the Organ Meridian theory, which also benefits in the TCM theory world. Here we only talk about my understanding of the Shaoyang disease. Hope that it is useful to others in TCM society.

Here we discuss the difference between Organ Meridian theory and the half-surface half-inner disease location theory (hereafter as Half-half theory) in the explanation of *Shanghan Lun*.

In Organ Meridian theory, Shaoyang refers to the gallbladder and the Triple Jiao. Because many of the symptoms mentioned in the book *Shanghan Lun* are not limited to these locations, doctors use the Liver-gallbladder relationship, and the gallbladder disease must have an impact on the liver, to explain it. So there is a saying that Shaoyang disease also involves the Liver. Also, they applied Five-element theory too, saying that the Wood (Liver) inhibits the Soil (Spleen) so that the disease in the gallbladder and liver can also affect the stomach. Moreover, the Shaoyang diseases involve many other parts of the body, such as lungs, heart, and spleen.

Though previous doctors have tried and indeed completed the explanation of the links between all the locations for the Shaoyang diseases, in clinical work, doctors feel confused and puzzled. Such a situation left a lot of misdiagnoses, improper treatments and prevented the healing of many diseases. The reason for such results is that, in the mind of many doctors, Shaoyang is the gallbladder and the three cavities. It does not matter whether we use Classical literature or the textbook, the definition of the Gallbladder and the Triple Jiao is blurred. Now we can see the weakness of the Organ Meridian theory in the explanation of the disease locations of Shaoyang diseases.

For example, for pain in the stomach region, if the pulse feels like string, using Organ Meridian theory, it is diagnosed as Liver-Stomach disharmony. However, in clinics, such treatment may or may not work.

Another example is asthma. If the pulse feels like string, slippery and strong, with the Organ Meridian theory, it is hard to tell which disease pattern the disease condition here belongs to. Even if all the formulas that are commonly used for the treatment of asthma are tried, the asthma is still there. There are many such examples. Of course, this is only the incomplete part of the Organ Meridian diagnosis system. It is where we need to modify and to improve. With improvement, our treatment can be more effective.

With the Half-half theory to explain Shaoyang disease, the explanation is more flexible. That is, no matter what the diseases are, and no matter where the disease is located, once it matches the diagnosis parameter for the Shaoyang disease, treat it as a Shaoyang disease. This is true, even if the disease is a body surface condition. Some say that this way might be too general, too vague. Then, what is the parameter to diagnose Shaoyang disease? It is in the book *Shanghan Lun*: once there is one indication, then diagnose as Shaoyang disease. There is no need to have all the indications show up at the same time. This is the essence of Shaoyang disease.

My experience is that, with one symptom plus string pulse, the disease condition can be diagnosed as Shaoyang disease.

For example, the patient has dry throat and string pulse. Xiao Chaihu Tang can be used for the treatment. This is my own experience that has been tested and verified for many years. I am not wagging my tongue too freely. Such explanations though do not link to particular disease locations, and they include all the organs and meridians. This mostly expands the target region of the Shaoyang disease. During the diagnosis of Shaoyang disease, Dr. Hu Xishu used an exclusive method. Among the Yang disease conditions, if there is no body surface condition or inner condition, it is Half-half condition. I disagree with this way of diagnosis. In clinics, there are some diseases which are not body surface condition, or inner condition, and neither are they Half-half Shaoyang condition. Therefore I use *one symptom plus pulse* indication for the diagnosis of Shaoyang disease.

For example, for the case above with pain in the stomach region, the pulse feels like string, so that the disease condition can be diagnosed as Shaoyang disease and the disease condition can be treated with Chaihu Tang. It indeed works well. Also, in the asthma case, with string, slippery and strong pulse, it is diagnosed as Da Chaihu Tang condition in the Shaoyang disease. It also works well. From these two cases, we can see the flexibility and practical nature of the Half-half Shaoyang theory in the diagnosis.

Dr. Xing Bin (邢斌): [47]

In the education system in TCM universities, there is no "Indication diagnosis system". What does *Indication* mean? It means the index and the indication for the use of the herbal formula. It is to use the name of an herbal formula to name a syndrome. The Indication diagnosis is to verify which indication the clinic manifestation belongs to. After the diagnosis, the herbal formula can be used directly for the treatment. The advantage of such a diagnosis is that, if the indication and the herbal formula match well, the healing effect is marvelous. Such a diagnosis is different from the commonly used Organ Meridian diagnosis system. The latter needs to find out the reason, and mechanism of the disease then set up the principle of the treatment, and then group herbs for the treatment. There are more steps during the diagnosis and prescriptions. Once there is any mistake in any step, the healing effect is questionable.

Commonly used Classical herbal formulas

Herbal formulas	Treatment targets	Ingredients
Bai Tong Tang (白通汤)	Shaoyin disease. Diarrhea. Jue syndrome. Face looks pink. Pulse feels not very weak (Yang-wearing syndrome).	Scallion, 4 stems; dried ginger 1 *liang* (3g); raw Fuzi (peeled, cut into 8 pieces) 1 granule (10g).
Baihe Dihuang Tang (百合地黄汤)	Baihe syndrome.	Baihe 7 granules (30g); Shengdi juice 1 *shen* (60g).
Baihe Jizihuang Tang (百合鸡子黄汤)	Baihe syndrome. Got after heavy vomiting.	Baihe 7 granules; Egg yolk, 1.
Baihe Zhimu Tang (百合知母汤)	Baihe syndrome. Got after heavy sweating.	Baihe 7 granules; Zhimu 3 *liang* (9g).
Baihu with Guizhi Tang (白虎加桂枝汤)	Baihu Tang condition, with Air up-rushing syndrome, Wind-disliking. Pain in bone and joints.	Zhimu 6 *liang* (18g); Shigao 1 *jin* (50g); Zhigancao 2 *liang* (6g); Glutinous rice 2 *he* (30g); Guizhi (peeled) 3 *liang* (9g).
Baihu with Ginseng Tang (白虎加人参汤)	Yangming disease, with strong inner Fire, Qi-Yin deficiency. Dry mouth and throat. Fullness in stomach region.	To the Baihu Tang, add Ginseng 3 *liang* (9g).
Baihu Tang (白虎汤)	Yangming Qi phase. Strong Fire condition. Dry mouth and tongue. Annoying thirst and wants large cold drink. Face is red. Dislikes heat. Sweats. Pulse feels floating-slippery.	Shigao (break) 1 *jin* (45g); Zhimu 6 *liang* (18g); Zhigancao 2 *liang* (6g); Glutinous rice 6 *he* (18g).
Baitouwen with Gancao and Ajiao (白头翁加甘草阿胶汤)	Jueyin disease. Hotness-Dampness diarrhea, with pus and blood in stool. Qi-blood deficiency.	Baitouwen 2 *liang* (6g); Huanglian 3 *liang* (9g); Huangbo 3 *liang* (9g); Qinpi 3 *liang* (9g); Gancao 2 *liang* (6g); Ajiao 2 *liang* (6g).
Baitouwen Tang (白头翁汤)	Jueyin disease. Hotness-Dampness diarrhea. Fever, thirst, diarrhea, pus and blood in stool, stool-retention feeling inside anus. Or, stomach pain, burning sensation inside anus. Short urination. Tongue is red. The tongue coating is yellow. Pulse	Baitouwen 2 *liang* (15g); Huanglian 3 *liang* (6g); Huangbo 3 *liang* (12g); Qinpi 3 *liang* (12g).

feels fast.

Banxia Ganjiang San (半夏干姜散)	Coldness in stomach. Spits. Nausea.	Banxia and dried ginger, in equal amounts.
Banxia Houpu Tang (半夏厚朴汤)	1. Shaoyang disease. Feeling of phlegm or foreign material choking throat. Difficulty spitting or swallowing. Not affecting eating or drinking. Emotional variation or dry weather can trigger it or make it worse. 2. Asthma with phlegm noise in throat. Cough causes low voice. Nausea with heavy cough. Phlegm is easy to cough up. Cough and asthma subside after phlegm comes out.	Banxia 1 *shen* (15g); Houpu 3 *liang* (9g); fresh ginger 5 *liang* (15g); Zisu leaves 2 *liang* (6 g).
Banxia San and Banxia Tang (半夏散及半夏汤)	Shaoyin disease. Cold-exposure history. Pain in throat. Voice is hoarse. Dislikes cold. Pulse feels floating.	Banxia (washed); Guizhi; Zhi Gancao; all in equal amounts.
Banxia Xiexin Tang (半夏泻心汤)	Jueyin disease. Upper Hotness and lower Coldness. Stomach Hotness and bowel Coldness. Hardness feeling in stomach, nausea and diarrhea.	Banxia 0.5 *shen* (12g); Huangqin 3 *liang* (9g); dried ginger (9g); Ginseng 3 *liang* (9g); Zhi Gancao 3 *liang* (9g); Huanglian 1 *liang* (3g); jujube 12 granules (6g).
Da Banxia Tang (大半夏汤)	Stomach Weakness. Spleen Yin deficiency. Vomits food that was eaten in previous meal. Poor digestion. Difficult to eat. Hardness feeling in stomach. Constipation. Tongue is thick with teeth index on sides.	Banxia (washed) 2 *shen* (15g); Ginseng 3 *liang* (9g); white honey 1 *shen* (30g).
Da Chaihu Tang (大柴胡汤)	Shaoyang-Yangming co-existing condition. Upper hotness and redness in face. Stomach has hardness, fullness, and bloating. Pressing pain and resistance feeling when pressing abdomen. Abdomen is full, big, and thick. Annoyed and nauseous. Shifting hot and cold feeling. The tongue coating is thick and yellow.	Chaihu 8 *liang* (15g); Huangqin 3 *liang* (9g); Banxia 0.5 *shen* (9g); Zhishi (processed) 4 granules (9g); Dahuang 2 *liang* (6g); Shaoyao 3 *liang* (9g); fresh ginger (cut in to slices) 5 *liang* (15g); jujube (cut open) 12 granules (4 granules).

Da Jianzhong Tang (大建中汤)	Weakness in digestive system. Spleen-Stomach Yang deficiency. Nausea. Cannot eat. Strong coldness pain; refuses to press the painful region. Abdomen is with big and fierce up-down, left-right impulse.	Shujiao 2 *he* (6g); dried ginger 4 *liang* (15g); Ginseng 2 *liang* (10g).
Da Qinglong Tang (大青龙汤)	1. Cold-exposure history. Outside Coldness, inner Hotness. Fever, chills, body pain, no sweat, annoyed. Hard to fall asleep. Coughing and chest pain. Phlegm is yellow and sticky. 2. Body heaviness feeling, sometimes severe and other times less. 3. Body swelling. Difficulty turning body. Body constitution is strong.	Dried ginger 4 *liang* (15g); Ginseng 2 *liang* (10g); Yitang 1 *shen* (60g).
Da Wutou Jiang (大乌头煎)	Strong Coldness inside the body. Coldness hernia. Pain around navel. Cold sweats. Deep and tight pulse.	Wutou (big size, peeled) 5.
Da Xianxiong Tang (大陷胸汤)	Water-Hotness Jie-xiong syndrome. Hardness, fullness and strong pain in whole abdomen. Refuses to press the abdomen, which feels stone-firm. Strongly annoyed feeling. No strong fever.	Dahuang (peeled) 6 *liang* (10-20g); Mangxiao 1 *shen* (12-15g); Gansui (grind into powder) 1 *qianbi* (1-3g).
Da Xianxiong Wan (大陷胸丸)	1. Water-Hotness Jie-Xiong syndrome. Stiffness in neck. 2. With Da Xiangxiong Tang condition, but the disease is less severe or body is weak.	Dahuang (peeled) 0.5 *jin* (24g); Mangxiao 0.5 *jin* (30g): Qinglizi (processed) 0.5 *jin* (18g); almond (remove peel and tip, processed to dark) 0.5 *jin* (18g); Gansui 1 *qianbi* (1.5 to 3g).
Boye Tang (柏叶汤)	Various bleeding due to Weakness-Coldness in Spleen system.	Boye 3 *liang* (9g); dried ginger 3 *liang* (9g); Aye 3 handles (9g).
Chai Bai Tang (柴白湯)	Taiyang-Yangming-Shaoyang co-existing condition. Strongly annoyed. Strong thirst.	Xiao Chaihu Tang, but subtracting Banxia; fresh ginger; Shigao; Zhimu; glutinous rice.
Chai Xian He Fang (柴陷合方)	Shaoyang disease with annoyed feeling. Not-smooth bowel movement. Or with chest pain or upper abdominal pain (due to	Banxia (6g); Gualou kernel (4g); Chaihu (4g); Huanglian (2g); Huangqin (2g); Ginseng

	Phlegm, Qi, Fire entanglement).	(1.4g); Gancao (1g); fresh ginger (1g); jujube 1 granule.
Chaihu Biejia Tang (柴胡鳖甲汤)	Withered condition. Night sweats. Continuous coughing. Withered yellow color in face. Weakness in arms and legs. No desire to eat.	Chaihu (30g); turtle shell (processed) (30g); Digupi (45g); Zhimu (baked to dry) (30g).
Chaihu Guizhi Ganjiang Tang (柴胡桂枝干姜汤)	1. Shaoyang disease with inner Weakness-Coldness, or Gallbladder Hotness-Spleen Weakness. Slight fullness in chest and under rib-arches. Thirst. Difficulty in urination. Shifting hot and cold feeling. Annoyed feeling. Loose stool. 2. Cold type malaria. More cold feeling, with slight, or even no, hot feeling.	Chaihu 0.5 *jin* (24g); Guizhi (peeled) 3 *liang* (9g); dried ginger 2 *liang* (6g); Gualou root 4 *liang* (12g); Huangqin 3 liang (9g); oyster shell 2 *liang* (6g); Zhi Gancao 2 *liang* (6g).
Chaihu Guizhi Tang (柴胡桂枝汤)	1. Shaoyang-Taiyang co-existing condition. Chilly, hot, sweaty, or hot-chilly shifting feeling. Stuffy nose and belch. Headache and stiff neck. 2. Common cold with pain and fullness in chest and under rib-arches. Annoying pain in arms and legs. Symptoms are more severe in the morning and less in afternoon. 3. Sweats more in the morning. 4. Specifically used in the treatment of epilepsy, or high fever, or common cold in weak person.	Chaihu 4 *liang* (12g); Guizhi 1.5 *liang* (4.5g); Ginseng 1.5 *liang* (4.5g); Zhi Gancao 1 *liang* (3g); Banxia (washed) 2.5 he (6g); Huangqin 1.5 *liang* (4.5g); Shaoyao 1.5 *liang* (4.5g); jujube 6 granules (3 granules); fresh ginger (cut into slices) 1.5 *liang* (4.5g).
Chaihu Jiang Wei Tang (柴胡姜味湯)	Shaoyang disease with Cold-choking on the lung. Lung is in Coldness. Coughing.	This formula is developed from Xiao Chaihu Tang by subtracting Ginseng, jujube, and fresh ginger, but adding dried ginger and Wuweizi.
Chaihu Jiedu Tang (柴胡解毒湯)	Long term Dampness-Hotness in the Liver and Gallbladder. Toxic-poisoning formed. Pain in the liver region. Dislikes oily food. Frequent nausea. Fatigue. Short and yellow urine. The tongue coating is thick-greasy.	This formula is developed from Xiao Chaihu Tang, but subtracting Ginseng, Gancao, and jujube, and with the addition of Yinchen, Tufuling, Fengweicao, and

Caoheche.

Chaihu with Longgu Muli Tang (柴胡加龙骨牡蛎汤)	Jueyin disease. Chest fullness, annoyed feeling, poor sleep, scared or frightened, delirious speech, depression, dislikes cold.	Chaihu 5 *liang* (12g); Longgu 1.5 *liang* (5g); Huangqin 1.5 *liang* (5g); fresh ginger 1.5 *liang* (5g); Qiandan (red lead) 1.5 *liang* (5g); Ginseng 1.5 *liang* (5g); Guizhi (peeled) 1.5 *liang* (5g); Fuling 1.5 *liang* (5g); Banxia (washed) 2.5 *he* (6g); Dahuang 2 *liang* (6g); oyster shell 1.5 *liang* (6g); jujube (cut open) 6 granules (3 granules).
Chaihu with Mangxiao Tang (柴胡加芒硝汤)	Shaoyang disease with Dryness-Hotness in stomach. Wave-fever in later evening. Discomfort under rib-arches. Bitter taste in mouth and annoyed and perturbed feelings.	Add Mangxiao (6 *liang*) to Xiao Chaihu Tang.
Chaihu without Banxia but add Gualou Tang (柴胡去半夏加栝蒌汤)	Xiao Chaihu Tang condition. No nausea but with strong thirst.	Chaihu 8 *liang* (24g); Ginseng 3 *liang* (9g); Huangqin 3 *liang* (9g); Zhi Gancao 3 *liang* (9g); Gualou root 4 *liang* (12g); fresh ginger 2 *liang* (6g); jujube 12 granules (4 granules).
Chi Wan (赤丸)	Spleen-Stomach Yang deficiency. Cold pathogenic Qi and thin-phlegm rush-up to cause abdominal pain.	Fuling 4 *liang* (12g); Wutou (processed) 2 *liang* (6g); Banxia (washed) 4 *liang* (12g); Xixin 1 *liang* (3g).
Chishizhi Yuyuliang Tang (赤石脂禹余粮汤)	Spleen-Kidney Yang deficiency. Coldness-Dampness blockage in the middle part of the body. Yang cannot hold the bowel movement. Patient has Slippery diarrhea.	Chishizhi (break) 1 *jin* (30g); Yuyuliang (break) 1 *jin* (30g).

Chixiaodou Danggui San (赤小豆当归散)	Fox-puzzling syndrome (similar to Behcet's syndrome). Dampness-Hotness-toxic in Blood phase. Eyes are red like a bird's. Hot diarrhea with blood in stool due to Hotness-toxic in large intestine.	Chixiaodou 3 *shen* (rinsed in water to get sprouts, then dried (150g); Danggui (30g).
Dahuang Fuzi Tang (大黄附子汤)	Yang deficiency and Coldness-Excessiveness inside. Pain on one side of the body. Pulse feels tight-string. Pain is triggered by eating or drinking cold foodstuffs or cold environment.	Dahuang 3 *liang* (9g); processed Fuzi 3 granules (15g); Xixin 2 *liang* (6g).
Dahuang Gancao Tang (大黄甘草汤)	1. Stomach-Bowel Hotness but not with more Dryness-Firmness. Stool is difficult to pass. 2. Vomits soon as after eating (due to Stomach Hotness and Excessiveness).	Dahuang 4 *liang* (12g); Zhibancao 1 *liang* (3g).
Dahuang Gansui Tang (大黄甘遂汤)	Water-blood entanglement in Bloodroom. Fullness and pain in lower abdomen. Refuses to press the lower abdomen. Difficulty in urination. Constipation.	Dahuang 4 *liang* (12g); Gansui 2 *liang* (6g); Ajiao 2 *liang* (6g).
Dahuang Huanglian Xiexin Tang (大黄黄连泻心汤)	1. Hotness Pi syndrome in stomach region. Pulse feels floating in the Cun and Guan positions on the wrist. 2. Hotness in all three Jiao.	Dahuang 2 *liang* (6g); Huanglian 1 *liang* (3g); Huangqin 1 *liang* (3g).
Dahuang Mudanpi Tang (大黄牡丹皮汤)	Hotness-Stagnation, swelling and knob in lower abdomen. Inflammation in lower part of the abdomen. Area is red with swelling, heat, pain.	Dahuang 4 *liang* (10g); Danpi (peony tree bark) 1 *liang* (5g); peach kernel 15 granules (12g); Dongguaren (winter melon kernel) 0.5 *jin* (20g); Mangxiao 3 *he* (5g).
Dahuang Xiaoshi Tang (大黄硝石汤)	Jaundice. More Hotness than Dampness.	Dahuang 4 *liang* (12g); Huangbo 4 *liang* (12g); Xiaoshi 4 *liang* (12g); Zhizi 15 granules (9g).

Dahuang Zhechong Wan (大黄蛰虫丸)	Withered condition. Abdomen looks full. Has no desire to eat. Skin is dry as fish scales. Eyes look dark and dim. Very dry on some regions of skin, with dander easily falling.	Dahuang 10 *liang* (300g); Gancao 3 *liang* (90g); peach kernel 1 *shen* (120g); almond (fried) 1 *shen* (120g); Shaoyao 4 *liang* (120g) Dihuang 10 *liang* (300g); dried lacquer 1 *liang* (30g); Zhechong (fired) 1 *shen* (30g); Shuizhi 100 bodies (60g); Qicao 1 *shen* (45g); Zhechong 0.5 *shen* (90g).
Danggui Beimu Kushen Wan (当归贝母苦参丸)	1. Difficulty in urination or bowel movement in pregnant women. Urination is spontaneous, continuous, drop by drop; coarse pain in urinary duct; urine is short and yellow. Constipation. (Urinary infection in weak body condition). 2. Dampness-Hotness type skin rash.	Danggui 4 *liang* (12g); Beimu 4 *liang* (12g); Kushen 4 *liang* (12g).
Danggui Jianzhong Tang (当归建中汤)	1. Withered condition. Body is thin and weak with abdominal pain. Short of breath. Pain in lower abdomen which can move to the lower back. Spontaneous sweating. No desire to eat. 2. Body pain due to Blood stagnation.	Danggui 4 *liang* (12g); Guizhi 3 *liang* (9g); Shaoyao 6 *liang* (18g); fresh ginger 3 *liang* (9g); Zhigancao 2 *liang* (6g); jujube 6 granules.
Danggui Shaoyao San (当归芍药散)	Various abdominal pains in women. Liver-Spleen disharmony. Disease in Blood-water phase. Basic condition is anemia with water accumulation in the body. Weakness in body constitution and inner organs, but less symptoms in digestive system.	Danggui 3 *liang* (9g); Shaoyao 1 *jin* (50g); Fuling 4 *liang* (12g); Chuanxiong 8 *liang* (24g); Baizhu 4 *liang* (12g); Zexie 8 *liang* (24g).
Danggui Shengjiang Yangrou Tang (当归生姜羊肉汤)	Blood deficiency with Coldness inside. Abdominal pain. Abdomen likes warm and dislikes cold. Cold body constitution. Not easy to sweat usually. Cold hands and feet. Used as Blood-nourishing therapy for patients after chemotherapy or radiation therapy.	Danggui 3 *liang* (9g); fresh ginger 5 *liang* (15g); mutton 2 *jin* (50g).

Danggui Si Ni with Wuzhuy Shengjing Tang (当归四逆加吴茱萸生姜汤)	Similar to Danggui Si Ni Tang condition but much worse. Pulse feels faint.	To Danggui Si Ni Tang, add Wuzhuyu 2 *shen* (5g); fresh ginger (cut) 8 *liang* (15g).
Danggui Si Ni Tang (当归四逆汤)	Blood deficiency with Coldness. Cold hands and feet and pain due to contracting of micro blood vessels in hands, feet, nose, ears, etc. Pulse feels thin and weak.	Danggui 3 *liang* (10-20g); Guizhi (peeled) 3 *liang* (10-20g); Baishao 3 *liang* (10-30g); Xixin 3 *liang* (3-10g); Zhigancao 2 *liang* (6-10g); Tongcao 2 *liang* (6g); jujube 25 granules (10-30g).
Dangui San (当归散)	Early signs of abortion due to Blood Hotness. Irregular and irritated fetus movement. Pain in chest or abdomen from time to time. Fullness or stagnation feeling under rib-arch. Spit water-like saliva.	Danggui 1 *jin* (50g); Huangqin 1 *jin* (50g); Shaoyao 1 *jin* (50g); Chuanxiong 1 *jin* (50g); Baizhu 8 *liang* (25g).
Didang Tang (抵挡汤)	Long term Blood stagnation in lower abdomen region. Lower abdomen feels stiff, hard, full, painful. Strongly annoyed and perturbed feeling, or madness. Constipation or black stool. Urination is normal.	Leech (dried) 30 bodies (5g); gadfly (removal of feet and wings, dried) 30 bodies (10g); Dahuang (peeled, washed with wine) 3 *liang* (10g); peach kernel (peeled, dried) 30 granules (10g).
Didang Wan (抵挡丸)	Similar to Didang Tang condition, but not severe. Lower abdomen is full but not hard.	Leech (dried) twenty bodies (6g); gadfly (dried, removal of feet and wings) 20 bodies (3g); peach kernel (removal of peel and tip) 25 granules (9g); Dahuang (washed with wine) 3 *liang* (9g).
Fangji Dihuang Tang (防己地黄汤)	Shaoyin disease. Blood deficiency, which results in inner Hotness. The Hotness disturbs emotions and mood, causing madness, talking-to-self, running here and there. Very difficult and very poor sleep. Pulse feels floating.	Fangji 1 *qian* (0.3g); Guizhi 3 *qian* (0.9g); Fangfeng 3 *qian* (0.9g); Gancao 2 *qian* (0.6g).

Fangji Fuling Tang (防己茯苓汤)	Spleen deficiency. Spleen fails to transport water and to conduct water metabolism. Water accumulated under skin, with sunken skin when pressed. Muscles quiver or tremble. Urination is difficult.	Fangji 3 *liang* (9g); Huangqi 3 *liang* (9g); Guizhi 3 *liang* (9g); Fuling 6 *liang* (18g); Gancao 2 *liang* (6g).
Fangji Huangqi Tang (防己黄芪汤)	Spleen deficiency. Spleen fails to transport water and to conduct water metabolism. Swelling, which is more down towards the lower back. Sweating and joint pain. Huangqi body constitution.	Fangji 1 *liang* (12g); Huangji 1 *liang* and 1 *fen* (15g); Baizhu 7 *qian* and 0.5 (9g); Gancao (fried) 0.5 *liang* (6g).
Fanshi Tang (矾石汤)	Dampness-toxic rinse in the meridians and tissues. Swelling or ulcer or very itchy on feet. Tongue is thin-yellow. Pulse feels deep or slippery. (The odor of lesion is not very bad.)	Fanshi 2 *liang*.
Fengyin Tang (风引汤)	Strong Hotness and Fire in Heart and Liver. Fire produces Wind. Stroke, epilepsy, muscle spasms, stiffness.	Dahuang 4 *liang* (12g); dried ginger 4 *liang* (12g); Longgu 4 *liang* (12g); Guizhi 3 *liang* (9g); Gancao 2 *liang* (6g); Muli 2 *liang* (6g); Hanshuishi 6 *liang* (18g); Huashi 6 *liang* (18g); Chishizhi 6 *liang* (18g); Baishizhi 6 *liang* (18g); Zishiying 6 *liang* (18g); Shigao 6 *liang* (18g).
Fuling Gancao Tang (茯苓甘草汤)	Garbage water retention in stomach. Palpitations. Cold hands and feet (Water Jue syndrome). Poor sleep due to water in stomach.	Fuling 2 *liang* (6g); Guizhi (peeled) 2 *liang* (6g); Zhigancao 1 *liang* (3g); fresh ginger 3 *liang* (9g).
Fuling Si Ni Tang (茯苓四逆汤)	Shaoyin disease. Heart Yang Qi is very weak. Yang Qi escapes. Water rushes up to attack the Heart to disturb Heart. Patient feels palpitations and annoyed.	Fuling 6 *liang* (12g); Ginseng 1 *liang* (3g); raw Fuzi 1 granule; Zhigancao 2 *liang* (6g); dried ginger 1.5 *liang* (4.5g).
Fuling Xingren Gancao Tang (茯苓杏仁甘草汤)	Thin-phlegm blockage in chest causes Chest Bi syndrome. Fullness and bloating feeling in chest.	Fuling 3 *liang* (9g); almond fifty granules (9g); Gancao 1 *liang* (3g).

Fuling Yin (茯苓饮)	Taiyin inner Weakness and Coldness. Spleen-Stomach weakness. Garbage water accumulated. Fullness or bloating feeling in stomach region. After vomiting, feel bloated. Cannot eat.	Fuling 3 *liang* (9g); Ginseng 3 *liang* (9g); Baizhu 3 *liang* (9g); Zhishi 2 *liang* (6g); orange peel 2.5 *liang* (7.5g); fresh ginger 4 *liang* (12g).
Fuling Zexie Tang (茯苓泽泻汤)	Thin-phlegm accumulation. Thirst for water. The water blocks the Stomach Yang Qi, causing vomit. After vomiting, desires more water.	Fuling 0.5 *jin* (24g); Zexie 4 *liang* (12g); Guizhi 2 *liang* (6g); Baizhu 3 *liang* (9g); fresh ginger 4 *liang* (12g).
Fuzi Jingmi Tang (附子粳米汤)	Spleen-Stomach Yang deficiency. Water-Dampness accumulation inside. The garbage water brings Coldness air, rushes and jostles in between the intestines. Feel cold and severe pain in abdomen. Thunderous noise in the abdomen. Reversing fullness feeling in chest and nausea.	Fuzi (processed) 1 granule (5g); Banxia 0.5 *shen* (12g); Zhigancao 1 *liang* (3g); jujube 10 granules (4 granules); Glutinous rice 0.5 *shen* (15g).
Fuzi Tang (附子汤)	Shaoyin disease. Weakness and Coldness. Pain in bone and joints. Back is cold. Cold hands and feet. Or cold pain in whole body.	Processed Fuzi (peeled, cut into 8 slices) 2 granules (15g); Fuling 3 *liang* (9g); Ginseng 2 *liang* (6g); Shaoyao 3 *liang* (9g).
Gan Mai DazaoTang (甘麦大枣汤)	Organ Restless syndrome. Heart-Spleen impairment, Liver Qi disharmony. Easily feels sad. Easily cry. Easily yawn a lot. Continuous laughing or crying. More like hysteria.	Gancao 3 *liang* (9g); wheat 1 *shen* (15-30g); jujube 10 granules (5 granules).
Gancao Fengmi Tang (甘草粉蜜汤)	Worm disease. Abdominal pain, which comes and goes. Spits.	Gancao 2 *liang* (6g); Glutinous rice powder 1 *liang* (3g); honey 4 *liang* (12g).
Gancao Ganjiang Tang (甘草干姜汤)	1. Spleen Yang deficiency, then Stomach Coldness and Weakness. Vomiting. Cold hands and feet. Dry throat. Spasms in calf, Annoyed feeling. Chilly. 2. Lung withered syndrome. Spits.	Zhigancao 4 *liang* (12g); dried ginger 2 *liang* (6g).
Gancao Mahuang Tang (甘草麻黄汤)	Wind-Cold choking in body surface. No sweat. Swelling. The swelling starts from upper part of the body. No sunken skin when pressing on swelling skin.	Gancao 2 *liang* (6g); Mahuang 4 *liang* (12g).

196

Gancao Tang (甘草汤)	1. Shaoyin disease. Sore throat. 2. Lung withered syndrome. Spits.	Gancao 2 *liang* (6g).
Gancao Xiexin Tang (甘草泻心汤)	1. Coldness-Hotness condition. Upper Hotness and lower Coldness. Stomach Hotness and bowel Coldness. Fullness and Hardness in stomach region. Vomiting and diarrhea. Undigested food in stool. Thunder noise in abdomen. Annoyed and perturbed feeling. Child night crying. Oral ulcer but diarrhea too. 2. Fox puzzling syndrome (Behcet's syndrome).	Banxia 0.5 *shen* (10g); Huangqin 3 *liang* (15g); dried ginger 3 *liang* (10g); Ginseng 3 *liang* (15g); Zhigancao 4 *liang* (20g); Huanglian 1 *liang* (5g); jujube 12 granules (20g).
Ganjiang Banxia Renshen Wan (干姜半夏人参丸)	1. Spleen-Stomach Weakness, garbage water accumulation in stomach. Nausea and continuous vomiting. Hardness and fullness in stomach region. Cold hands and feet. Pulse feels thin. 2. Pregnancy vomit due to Spleen-Stomach Weakness and Coldness.	Dried ginger 1 *liang* (9g); Ginseng 1 *liang* (9g); Banxia 2 *liang* (18g); fresh ginger 1 *liang* (10g).
Ganjiang Fuzi Tang (干姜附子汤)	Shaoyin disease. Yang Qi floats to disturb Heart and cause annoyed and perturbed feeling, restless feeling, hard to be calm down, but pretty quiet at night.	Dried ginger 1 *liang* (9g); Fuzi (cut into 8 slices) 1 granule (9g).
Ganjiang Huangqin Huanglian Ginseng Tang (干姜黄连黄芩人参汤)	Spleen-Stomach Weakness. Coldness and Hotness reject each other. Vomits after eating. Pregnancy vomit due to the Hotness-Coldness rejection syndrome.	Dried ginger 3 *liang* (9g); Huangqin 3 *liang* (9g); Huanglian 3 *liang* (9g); Ginseng 3 *liang* (9g).
Gegen Huangqin Huanglian Tang (葛根芩连汤)	Body Exterior condition remains when pathogenic Qi invades into bowel. Diarrhea with very bad odor in stool. Hot feeling inside anus. (Hotness diarrhea). Hardness and fullness in stomach. Annoying heat in chest. Asthma and sweating. Dry mouth and thirst. Tongue is yellow and pulse feels fast.	Gegen 0.5 *jin* (15g); Huangqin 3 *liang* (9g); Huanglian 3 *liang* (9g); Gancao 2 *liang* (6g).
Gegen with Banxia Tang (葛根加半夏汤)	Taiyang-Yangming co-existing. No diarrhea, but nausea.	To Gegen Tang, add Banxia (3 *liang*) (9g).

Gegen Tang (葛根汤)	1. Taiyang disease. No sweat, but dislikes wind. Stiffness in neck and back. 2. Taiyang-Yangming co-existing. Diarrhea. 3. Early stage of Warm disease. Chilly, fever, no sweat. Stiffness in neck. Sore throat. Swelling under lower jaw. Swelling and pain in eyes, etc.	Gegen 4 *liang* (12g); Mahuang 3 *liang* (9g); Guizhi 2 *liang* (6g); Shaoyao 2 *liang* (6g); Zhigancao 2 *liang* (6g); fresh ginger 3 *liang* (cut into slices) (9g); jujube (cut open) 12 granules.
Guadi San (瓜蒂散)	Vomiting therapy. Fullness in chest with phlegm, garbage water, thin-phlegm, and Hotness. Fullness and hardness in chest and in upper abdomen. Annoyed and perturbed feeling. Feels hungry but cannot eat. Air rushes up to punch chest and the throat, so that it's difficult to breathe.	Sweet Guadi (muskmelon pedicles fried to yellow) 1 *fen*; Chixiaodou (red phaseolus bean) 1 *fen*. (The ratio between these two is 1:1.)
Gualou Guizhi Tang (瓜蒌桂枝汤)	Wind-Hotness attack. Hotness hurts body liquid to cause spasm diseases. With Guizhi Tang condition, plus body spasm, hot, sweaty, dry mouth and thirsty.	Gualou root 2 *liang* (6g); Guizhi 3 *liang* (9g); Shaoyao 3 *liang* (9g); Gancao 2 *liang* (6g); fresh ginger 3 *liang* (9g); jujube 12 granules.
Gualou Jumai Wan (瓜蒌瞿麦丸)	Shaoyin disease with thin-phlegm. Dryness and Dampness mixture. Yang deficiency. Difficulty in urination. Annoying thirst.	Gualou root 2 *liang* (6g); Fuling 3 *liang* (9g); Shuyu 3 *liang* (9g); Fuzi (processed) 1 granule (6g); Jumai 1 *liang* (3g).
Gualou XieBai Baijiu Tang (瓜蒌薤白白酒汤)	Chest Bi syndrome, due to Chest Yang Qi deficiency, Yinqi overwhelming up-rushes to attack heart. Severe pain in heart and back of chest. Short of breath, cough and spit phlegm.	Gualou kernel 1 granule (24g); Xiebai half *shen* (12g); alcohol 7 *shen* (1400 ml).
Gualou Xiebai Banxia Tang (瓜蒌薤白半夏汤)	Chest Bi syndrome, due to Excessiveness and accumulation of phlegm, which blocks Heart Yang Qi to cause severe pain in front and back of chest.	Gualou (whole, chop broken) 1; Xiebai 3 *liang* (12g); Banxia 0.5 *shen* (12g); alcohol 1 *dou*.

Gui Shao Zhimu Tang (桂芍知母汤)	Long-term joint pain. Wind-Cold-Dampness invades and entangles inside the joint. Body defense ability is weak. Joints are swollen, painful, malformed. Dizziness and shortness of breath.	Guizhi 4 *liang* (12g); Shaoyao 3 *liang* (9g); Gancao 2 *liang* (6g); Mahuang 2 *liang* (6g); fresh ginger 5 *liang* (15g); Baizhu 5 *liang* (15g); Zhimu 4 *liang* (12g); Fangfeng 4 *liang* (12g); and Fuzi 2 granules (12g).
Guizhi Fuling Wan (桂枝茯苓丸)	Blood stagnation syndrome. 1. Lower abdomen has a mass and abdominal pain which patient refuses to press. Tongue is purple. Pulse feels deep and slow. 2. Asthma or chest pain due to blood stagnation.	Equal amounts of Guizhi, Fuling, Danpi (the root bark of the peony tree), Shaoyao, Taoren (peach kernel, removal of tip and peel).
Guizhi Fuzi Tang (桂枝附子汤)	Taiyang disease. Body surface weakness, Wind-Dampness entanglement. Sweat. Dislikes wind. Annoying pain in the body. Hard to turn the body.	Guizhi (peeled) 4 *liang* (12g); Paofuzi (peeled, cut into 8 slices) 3 granules (15g); fresh ginger (cut) 3 *liang* (9g); jujube 12 granules; Zhigancao 2 *liang* (6g).
Guizhi Gancao Fuling Dazao Tang (桂枝甘草茯苓大枣汤)	Shanghan disease, after Sweating therapy. Palpitations in lower abdomen (under the navel). Air is about to rush up (to start Bentun disease).	Fuling 0.5 *jin* (25g); Zhigancao 2 *liang* (6g); jujube 15 granules (3 granules); Guizhi 3 *liang* (12g).
Guizhi Gancao Longgu Muli Tang (桂枝甘草龙骨牡蛎汤)	Heart Yang Qi deficiency. Annoyed and restless feeling (mostly caused by burning or fire).	Guizhi 1 *liang* (peeled) (15g); Zhigancao 2 *liang* (30g); Longgu 2 *liang* (30g); Muli 2 *liang* (30g).
Guizhi Gancao Tang (桂枝甘草汤)	Heart Yang Qi is hurt from over sweating. Palpitations. Desire to press and to hold heart area.	Guizhi (peeled) 4 *liang* (12g); Zhigancao 2 *liang* (6g).
Guizhi Mahuang Half-half Tang (桂枝麻黄各半汤)	Taiyang disease. Fever then chilly, or fever and chilly at the same time. Repeats fever and chills twice or more times. Face is red. No sweat. Skin itchy.	Guizhi (peeled) 1 *liang* and 16 *zhu* (5g); Shaoyao 1 *liang* (3g); fresh ginger 1 *liang* (3g); Zhigancao 1 *liang* (3g); Mahuang (removal of branch section) 1 *liang* (3g); jujube (cut open) 4 granules; almond 24 granules (removal of tip and peel).

Guizhi Jia Dahuang Tang (桂枝加大黄汤)	Taiyang-Yangming co-existing. Guizhi Tang condition with abdominal pain.	Guizhi 3 *liang* (peeled) (9g); Shaoyao 6 *liang* (18g); Zhi Gancao 2 *liang* (6g); jujube 12 granules; fresh ginger 3 *liang* (cut into slices) (9g); Dahuang 2 *liang* (6g)
Guizhi Jia Fuzi Tang (桂枝加附子汤)	Taiyang-Shaoyin co-existing. Sweat, or continuous sweat. Dislikes wind. Difficult urination. Slight spasms in arms and legs, which are difficult to bend or stretch.	Guizhi (peel) 3 *liang* (9g); Shaoyao 3 *liang* (9g); Zhigancao 3 *liang* (9g); fresh ginger 3 *liang* (9g); jujube 12 granules; Paofuzi (peel, cut open into 8 pieces) one granule.
Guizhi Jia Gegen Tang (桂枝加葛根汤)	Guizhi Tang condition, with stiffness in neck and back. Sweats. Dislikes wind.	Gegen 4 *liang* (12g); Guizhi (peeled) 2 *liang* (6g); Shaoyao 2 *liang* (6g); fresh ginger 3 *liang* (9g); Zhigancao 2 *liang* (6g); jujube (cut open) 12 granules.
Guizhi Jia Gui Tang (桂枝加桂汤)	Taiyang disease, Heart Yang Qi deficiency due to fire needle (or other fire therapy). Cold air rushes up from lower abdomen to punch chest and heart. (Bentun syndrome).	Guizhi (peeled) 5 *liang* (15g); Shaoyao 3 *liang* (9g); Zhi Gancao 2 *liang* (6g); fresh ginger (cut into slices) 3 *liang* (9g); and jujube 12 granules.
Guizhi Jia Houpu Xingze Tang (桂枝加厚朴杏子汤)	Guizhi Tang condition, with coughing or asthma, shortness of breath.	Guizhi 3 *liang* (9g); Baishao 3 *liang* (9g); Zhigancao 3 *liang* (6g); fresh ginger 3 *liang* (9g); jujube 12 granules (4 granules); Houpo (peeled, processed) 2 *liang* (6g); almond (peeled, tip removed) 50 granules (10g).
Guizhi Jia Huangqi Tang (桂枝加黄芪汤)	Guizhi Tang condition, with sharp pain or dragging pain in hip and lower back. Heaviness and pain in body. Sweat.	Guizhi 3 *liang* (9g); Shaoyao 3 *liang* (9g); Gancao 2 *liang* (6g); fresh ginger 3 *liang* (9g); jujube 12 granules; Huangqi 2 *liang* (6g).

Guizhi Jia Longgu Muli Tang (桂枝加龙骨牡蛎汤)	Withered condition. Dragging pain in lower abdomen. Cold feeling in perinea region. Blurring vision. Loss of hair. Loss of essence. Sexual dreams or palpitations. Easily sweats and gets nervous.	Guizhi 3 *liang* (9g); Shaoyao 3 *liang* (9g); fresh ginger 3 *liang* (9g); Gancao 2 *liang* (6g); jujube 12 granules; Longgu 3 *liang* (9g); Muli 3 *liang* (9g).
Guizhi Jia Shaoyao Tang (桂枝加芍药汤)	Guizhi Tang condition, with abdominal pain, fullness.	Guizhi 3 *liang* (peeled) (9g); Shaoyao 6 *liang* (18g); Zhigancao 2 *liang* (6g); jujube 12 granules; fresh ginger 3 *liang* (cut into slices) (9g).
Guizhi Ginseng Tang (桂枝人参汤)	Taiyang disease. Body Exterior condition with inner Coldness. Body Exterior condition with continuous diarrhea. Hardness and fullness feeling in stomach region.	Guizhi (peeled) 4 *liang* (12g); Zhigancao 4 *liang* (12g); Baizhu 3 *liang* (9g); Ginseng 3 *liang* (9g); dried ginger 3 *liang* (9g).
Guizhi Shengjiang Zhishi Tang (桂枝生姜枳实汤)	Coldness or garbage water accumulation in stomach. Hardness and fullness feeling in stomach region. Feel as if something drags heart downwards (inner organ prolapse syndrome).	Guizhi 3 *liang* (9g); fresh ginger 3 *liang* (9g); Zhishi 5 granules (15g).
Guizhi Tang (桂枝汤)	1. Taiyang body surface weakness condition. Fever, headache, sweat, dislike wind, nose stuffiness, belch, floating-soft pulse. 2. Ying-Wei (nutrition Qi and defense Qi) disharmony.	Guizhi (removal of bark) 3 *liang* (9g); Baishao 3 *liang* (9g); Zhiancao 2 *liang* (6g); fresh ginger 3 *liang* (9g); jujube 12 granules.
Guizhi Two Mahuang One Tang (桂枝二麻黄一汤)	Taiyang disease. Fever, headache, sweat, chilly, floating pulse. Such feelings come more than once per day.	Guizhi (peeled) 1 *liang* 17 *zhu* (5.4g); Shaoyao 1 *liang* 6 *zhu* (3.7g); Mahuang (removal of branch section) 16 *zhu* (2.1g); fresh ginger (cut into pieces) 1 *liang* 6 *zhu* (3.7g); almond (removal of tip and peel) 16 granules (2.5g); Zhigancao 1 *liang* 2 *zhu* (3.2g); jujube (cut open) 5 granules.

Guizhi Two Yuebi One Tang (桂枝二越婢一汤)	Taiyang disease. Pathogenic Qi penetrates inside to transform into Hotness. More fever than chills, slightly fast and weak pulse. Tongue is slightly yellow. The severity of body condition is between the Guizhi Tang and Yuebi Tang.	Guizhi (peeled) 18 *zhu* (2.3g); Shaoyao 18 *zhu* (2.3g); Mahuang 18 *zhu* (2.3g); Zhigancao 18 *zhu* (2.3g); jujube 4 granules; fresh ginger (cut into slices) 1 *liang* 2 *zhu* (3.1g); Shigao (grind into small pieces, fold in cotton cloth) 1 *liang* (3g).
Guizhi Qui Shaoyao Jia Fuzi Tang (桂枝去芍药加附子汤)	Chest Yang Qi is insufficient. Chest fullness, pulse feels hurried and slightly weak. No sign of Fire on tongue.	Guizhi (peeled) 3 *liang* (9g); Zhigancao 2 *liang* (6g); fresh ginger (cut) 3 *liang* (9g); jujube 12 granules; Fuzi (cook first) 1 granule (3g).
Guizhi Qui Shaoyao Jia Mahuang Fuzi Xixin Tang (桂枝去芍药加麻辛附)	Coldness-thin-phlegm entanglement in stomach area. Chest fullness. Hurried pulse. Hardness and fullness in stomach region. Diarrhea and difficulty in urination.	Guizhi 3 *liang* (9g); fresh ginger 3 *liang* (9g); Gancao 2 *liang* (6g); jujube 12 granules; Mahuang 1 *liang* (6g); Xixin 1 *liang* (3g); Paofuzi 1 granule (5g).
Guizhi Qui Shaoyao Jia Zaojia Tang (桂枝去芍药加皂荚汤)	Lung withered syndrome. Chest fullness. Coughing and shortness of breath. Difficult to lie down. Spits sticky phlegm and saliva. Pulse feels fast or slippery.	Guizhi 3 *liang* (9g); fresh ginger 3 *liang* (9g); jujube 12 granules; Gancao 2 *liang* (6g); Zaojia (peel, baked) 1 granule.
Guizhi Qui Shaoyao Jia Shuqi Longgu Muli Tang (桂枝去芍药加蜀漆龙牡汤)	Heart Yang Qi is hurt by fire therapy or fire disaster. Heart Yang Qi floats to cause annoyed and perturbed feeling, palpitations, heavy sweating. Feel air up-rushing feeling. Pulse feels fast or knobbed.	Guizhi (peeled) 3 *liang* (9g); Zhigancao 2 *liang* (6g); fresh ginger 3 liang (9g); jujube (cut open) 12 granules; Longgu 4 *liang* (12g); Muli (cooked) 5 *liang* (15g); Shuti (removal of fishy smell) 3 *liang* (9g).
Guizhi Qui Shaoyao Tang (桂枝去芍药汤)	Taiyang disease wrongly treated with Purging therapy. Chest Yang Qi is hurt. Exogenous pathogenic Qi shrinks in the chest. Fullness and pain in chest. Pulse feels fast and hurried.	Guizhi (peeled) 3 *liang* (9g); Zhigancao 2 *liang* (6g); fresh ginger (cut) 3 *liang* (9g); jujube 12 granules.

Guizhi Xin Jia Tang (桂枝新加汤)	Taiyang disease after Sweating therapy. Qi-Yin both deficiency. Guizhi Tang condition with more pain in the body. Poor appetite. Pulse feels deep and slow.	Guizhi (peeled) 3 *liang* (9g); Shaoyao 4 *liang* (12g); Zhigancao 3 *liang* (9g); Ginseng 3 *liang* (9g); jujube 12 granules, fresh ginger 4 *liang* (12g).
Gualou Muli San (瓜蒌牡蛎散)	Baihe disease. Heart-Lung Yin deficiency. Hot, and annoying thirst.	Gualou and oyster shell (processed) in equal amounts.
Hou Jiang Xia Cao Renshen Tang (厚姜半夏甘草人参汤)	1. Tangyang disease after Sweating therapy. Middle Qi is hurt. Abdominal fullness and bloating. 2. Spleen deficiency, with Phlegm-Dampness accumulation. Fullness in abdomen (mixed Weakness and Excessiveness condition).	Houpu (24g); fresh ginger (24g); Banxia (15g); Zhiganao (6g); Ginseng (3g).
Houpu Mahuang Tang (厚朴麻黄汤)	1. Xiao Qinglong Tang condition plus dry nose and thirst. Fullness in chest. Palpitations and sweat. Difficulty in urination. 2. Coughing, strong air up-rushing feeling. Chest fullness. Sticky feeling in throat, which sounds like birds. Pulse feels floating.	Houpu 5 *liang* (15-30g); Mahuang 4 *liang* (10-256g); Shigao (size of chicken egg) (50-150g); almond 0.5 *shen* (15-20g); Banxia 0.5 *shen* (12-20g); Wuweizi 0.5 *shen* (12-15g); wheat 1 *shen* (20-50g); dried ginger 2 *liang* (10-15g); Xixin 2 *liang* (10-15g).
Houpu Qi Wu Tang (厚朴七物汤)	Spleen deficiency with Qi sluggishness, Phlegm-Hotness entanglement. Dirty air, dry stool and hotness in bowel. Abdominal fullness. Bowel movement is sluggish. Tongue is pale. Pulse feels deep.	Houpu 8 *liang* (24g); Gancao 3 *liang* (9g); Dahuang 3 *liang* (9g); jujube 10 granules; Zhishi 5 granules (12g); Guizhi 2 *liang* (6g); fresh ginger 5 *liang* (15g).
Houpu San Wu Tang (厚朴三物汤)	Similar to Xiao Qinglong Tang condition. Stool is retarded and can't pass out. Strong fullness in abdomen. More fullness (Qi sluggish) than stool accumulation.	Houpu 8 *liang* (18g); Dahuang 4 *liang* (9g); Zhishi 5 granules (11g).

Houshi Hei San (侯氏黑散)	Blood deficiency, Meridians are hollow (empty). Wind-attacked. Annoying heaviness feeling in arms and legs. Wind type epilepsy. Cold feeling in paralysis arm or leg.	Juhua 40 *fen* (30g); Fangfeng 10 *fen* (7.5g); Baizhu 10 *fen* (7.5g); Jiegen 8 *fen* (6g); Ginseng 3 *fen* (2.25g); Fuling 3 *fen* (2.25g); Danggui 3 *fen* (2.25g); Chuanxiong 3 *fen* (2.25g); dried ginger 3 *fen* (2.25g); Guizhi 3 *fen* (2.25g); Xixin 3 *fen* (2.25g); Muli 3 *fen* (2.25g); Panshi 3 *fen* (2.25g); Huangqin 5 *fen* (2.25g).
Huanglian Ajiao Tang (黄连阿胶汤)	1. Shaoyin disease, Hotness transform phase. Inner Hotness and blood insufficient. Palpitations, annoyed. Difficult to fall asleep. 2. Bleeding condition. Blood is fresh red, small in volume and sticky.	Huanglian 4 *liang* (12g); Ajiao 3 *liang* (9g); Huangqin 2 *liang* (6g); Baishao 2 *liang* (6g); Chicken egg yolk, 2.
Huanglian Tang (黄连汤)	Stomach Weakness and Coldness, Hotness in chest. Abdominal pain and nausea. Annoying fullness in chest. Air up-rushing feeling in abdomen. The tongue coating is white-greasy. Pulse feels like string.	Huanglian 3 *liang* (9g); Guizhi 3 *liang* (9g); dried ginger 3 *liang* (9g); Gancao 3 *liang* (9g); Ginseng 2 *liang* (6g); Banxiao half *shen* (12g); jujube 12 granules (4 granules).
Huangqi Guizhi Wu Wu Tang (黄芪桂枝五物汤)	Blood Bi syndrome. Body feels weak, heavy, has difficulty moving. Feels numb, sore or pain in body. Muscle is withered. Huangqi body constitution.	Huangqi 3 *liang* (9g); Shaoyao 3 *liang* (9g); Guizhi 3 *liang* (9g); fresh ginger 6 *liang* (18g); jujube 12 granules (4 granule).
Huangqi Jianzhong Tang (黄芪建中汤)	Withered syndrome. Deficiency in Yin, Yang, Qi and blood. Abdominal region has urgent and sharp pain. Desire for warmth and pressing on abdomen. Sweat and Wind-disliking.	Guizhi (peeled) 3 *liang* (9g); Shaoyao 6 *liang* (16g); Zhigancao 2 *liang* (6g); fresh ginger 3 *liang* (9g); jujube (cut open) 12 granules; Yitang 1 *shen* (30g); Huangqi 1.5 *liang* (4.5g)
Huangqi Shaoyao Guizhi Kujiu Tang (黄芪芍药桂枝苦酒汤)	Yellow sweat syndrome. Body is swollen or heavy. Fever and sweating. Sweat is yellow in color. Pulse feels deep.	Huangqi 5 *liang* (30-100g); Shaoyao 3 *liang* (10-20g); Guizhi 3 *liang* (10-20g); wine 30-100ml.

Huangqin Jia Banxia Shengjiang Tang (黄芩加半夏生姜汤)	Shaoyang-Yangming co-existing. Hot diarrhea with nausea (or Huangqin Tang condition with nausea).	This formula adds Banxai and fresh ginger to Huangqin Tang.
Huangqin Tang (黄芩汤)	Shaoyang-Yangming co-existing. Shaoyang Fire pushes Yangming, causes Hot diarrhea, abdominal pain. (Shaoyang condition with hot diarrhea.)	Huangqin 3 *liang* (9g); Zhigancao 2 *liang* (6g); Shaoyao 2 *liang* (6g); jujube 12 granules (4 granules).
Huangtu Tang (黄土汤)	Bleeding in stool due to Coldness-Weakness. Blood is dim red. Body is cold. Face is withered yellow in color. Tongue is pale and pulse feels deep, thin, and weak.	Gancao 3 *liang* (9g); Shoudi 3 *liang* (9g); Baizhu 3 *liang* (9g); Processed Fuzi 3 *liang* (9g); Ajiao 3 *liang* (9g); Huangqin 3 *liang* (9g); yellow soil collected from inner wall of a soil oven 0.5 *jin* (24g).
Huashi Daizhe Tang (滑石代赭汤)	Baihe Syndrome. Occurred after wrong use of Purging therapy.	Baihe (cut open) 7 granules (30g); Huashi (broken, fold with cotton cloth) 3 *liang* (9g); Daizheshi (broken, fold with cotton cloth) 1 granule (9g).
Ji Jiao Li Huang Wan (己椒苈黄丸)	Phlegm or thin-phlegm accumulates and hurries in bowel. Fullness and bowel noise in abdomen. Dry mouth. Constipation. Pulse feels deep and stringy.	Fangji 1 *liang* (15g); Huajiao 1 *liang* (15g); Tinglizi (cooked) 1 *liang* (15g); Dahuang 1 *liang* (15g).
Jiegen Bai San (桔梗白散)	1. Lung abscess. Fullness in chest. Coughing and spitting pus-like phlegm, which is sticky and with bad odor. Dry throat but not thirsty. Shaking with chills. Pulse feels fast. 2. Coldness-Excessiveness Jie-xiong syndrome. No sign of Hotness.	Jiegen 3 *fen*; Beimu 3 *fen*; Badou (peeled, bake to take oil out, remove oil) 1 *fen*. (The *fen* here means the ratio, not the weight.)
Jiegen Tang (桔梗汤)	1. Shaoyin disease. Sore throat. 2. Lung abscess.	Jiegen 1 *liang* (3-6g); Gancao 2 *liang* (6-12g).
Jupi Tang (橘皮汤)	Stomach Weakness. Belching, nausea. Cold hands and feet.	Orange peel 4 *liang* (12g); fresh ginger 8 *liang* (24g).

Formula	Indication	Ingredients
Jupi Zhishi Shenjiang Tang (橘皮枳实生姜汤)	Chest Bi syndrome due to Qi sluggish. Fullness in chest. Short of breath. Fullness and bloating in stomach region too.	Orange peel 1 *jin* (50g); Zhishi 3 *liang* (10g); fresh ginger 0.5 *jin* (24g).
Jupi Zhuru Tang (橘皮竹茹汤)	Stomach Weakness. Urgent and violent nausea, belching, and coughing. Symptoms are more violent and worse than in Jupi Tang condition.	Orang peel 2 *jin* (90g); Zhuru 2 *jin* (10g); jujube 30 granules (10 granules); Dangshen 1 *liang* (3g); Gancao 5 *liang* (15g); fresh ginger 8 *liang* (25g).
Kuizi Fuling San (葵子茯苓散)	1. Yang Qi sluggish and water accumulation in urine bladder. Pregnant women feel heaviness in the body. Difficulty in urination. Chilly. Dizziness when getting up. 2. Menopause syndrome with frequent urination.	Kuizi (sunflower seed) 1 *shen* (500g); Fuling 3 *liang* (90g).
Kujiu Tang (苦酒汤)	Shaoyin disease. Sore throat with ulcer . Cannot speak. Symptoms are more severe than in Gangao Tang condition.	Banxia (wash in boiling water 7 times) 6g; egg white, one; kujiu (vinegar) 100ml.
Ling Gan Wuwei Jiang Xin Tang (苓甘五味姜辛汤)	Coughing, short of breath. Large volume of phlegm. Phlegm is clear as water, white in color. No body Exterior condition (Xiao Qinglong Tang condition without body surface condition).	Fuling 4 *liang* (12g); Gancao 3 *liang* (9g); dried ginger 3 *liang* (9g); Xixin 3 *liang* (9g); Wuweizi half *shen* (5g).
Ling Gan Wuwei Jiang Xin Xia Tang (苓甘五味姜辛夏汤)	Ling Gan Wuwei Jiang Xin Tang condition with more dizziness and nausea.	This formula adds Banxia to Ling Gan Wuwei Jiang Xin Tang.
Ling Gan Wuwei Jiang Xin Xia Xing Dahuang Tang (苓甘五味姜辛夏杏大黄汤)	Ling Gan Wuwei Jiang Xin Xia Xing Tang condition with warm face, red face as if drunk, difficulty in bowel movement.	Add Dahuang to Ling Gan Wuwei Jiang Xing Xia Xin Tang.
Ling Gan Wuwei Jiang Xin Xia Xing Tang (苓甘五味姜辛夏杏汤)	Ling Gan Wuwei Jiang Xin Xia Tang condition with swelling in face, arms or legs.	To Ling Gan Wuwei Jiang Xin Xia Tang, add almond.
Ling Gui Wei Gan Tang (苓桂味甘汤)	Water up-rushing feeling. Violent up-rushing from lower abdomen to chest and to throat. Face is hot as if drunk (Bentun syndrome).	Fuling 4 *liang* (12 -30g); Guizhi (peeled) 4 *liang* (12-30g); Zhigancao 3 *liang* (6-10g); Wuweizi 0.5 *shen* (10-15g).

Ling Gui Zao Gan Tang (苓桂枣甘汤)	Water up-rushing from lower abdomen up to chest and to heart. Palpitations in lower abdomen. Bentun syndrome is about to occur.	Fuling 0.5 *jin* (40g); Guizhi (peeled) 4 *liang* (20g); Zhigancao 2 *liang* (10g); jujube 15 granules (5 granules).
Ling Gui Zhu Gan Tang (苓桂术甘汤)	Reversing up-rushing from middle abdomen to stomach region and to chest. Dizziness when getting up. Body shaking. Pulse feels deep and tight.	Fuling 4 *liang* (12g); Guizhi (peeled) 3 *liang* (9g); Baizhu 2 *liang* (6g); Zhigancao 2 *liang* (6g).
Liu Wu Huangqin Tang (六物黄芩汤)	Belching and diarrhea. Fullness and hardness in stomach region.	Huangqin (5.5g), Ginseng (5.5g), dried ginger (5.5g); jujube (5.5g); Guizhi (1.8g); Banxia (11g).
Lizhong Tang (理中汤)	1. Middle part Weakness and Coldness. 2. Chest Bi syndrome. Or spits saliva after a severe disease. 3. Bleeding condition due to Weakness and Coldness.	Chao Baizhu 2 *liang* (12g); Ginseng 1 *liang* (6g); dried ginger 1 *liang* (9g); Zhigancao 1 *liang* (6g).
Ma Xing Shi Gan Tang (麻杏石甘汤)	Wind-cold attack Taiyang disease. Body surface Cold but inner Hotness (in lungs). Fever, urgent coughing and short of breath (asthma). Dry mouth. Tongue is thin-yellow. Pulse feels floating, fast, and slippery. (The Lung is dry and hot.)	Mahuang (removal of knot) 4 *liang* (9g); almond (removal of tip and peel) 50 granules (9g); Zhigancao 2 *liang* (6g); Shigao (fold, break into smaller pieces); 18 *liang* (18g).
Ma Xing Yi Gan Tang (麻杏薏甘汤)	Wind-Dampness in body surface. Pain in joints and in whole body. Fever is severe in the afternoon. This formula is also a TCM beauty formula.	Mahuang (removal of knot) 0.5 *liang* (7g); Zhigancao 1 *liang* (14g); Yiyiren 0.5 *liang* (7g); almond (removal of tips and peel) 10 granules (3g).
Mahuang Fuzi Gancao Tang (麻黄附子甘草汤)	Shaoyin body surface condition. Chilly, pain in the body. No sweat. Slight fever. Pulse feels deep and weak.	Mahuang 2 *liang* (6g); Zhigancao 2 *liang* (6g); Pao Fuzi (peeled, cut into 8 pieces) 1 granule (3g).
Mahuang Fuzi Xixin Tang (麻黄附子细辛汤)	Shaoyin body surface condition. Severe chills, fever. Desire to lie down on bed. No sweat. Pulse feels deep. Sudden deafness, suddenly mute, or suddenly blind, all of which are due to exposure to very cold environment.	Mahuang 2 *liang* (6g); Paofuzi (peeled, broken into 8 pieces) 1 granule (9g); Xixin 2 *liang* (6g).

Mahuang Lianqiao Chixiaodou Tang (麻黄连翘赤小豆汤)	1. Coldness in body surface, Dampness-Hotness under skin. Skin lesion or itchiness. Annoyed and perturbed feeling. Difficulty in urination. 2. Dampness-Hotness jaundice (in blood phase).	Mahuang 2 *liang* (remove knot) (5-20g); Lianqiao 2 *liang* (10-15g); almond (removal of tips and peel) 40 granules; Chixiaodou 1 *shen* (30-50g); jujube (cut open) 12 granules; fresh ginger 2 *liang* (10g); fresh Chinese catalpa bark 1 *shen* (15-25g); Gancao 2 *liang* (10-15g).
Mahuang p lus Zhu Tang (麻黄加术汤)	Dampness person. No sweat. Feels annoying pain in whole body. Body is strong.	Mahuang 3 *liang* (45g); Guizhi 3 *liang* (30g); almond 70 granules (20g); Zhigancao 1 *liang* (15g); and Baizhu 4 *liang* (60g).
Mahuang Shengma Tang (麻黄升麻汤)	Jueyin disease. Upper Hotness and lower Coldness. Body defense force is weak, Yang Qi is choked. Sore throat and esophagus. Spits pus and blood. Continuous diarrhea.	Mahuang 2.5 *liang* (7.5g); Shengma 1 *liang* and 6 *zhu* (3.5g); Danggui 1 *liang* and 6 *zhu* (3.5g); Zhimu 18 *zhu* (2.5g); Huangqin 18 *zhu* (2.5g); Weirui 18 *zhu* (2.5g); Shigao 6 *zhu* (3g); Baizhu 6 *zhu* (2g); dried ginger 6 *zhu* (2g); Shaoyao 6 *zhu* (2g); Tianmendong 6 zhu (2g); Guizhi 6 *zhu* (2g); Fuling 6 *zhu* (2g); Zhigancao 6 *zhu* (2g).
Mahuang Tang (麻黄汤)	1.Taiyang body surface Excessiveness condition. Headache and pain in body and joints. Chilly and no sweat. With or without fever. Pulse feels floating-tight. 2. Taiyang-Yangming co-existing condition with asthma and fullness in chest. 3. Yangming disease, no sweat. Asthma. Pulse feels floating. 4. Sudden loss of voice due to Cold choking.	Mahuang (remove the knot) 3 *liang* (45g); Guizhi 2 *liang* (30g); Zhigancao 1 *liang* (15g); almond 70 granules (remove peel and tips) (20g).

Maimendong Tang (麦门冬汤)	Lung withered condition (due to Weakness-Hotness). Body water cannot be distributed by the lung, so feels thirsty. Spits sticky and thick saliva.	Maimendong 7 shen (21g); Banxia 1 shen (3g); Ginseng 3 liang (9g); Gancao 2 liang (6g); Glutinous rice 3 he (15g); jujube 12 granules (4 granules).
Maziren Wan (麻子仁丸)	Hotness and dryness in digestive duct. Stool is firm and difficult to pass. Frequent urination. Skin is wet.	Maziren 2 *shen* (10-30g); Shaoyao 0.5 *jin* (10-20g); Zhishi (processed) 0.5 *jin* (10-15g); Dahuang (peeled) 1 *jin* (10-20g); Houpu (processed, peeled) 1 *chi* (10-20g); almond (remove peel and tip, processed) 1 *shen* (10-20g).
Mi Jian Dao (蜜煎导)	Habitual constipation. Stool is in colon and near anus. This is external way to conduct stool passing.	Honey 150g.
Mufangji Tang (木防己汤)	Branch Thin-phlegm accumulation in chest and diaphragm. Asthma and fullness in chest. Hardness and fullness in stomach region. Black and dim color of face. Pulse feels deep and tight.	Mufangji 3 *liang* (10-15g); Shigao 12 granules (30-50g); Guizhi 2 *liang* (6-10g); Ginseng 4 *liang* (10-15g).
Mufangji Tang without Shigao but with Fuling and Mangxiao (木防己去石膏加茯苓芒硝汤)	Mufangji Tang condition but with much stronger hardness and fullness in stomach region. Difficulty in urination and bowel movement.	Use Mufangji Tang, but omit Shigao, and add Fuling (18g); Mangxiao (27g).
Muli Tang (牡蛎汤)	Malaria-like disease with more chills.	Muli (oyster shell) (processed) (1.2g); Mahuang (remove stem) (12g); Zhigancao (9g); Shuqi (9g) (it can be replaced with Changshan).
Muli Zexie San (牡蛎泽泻散)	Swelling from lower back to legs. Mostly used if such swelling occurs after a severe disease.	Equal amounts of: Muli (fried); Zexie; Shuqi (washed in warm water); Tinglize (fried); Shanglugent (Pokeweed root, fried); Haizao (washed); Gualougen.

Painong San (排脓散)	Purulent diseases. The lesions are painful, hard and open. No clear whole body symptoms.	Zhishi 16 granules (2g); Shaoyao 6 *fen* (2g); Jiegen 2 *fen* (1g).
Painong Tang (排脓汤)	Similar to Painong San. Used more in chronic stage.	Gancao 2 *liang* (6g); Jiegen 3 *liang* (9g); fresh ginger 1 *liang* (3g); jujube 10 granule (3 granules).
San Huang Tang (三黄汤)	Hotness in all the three Jiao (body cavities). Annoyingly restless. Fullness and pain in abdomen. Constipation. Delirious speech, or madness. Oral ulcer.	Dahuang 3 *liang* (9g); Huanglian 3 *liang* (9g); Huangqin 3 *liang* (9g).
San Wu Bei Ji Wan (三物备急丸)	Coldness-Excessiveness syndrome. Sudden severe pain in heart, stomach, with urgent breathing. Hard to speak. Difficult to pass stool.	Badou 1 *liang* (30g); dried ginger 1 *liang* (30g); Dahuang 1 *liang* (30g).
San Wu Huangqin Tang (三物黄芩汤)	1. Wind attack after birth delivery. Annoyingly hot on arms and legs. No headache but feels annoyed and perturbed. 2. Annoyingly hot with headache.	Huangqin 1 *liang* (15-50g); Kushen 2 *liang* (15-30g); Shengdi 4 *liang* (30-100g).
Shaoyao Gancao Tang (芍药甘草汤)	1. Muscle spasms in arms, legs or calves. 2. Inner organ spasms and pain. 3. Restless leg syndrome. 4. Child crying at night.	Shaoyao 4 *liang* (20-60g); Zhigancao 4 *liang* (10-30g).
Shechuangzi San (蛇床子散)	Coldness-Dampness in lower abdomen. Itching in perinea region. Lots of discharge of white color. Weak and sore on lower back and knee. Or with eczema, or wet ulcer.	Grind Shechuangzi into powder. Mix it with rice powder. Make a pill as big as a jujube, and fold with cotton cloth.
Shegan Mahuang Tang (射干麻黄汤)	Cold thin-phlegm accumulation in lung. Cough with water noise in throat like a bird singing. Similar to Xiao Qinglong Tang condition, but with more phlegm, heat in eyes, dry mouth, bad odor in mouth. Stool is dry.	Shegan 3 *liang* (10-15g); Mahuang 4 *liang* (12-20g); fresh ginger 4 *liang* (15g); Xixin 3 liang (5-15g); Wuweizi 0.5 *jin* (12-20g); Banxia (wash) 0.5 *shen* (15-20g); Ziquan 3 *liang* (10-15g); Kuandonghua 3 *liang* (10-15g); jujube 7 granules (7-12 granules)

Shen Qi Wan (肾气丸)	Kidney Yang deficiency. Weak and sore in lower back. Spasm in lower abdomen. short of breath. Slight cough. Swelling in ankle. Annoying thirst or long-term diarrhea.	Dried Dihuang 8 *liang* (24g); Shuyu 4 *liang* (12g); Shanzhuyu 4 *liang* (12g); Zexie 3 *liang* (9g); Fuling 3 *liang* (9g); Mudanpi 3 *liang* (9g); Guizhi 1 *liang* (3g); Pao Fuzi one *liang* (3g).
Shengjiang Gancao Tang (生姜甘草汤)	Lung withered syndrome. Continuous spitting. Throat is dry and feels thirsty.	Fresh ginger 5 *liang* (15g); Ginseng 3 *liang* (10g); Gancao 4 *liang* (12g); jujube 15 granules (5 granules).
Shengjiang Xiexin Tang (生姜泻心汤)	Pi syndrome in upper abdomen. Hardness and fullness in stomach region. No pain upon pressing. Water noise in abdomen. Annoyed and perturbed feeling. Belching and bad odor from mouth. Diarrhea.	Fresh ginger (cut into pieces) 4 *liang* (12g); Zhigancao 3 *liang* (9g); Ginseng 3 *liang* (9g); dried ginger 1 *liang* (3g); Huangqin 3 *liang* (9g); Banxia (washed) 0.5 *shen* (9g); Huanglian 1 *liang* (3g); jujube (cut open) 12 granules (4 granules).
Shengma Gegen Tang (升麻葛根汤)	1. Yangming Wind-attack body surface condition. Headache. Pain in whole body. Fever, chills, no sweat. Thirsty. Pain in eyes. Dry nose. Hard to fall asleep. 2. During measles, child sneezes, cries, and has fever. Annoyed. Skin rash comes with difficulty.	Shengma; Baishao; Zhigancao; 10 *liang* for each (6g for each); Gegen 15 *liang* (9g).
Shenma Biejia Tang (升麻鳖甲汤)	1. Jueyin disease. Yang-toxic disease. Face has patches of redness. Sore throat. Spits pus and blood. 2. Skin disease due to Hotness in blood phase. 3. Leukemia.	Shenma 2 *liang* (18g); Danggui one *liang* (9g); Shujiao (fried) one *liang* (9g); Gancao 2 *liang* (18g); Biejia (turtle shell) 8-10cm diameter; Xionghuang (regular) 0.5 *liang*.
Shi Zao Tang (十枣汤)	1. Pending thin-phlegm syndrome. Coughs and spits. Chest pain dragging to rib-arch. Or severe chest pain. Hardness in stomach region. Belches and short of breath. Headache and dizziness. 2. Swelling in whole body, especially in lower part of the body. Asthma. Fullness in abdomen. Difficulty in urination	Equal amounts of Yanhua (processed); Gansui; Daji.

and bowel movement.

Shuqi San (蜀漆散)	Malaria-like disease, more cold than fever.	Equal amounts of Shuqi (washed); Yunmu (burning for 2 days and nights); Longgu.
Si Ni Jia Ginseng Tang (四逆加人参汤)	Yang deficiency and Yin damaged (due to wrong treatment). Palpitations. Heavy sweat on head, or on whole body. Annoyed and restless. Cold hands and feet (Jue syndrome). Cloudy mind or near loss of consciousness. Red face. Tongue is dim dark. Purple in mouth lips. Pulse feels faint. (This is shock condition).	Use Si Ni Tang. Add Ginseng 1 *liang* (3 g).
Si Ni San (四逆散)	Body Yang Qi is choked and sealed inside, cannot spread out to body surface. Cold hands and feet (Yang choked Jue syndrome). The cold feeling does not go up to the level of elbow or knee. Chest fullness and pain.	Chaihu 0.5 *Jin* (30g); Zhishi (processed) 4 granules (30g); Baishao 3 *liang* (30g); Zhigancao 3 *liang* (30g).
Si Ni Tang (四逆汤)	1. Yang Qi is weak to faint. Yin Coldness is Excessiveness. Cold hands and feet (Cold Jue syndrome). Chills and fatigue. Likes to lie down. Diarrhea with undigested food in stool. Cold pain in stomach. No thirst. Pulse feels deep and tiny. 2. Yang Qi is lost (Shock condition).	Zhigancao 2 *liang* (6g); dried ginger 1.5 *liang* (4.5g); raw Fuzi 1 granule (cut into 8 slices) (10g).
Xiao Banxia Jia Fuling Tang (小半夏加茯苓汤)	Garbage water accumulation in stomach. Nausea mostly, with fullness in stomach. Palpitations, dizziness and blurred vision.	Banxia 1 *shen* (18g); fresh ginger 8 *liang* (15g); Fuling 3 *liang* (9g).
Xiao Banxia Tang (小半夏汤)	Garbage water accumulation. Hardness and fullness in stomach region. Nausea. No thirst. Stomach Coldness. Coughing phlegm. Various types of nausea so it is difficult to eat.	Banxia 1 *shen* (18g); fresh ginger 0.5 *jin* (15g).

Xiao Chaihu Tang (小柴胡汤)	1. Shaoyang disease. Shifting cold and hot. Annoying fullness under rib arches. No desire to eat. Annoyed and perturbed. Frequent nausea or belching. Bitter taste in mouth and dry throat. The tongue coating is white. Pulse feels stringy and fast. 2. Hotness in Bloodroom in women. 3. Early stage of Wind-Warm disease, Dampness-Warm disease and plague.	Chaihu 0.5 *jin* (24g); Huangqin 3 *liang* (9g); Ginseng 3 *liang* (9g); Banxia (washed) 0.5 *shen* (9g); Gancao 3 *liang* (9g); fresh ginger 3 *liang* (9g); jujube 12 granules (4 granules).
Xiao Chengqi Tang (小承气汤)	Yangming inner Excessiveness condition. Abdominal fullness. Difficulty in bowel movement.	Dahuang (washed in alcohol) 4 *liang* (12g); Houpu (peeled, processed) 2 *liang* (6g); Zhishi (processed) 3 big granules (9g).
Xiao Jianzhong Tang (小建中汤)	Withered condition. Abdominal pain, likes warmth and pressure on abdomen. Tongue is dry. The tongue coating is white. Pulse feels thin-stringy. Or, has palpitations. No-reason annoyed. Pale face. Or sore and weak in arms and legs, annoying heat on palms and sole. Dry mouth and throat.	Guizhi (peeled) 3 *liang* (9g); Baishao 6 *liang* (18g); Zhigancao 3 *liang* (9g); fresh ginger 3 *liang* (9g); jujube 12 granules; Yitang (Malt sugar) 1 *shen* (30g).
Xiao Qinglong Tang (小青龙汤)	1. Body surface Coldness and inner Coldness-thin-phlegm accumulation. Coughing, slightly short of breath, spits white foam-like phlegm. 2. Spilling swelling condition. Swelling in arms and legs.	Mahuang (removal of knot) 3 *liang* (45g); Shaoyao 3 *liang* (45g); Wuweizi 0.5 *shen* (40g); Ganjiang 2 *liang* (30g); Zhigancao 3 *liang* (45g); Banxia 0.5 *shen* (45g); Guizhi 3 *liang* (45g); Xixin 3 *liang* (45g).
Xiao Qinglong Tang Jia Shigao (小青龙加石膏)	1. Xiao Qinglong Tang condition with annoying Hotness inside, dry mouth, annoyed feeling. 2. Lung Fullness condition. Fullness feeling in chest, violent coughing and shortness of breath. Annoyed feeling.	Add Shigao to Xiao Qinglong Tang.
Xiao Xianxiong Tang (小陷胸汤)	Small Jie-xiong syndrome. Hardness and fullness in the upper abdomen, feels pain upon pressing. Pulse feels floating and	Huanglian 1 liang (6g); Banxia 0.5 shen (12g); Gualou 1 big granule (30g).

slippery.

Suanzaoren Tang (酸枣仁汤)	1. Withered condition. No-reason annoyed and perturbed feeling. Easy to have poor sleep after labor or mental work. Body is weak and thin. Easily feels scared and urgent. 2. Also works for craving sleep (too much sleep). This formula has double regulation effect. 3. Any diseases that occurs or become worse between 1 am and 3 am.	Suanzao kernel 2 *shen* (10-30g); Gancao 1 *liang* (3-6g); Zhimu 2 *liang* (6-12g); Fuling 2 *liang* (6-12g); Chuanxiong 2 *liang* (6-12g).
Taohe Chengqi Tang (桃核承气汤)	Dead blood accumulation in lower abdomen. It is early stage of the accumulation. Lower abdomen feels urgent, tight and pain. Fever at night. Delirious speech. Annoying thirst. Even madness. Urine is normal. Pulse feels deep, strong. Women can have cessation of menstruation, or painful menstruation.	Peach kernel (removal of peel and tips) 50 granules (12g); Dahuang 4 *liang* (12g); Guizhi 2 *liang* (6g); Zhigancao 2 *liang* (6g); Mangxiao 2 *liang* (6g).
Taohua Tang (桃花汤)	Shaoyin disease. Spleen-Kidney Yang Qi deficiency. Coldness-Dampness accumulation in middle of body. Long-term diarrhea with pus and blood in stool. Blood is not fresh red. No stool retention feeling inside the anus. Abdomen likes warmth and pressure. Urination is difficult.	Chishizhi 1 *jin* (25g) (with half ground into thin powder); dried ginger 1 *liang* (6g); Glutinous rice 1 *jin* (25g).
Tiaowei Chengqi Tang (调胃承气汤)	1.Yangming inner Excessiveness condition. Dislikes heat. Dry mouth and thirst. Constipation. Fullness in abdomen. Delirious speech. 2. After Vomiting therapy, patient feels abdominal bloating. 3. Yangming disease, no Vomiting therapy, or no Purging therapy yet, but patient feels annoyed.	Dahuang (peeled, washed with alcohol) 4 *liang* (12g); Zhigancao 2 *liang* (6g); Mangxiao (melted) 0.5 *shen* (10g).

Tinglizi Dazao Xiefei Tang (葶苈大枣泻肺汤)	1. Lung abscess. Coughs sticky purulent phlegm with very bad odor. Thirst. Tongue is red. The tongue coating is yellow. Or, lots of phlegm, coughs, asthma, short of breath. Fullness feeling in chest. Hard to lie down, or swelling of face. Urination is short. 2. Lung Fullness syndrome. Fullness in chest, short of breath. Hard to lie down. Swelling of face and body, loss of smell. Coughing and urgent sneezing.	Tinglizi (Processed to yellow color. Grind into pills 1cm in diameter.) twenty granules (10g); jujube (cut open) 12 granules.
Tongmai Si Ni Tang (通脉四逆汤)	Shaoyin disease. Body surface Hotness but inner Coldness. Cold hands and feet (Cold Jue condition). No cold-dislike feeling. Face is pink. Abdominal pain. Diarrhea with undigested food in stool. Belching or sore throat. Diarrhea stops but pulse cannot be felt. (Yang-wearing condition).	Use Si Ni Tang. Increase the amount of dried ginger to 3-4 *liang* (9g-12g). The Fuzi needs to be large.
Tongmai Si Ni Tang Jia pig gallbladder juice (通脉四逆加猪胆汁汤)	On the basis of the Tongmai Si Ni Tang condition, no more vomiting, nor further diarrhea. Body has sweat and Cold Jue condition. Arms and legs spasm without release. Pulse feels very faint and almost cannot be felt.	To Tongmai Si Ni Tang, add pig gallbladder juice 0.5 *he* (10ml).
Tuguagen San (土瓜根散)	Blood stagnation. It causes irregular menstruation. Blood volume is small. Color is dark red or purple with clots. Fullness and pain in lower abdomen. The pain is not reduced or patient refuses to press. Or, there is hard or firm mass in lower abdomen. Tongue is dim purple. Pulse feels deep or coarse.	Tuguagen; Shaoyao; Guizhi; Zhechong. 3 *liang* for each.
Weijing Tang (苇茎汤)	Lung abscess. Coughs and spits yellow, sticky pus phlegm. Slight fever with annoying fullness in chest. Chest skin is like fish scales.	Weijing (cut) 2 *shen* (30g); Yiyiren 0.5 *shen* (18g); Guaban 0.5 *shen* (24g); peach kernel 30 granules (9g).

215

Wen Jing Tang (温经汤)	Withered body condition. Coldness in uterus, which causes infertility. Hot feeling at later afternoon. Annoyingly hot on palms and soles. Dry mouth and rough lips. Cold feet. Urgent and fullness feeling in lower abdomen. Tongue tip is red, and The tongue coating is white. (Upper Hotness, lower Coldness, with middle stagnation).	Wuzhuyu 3 *liang* (6g); Ginseng 2 *liang* (6g); Guizhi 2 *liang* (6g); Chuanxiong 2 *liang* (6g); fresh ginger 2 *liang* (6g); Banxia 0.5 *shen* (6g); Gancao 2 *liang* (6g); Danggui 2 *liang* (6g); Shaoyao 2 *liang* (6g); Ajiao 2 *liang* (9g); Danpi 2 *liang* (9g); Maidong (remove kernel) 1 *shen* (9g).
Wenhe San (文蛤散)	1. Dampness-Hotness in Yin-Wei phase. Skin has small up-rising dots. Or skin is itchy. 2. Dampness-Hotness in Spleen-Stomach. If it is more Hotness than Dampness, patient feels thirst and desire to drink a lot of water. If Dampness is more than Hotness, patient has desire to drink water, but no thirsty feeling.	Clam 5 *liang*.
Wenhe Tang (文蛤汤)	1. After vomiting, patient feels thirsty and wants to drink a lot of water. 2. After Wind-attack, headache. Pulse feels tight.	Wenhe 5 *liang* (70g); Mahuang 3 *liang* (42g); Gancao 3 *liang* (42g); fresh ginger 3 *liang* (42g); Shigao 5 *liang* (70g); almond 50 granules; jujube 12 granules (3 granules).
Wu Ling San (五苓散)	1. Body surface condition, with inner water accumulation. Headache, fever, annoying thirst. Desires to drink water, but vomits after. Difficulty in urination. 2. Water-Dampness accumulation. Swelling, diarrhea, difficulty in urination, and vomiting. 3. Phlegm and thin-phlegm accumulation in stomach region. Palpitations under the navel. Spits. Dizziness. Short of breath and coughs.	Fuling 18 *zhu* (9g); Guizhi (peeled) 0.5 *liang* (6g); Baizhu 18 *zhu* (9g); Zhuling 18 *zhu* (9g); Zexie 1 *liang* and 6 *zhu* (15g).

Wumei Wan (乌梅丸)	1. Jueyin disease, Liver Yang deficiency. Coldness-Hotness mixture. Upper vomiting, but lower diarrhea. The symptoms come and go. Symptoms are severe but the physical signs are less so. The patient looks very annoyed. Tongue looks "old", is dark red. Pulse feels stringy, big, or hard. Inner Hotness, outer coldness. Symptoms may be worse in middle of the night (1 to 3am). 2. Stomach is Coldness but bowel is Hotness. 3. Worm Jue syndrome (cold hands and feet due to very painful abdomen from attack of worm in the abdomen). 4. Organ Jue syndrome (due to degeneration of all organs).	Wumei (black plum) 300 granules (480g); Xixin 6 liang (180g); dried ginger 10 liang (300g); Huanglian 16 liang (480g); Danggui 4 liang (120g); Fuzi (processed, peeled) 6 liang (180g); Huajiao (fried) 4 liang (120g); Guizhi 6 liang (180g); Ginseng 6 liang (180g); Huangbo 6 liang (180g).
Wutou Guizhi Tang (乌头桂枝汤)	Cold hernia. Pain in abdomen. Cold hands and feet (Cold Jue syndrome). Numbness in hands and feet during the pain. Body pain.	Wutou (big size) 5 granules; Guizhi (peeled) 3 *liang* (9g); Shaoyao 3 *liang* (9g); Zhigancao 2 *liang* (6g); fresh ginger 3 *liang* (9g); jujube 12 granule (3 granules).
Wutou Tang (乌头汤)	Joint pain due to Coldness-Dampness. Body is with Qi deficiency too. Joints are very painful, hard to bend or stretch.	Mahuan, Shaoyao, Huangqi, Zhigancao, 3 *liang* (9 g) for each, Chuanwutou 5 granules (6 g).
Wuzhuyu Tang (吴茱萸汤)	Jueyin disease. Liver Coldness-Weakness. 1. Vomits after eating. 2. Vomiting and diarrhea, cold hands and feet (Cold Jue syndrome), annoyed so much so that the patient even wishes to die. 3. Belching, spits, headache. 4. Nausea and fullness feeling in chest.	Wuzhuyu (washed) 1 *shen* (10-15g); Ginseng 3 *liang* (10-15g); fresh ginger (cut into pieces) 6 *liang* (20-30g); jujube (cut open) 12 granules (12-20 granules).

Xia Yuxue Tang (下瘀血汤)	Dead blood accumulation in lower abdomen. Dried dead blood sticks under the navel. Pain in lower abdomen. Can feel firm knob in the lower abdomen. Feel pain and resistant feeling when pressing on it. Bloating in abdomen. Constipation.	Dahuang 2 *liang* (6g); peach kernel 20 granules (4g); Zhechong 20 bodies (10g).
Xiong Gui Jiao A Tang (芎归胶艾汤)	Loss of blood. Body is weakness. Abdominal pain. Used more in women, after threatening abortion, or after birth delivery, too early menstruation or too large volume of menstrual blood.	Chuanxiong 2 *liang* (6g); Ajiao 2 *liang* (9g); Gancao 2 *liang* (5g); Aye 3 *liang* (9g); Danggui 3 *liang* (9g); Baishao 4 *liang* (12-15g); Shengdi 6 *liang* (18-24g).
Xu Ming Tang (续命汤)	1. Paralysis, difficult to speak, difficult to tell the exact location of pain or numbness of the body. Stiffness of the body so much so that it is difficult to turn the body. 2. Da Qinglong Tang condition with more saliva or hardness and fullness in stomach region. Or headache, abdominal pain. 3. Coughs and up-rushing feeling. Urgent sneezing and cough. Swollen look to face. Dry mouth and annoying thirst. Can lie face down but not face up.	Mahuang 3 *liang* (10-30g); Guizhi 3 *liang* (10-30g); Danggui 3 *liang* (10-30g); Ginseng (10-30g); Shigao 3 *liang* (40-200g); dried ginger 3 *liang* (10-20g); Gancao 3 *liang* (5-15g); Chuanxiong 1 *liang* (10-20g); almond 40 granules (10-20g).
Xuanfu Daizhishi Tang (旋复代赭石汤)	Stomach Qi deficiency, Liver Qi up-rushing. Phlegm and thin-phlegm blockage in the stomach region. Hardness and firm feeling in stomach region. Continuous hiccup.	Xuanfuhua 3 *liang* (9g); fresh ginger 5 *liang* (15g); Ginseng 2 *liang* (6g); Daizheshi 1 *liang* (3g); Zhigancao 3 *liang* (9g); Banxia (washed) 0.5 *shen* (12g); jujube (cut open) 12 granules.
Xuanfuhua Tang (旋复花汤)	Liver Zhe syndrome. Fullness and bloating in chest, even bloating pain. Like the chest is being pressed or even wishes another person to stand on the chest.	Xuanfuhua 3 *liang* (9g); shallot 14 stems (6 stems); Xinjiang a little (a little).
Yinchenhao Tang (茵陈蒿汤)	Yangming Dampness-Hotness Jaundice. The Dampness and the Hotness are equal in intensity.	Yinchenhao 6 *liang* (10-80g); Zhizi (open) 14 granules (10-15g); Dahuang (peeled) 2 *liang* (6-10g).

Yiyi Fuzi Baijiang San (薏苡附子败酱散)	Bowel abscess. Body skin is like fish scales. Abdominal skin is tight, with drum-like surface. No fever. Pulse feels fast. Mostly used in chronic stage.	Yiyiren 10 *fen* (30g); Fuzi 2 *fen* (6g); Baijiancao (Patrinia) 5 *fen* (15g).
Yiyiren Fuzi San (薏苡附子散)	Chest Bi syndrome, due to Yang deficiency, Dampness accumulation. Pain in heart region and chest. The pain is worse with cold and damp weather. Face is pale. Cold hands and feet, chilly, dislikes cold. Fatigue. Poor appetite and poor sleep. Tongue is pale. The tongue coating is white-greasy. Pulse feels slow and soft. The pain comes and goes, sometimes worse, at other times there is no pain.	Yiyiren and Pao Fuzi in equal amounts.
Yuebi Jia Banxia Tang (越婢加半夏汤)	Lung Fullness syndrome. Fullness feeling in chest. Urgent coughing or sneezing, short of breath. Eyes bulge. Pulse feels floating and big.	To Yuebi Tang, add Banxia 0.5 *shen* (9g).
Yuebi Jia Zhu Tang (越婢加术汤)	Dampness and Hotness. 1. Face and whole body swelling. Pulse feels deep. Urination is difficult. 2. Body swelling and pain, but more swelling than pain. 3. Disease in Spleen-Stomach. Muscle is withered, thin, more sweat. 4. Yang choked and water accumulation. Swelling in face and body, big abdomen, heavy body, tired arms and legs. Annoyed feeling. Difficulty in urination. 5. Disease under skin. Sweat and swelling. With more sweat the swelling does not subside.	To Yuebi Tang, add Baizhu 4 *liang* (12g).
Yuebi Tang (越婢汤)	1. Wind-water syndrome. Swelling on face, arms and legs. The swelling develops very fast. Dislikes wind. Sweat and thirst. Pulse feels floating. 2. Early stage of Warm disease. Body surface hotness, not water accumulation.	Mahuang 6 *liang* (18g); Shigao 0.5 *jin* (24g); fresh ginger 3 *liang* (9g); Gancao 2 *liang* (6g); jujube 15 granules.

Zeqi Tang (泽漆汤)	Thin-phlegm rushes up with Hotness, to attack the lungs. Coughing and deep pulse. Tongue is red. The tongue coating is thick, while- or yellow-greasy. Eyes are red. Phlegm is sticky and yellowish. Long time coughing, which comes and goes. Coughs occur usually in the early morning.	Banxia 0.5 *shen* (9g); Zishen 5 *liang* (15g); Zeqi 3 *jin* (30g); fresh ginger 5 *liang* (15g); Baiqian 5 *liang* (15g); Gancao 3 *liang* (9g); Huangqin 3 *liang* (9g); Ginseng 3 *liang* (9g); Guizhi 3 *liang* (9g).
Zexie Tang (泽泻汤)	Branch thin-phlegm syndrome. Annoying dizziness, whether lying down or sitting up.	Zexie 5 *liang* (1 g); Baizhu 2 *liang* (6g).
Zhenwu Tang (真武汤)	1. Spleen-Kidney Yang deficiency. Garbage water accumulation. Arms and legs feel heavy. Difficulty in urination. Abdominal pain and diarrhea. Or swelling in arms and legs. The tongue coating is white. Pulse feels deep. 2. Taiyang disease, after Sweating therapy, the person still has fever. Palpitations, dizziness, shaking muscles. Body shakes as if about to fall to the ground.	Fuling 3 *liang* (9g); Fuzi (peeled, cut into 8 slices) 1 granule (12g); Shaoyao 3 *liang* (9g); Baizhu 2 *liang* (6g); fresh ginger 3 *liang* (9g).
Zhi Gancao Tang (炙甘草汤)	1. Withered condition. Yin and blood deficiency. Yang Qi is weak. Palpitations, short of breath. Tongue is smooth as mirror (with very little or no tongue cover), dry and small. Pulse feels irregular and as knob. 2. Lung withered syndrome. Coughs and spits. Body is weak and thin. Short of breath. Sweat anytime. No-reason annoyed feeling. Poor sleep. Dry mouth and throat. Constipation. Pulse feels weak and fast.	Zhigancao 4 *liang* (12g); fresh ginger 3 *liang* (9g); Ginseng 2 *liang* (6g); Shengdi 1 *jin* (50g); Guizhi (peeled) 3 *liang* (9g); Ajiao 2 *liang* (6g); Maimengdong (remove kernel) 0.5 *shen* (10g); Mazi kernel 0.5 *shen* (10g); jujube 30 granules (10 granules).
Zhi Zhu Tang (枳术汤)	Stomach function is impaired by improper diet. Qi stagnation and water accumulation in stomach. Feels hardness and fullness in the upper abdomen.	Zhishi 7 granules (15g); Baizhu 2 *liang* (5g).
Zhishi Shaoyao San (枳实芍药散)	After birth delivery, Qi-Blood stagnated or sluggish. Abdominal pain. Annoying fullness in abdomen, hard to lie down for	Zhishi (burn to black) and Shaoyao in equal amounts.

sleep.

Zhishi Xiebai Guuizhi Tang (枳实薤白桂枝汤)	Chest Bi syndrome due to Chest Yang Qi blockage. Phlegm and dirty Qi up-rushes to attack heart. More Qi stagnation. Pain in front and back of chest. Fullness in chest and in stomach region. Air up-rushing to punch the chest from under the rib arch. Fullness in abdomen. Firm stool. The tongue coating is thick, white-greasy. Pulse feels stringy and tight.	Zhishi 4 granules (9g); Houpu 4 *liang* (12g); Xiebai 8 *liang* (9g); Guizhi 1 *liang* (3g); Gualou kernel (grind to small pieces) 1 granule (15g).
Zhizi Baipi Tang (栀子柏皮汤)	Dampness-Hotness jaundice. More Hotness than Dampness.	Zhizi 15 granules (15g); Gancao 1 *liang* (5g); Huongbai 2 *liang* (10g).
Zhizi Chi Tang (栀子豉汤)	Yangming Hotness. Hotness in chest and stomach. Annoyed and perturbed feeling. Hard to fall asleep. In severe cases, the patient may turn left-right, right-left in bed.	Zhizi 12 granules (10-15g); Xiangchi (folded, Fermented soybean) 4 *liang* (10-15g).
Zhizi Dahuang Tang (栀子大黄汤)	Jaundice. Due to long-term alcoholism. Dampness-Hotness accumulated in stomach, steaming to skin. Feels annoyed and perturbed, or hot pain in stomach.	Zhizi 14 granules (9g); Dahuang 1 *liang* (3g); Zhishi 5 granules (12g); Douchi 1 *shen* (10g).
Zhizi Gancao Chi Tang (栀子甘草豉汤)	Zhizi Chi Tang condition with fatigue, shortness of breath.	Add Gancao 2 *liang* (6g) to Zhizi Chi Tang.
Zhizi Ganjiang Tang (栀子干姜汤)	Zhizi Chi Tang condition with diarrhea.	Zhizi (cut) 14 granules (9g); dried ginger 2 *liang* (6g).
Zhizi Houpu Tang (栀子厚朴汤)	Zhizi Chi Tang condition with fullness in abdomen, restlessness, hard to sit down or lie down.	Zhizi 12 granules (9g); Houpu (processed, peeled) 4 *liang* (12g); Zhishi (rinsed in water, processed) 4 granules (9g).
Zhizi Shengjiang Chi Tang (栀子生姜豉汤)	Zhizi Chi Tang condition with nausea and vomiting.	Add fresh ginger 5 *liang* (15g) to Zhizi Chi Tang.

Zhu Fa Gao Jian (猪膏发煎)	1. Dryness in stomach and bowel. Diet cannot nourish the skin. Skin is withered yellow in color. 2. Firm stool, the nutrition Qi goes to front of perinea region, feel as if wind blows in this region.	Zhugao 0.5 *jin* (24g); 3 lumps of hair (each the size of an egg) (9g).
Zhufu Tang (猪肤汤)	1. Shaoyin disease. Yin deficiency with dryness. Lower abdomen is Coldness, feet are cold. Acne on face. Hair is dry and withered. Face is wrinkled. Skin is coarse. 2. Shaoyin disease. Diarrhea, sore throat, fullness in chest, annoyed.	Zhufu (pig skin) 1 *jin*.
Zhuling Tang (猪苓汤)	Water-Hotness entanglement. Yin deficiency. 1. Fever, nausea and thirst. Annoyed and hard to fall asleep. Dry mouth, dry throat, and dry skin. Difficulty in urination. Urine is yellow and short. Pain in urinary duct. Bloating and fullness in lower abdomen. 2. Urgent urine, frequent urine, blood in urine or pain after urination. Tongue is red. The tongue coating is slippery. Pulse feels floating.	Zhuling (peel) 1 *liang* (9g); Fuling 1 *liang* (9g); Zexie 1 *liang* (9g); Ajiao 1 *liang* (9g); Huashi (break) 1 *liang* (9g).
Zhuye Shigao Tang (竹叶石膏汤)	1. Traditional stage of febrile diseases with slight hotness remaining in the body. Qi-Liquid both deficiency. Nausea, annoying thirst. Dry mouth and throat, and coughing. Annoying fullness in chest. Annoyed and hard to fall asleep. Tongue is red. The tongue coating is sparse. Pulse feels weak and fast. 2. Heatstroke. Qi-Liquid body deficiency. Hot, much sweating, short of breath, annoying thirst, wants to drink. Tongue is red. Pulse feels weak and fast.	Bamboo leaves (Zhuye) 2 handfuls (15g); Shigao 1 *jin* (30g); Banxia (washed) 0.5 *shen* (9g); Maidong (remove kernel) 5 *liang* (15g); Ginseng 2 *liang* (6g); Zhigancao 2 *liang* (6g); Glutinous rice 0.5 *shen* (15g).
Zou Ma Tang (走马汤)	Sudden onset of diseases. Acute and severe heart pain. Abdominal bloating. Stool is hard to pass. No sign of Hotness.	Badou (peeled, remove kernel, fried to deplete oil) 1 granule; almond 2 granules.

Note:

1. In the column of *Herbal Formulas, jin, liang,* and *fen,* are ancient Chinese units of weight. One *jin* is equal to 16 *liang.* One *liang* is equal to 10 *qian.* One *fen* is equal to four *qian.* *Shen, he and qianbi* are ancient units of volume. One *shen* is equal to ten *he.* One *shen* is equal to 200ml. One *he* is equal to 20ml (water). One *qianbi* is equal to 1.5-1.8ml.

2. In the column of *Herbal Formulas,* the *g* means weight in grams.

3. There is no standard agreement for the conversion of ancient units to modern ones. Current data from different sources suggests that one *liang* could be equal to 3 grams, 13 grams, or 15.625 grams. The amount of herbs listed in the formulas is mostly from current textbooks and used by most TCM doctors in China nowadays. However, it is only a reference.

4. Data here is far enough away to allow readers to apply it to clinical work. It is strongly recommended to refer to the book *Current Opinion on Classical Herbal Formula.* Different herbal formulas require different ways of preparation, drinking, and post-drinking precautions.

5. The data in the column *Treatment Targets* are a rough summary. Data are collected from either TCM textbook, online articles, or from various doctor's personal opinions. The data could be different from that in the TCM textbook.

6. Formulas in this table are collected mostly from the book *Shanghan Lun*; some are from *Jin Kui Yao Luo.*

Chinese and English names of herbs

Chinese Pinyin	Chinese name	English name
Ajiao	阿胶	Donkey-hide gelatin
Aye	艾叶	Mugwort
Badou	巴豆	Burging croton
Baibiandou	白扁豆	White lentils
Baihe	百合	Lily
Baihuasheshecao	白花蛇舌草	Herba Hedyotis
Baiji,	白芨	Common bletilla tuber
Baijiangcao	败酱草	Patrinia
Baijiezie	白芥子	Semen brassicae
Baijili	白蒺藜	Tribulus terrestris
Baimaogen	白茅根	Rhizoma imperatae
Baipi	柏皮	Cypress peel
Baiqian	白前	Cynanchum glaucescens
Baishao	白芍	Radices paeoniae alba
Baishizhi	白石脂	Halloysitum album
Baitouwen	白头翁	Windflower
Baiwei	白薇	Cynanchum atratum Bge.
Baixianpi	白鲜皮	Cortex dictam
Baiye	柏叶	Cypress leaf
Baizhi	白芷	Angelica dahurica benth. et hook
Baizhu	白术	White atractylodes rhizome
Baiziren	柏子仁	Semen boitae
Banlangen	板蓝根	Radix isatidis
Banxia	半夏	Pinellia ternata
Baodoukou	白豆蔻	Amomun kravanh
Beimu	贝母	Fritillaria
Biejia	鳖甲	Turtle shell
Binglang	槟榔	Areca catechu
Bingpian	冰片	Borneol
Bohe	薄荷	Mint
Buguzhi	补骨脂	Fructus psoraleae
Cangerzi	苍耳子	Cocklebur fruit
Caoheche	草河车	Bistortae,rhizoma
Cebaiye	侧柏叶	Cacumen biotae
Chaihu	柴胡	Radix Bupleuri
Changshan	常山	Antipyretic dichroa
Chanyi	蝉衣	Cicada sloughs

Chenpi	陈皮	Orange peel
Chenxiang	沉香	Eaglewood
Cheqianzi	车前子	Plantago seed
Chishao	赤芍	The (unpeeled) root of common peony
Chishizhi	赤石脂	Red halloysite
Chixiaodou	赤小豆	Red phaseolus bean
Chongweizi	茺蔚子	Fructus leonuri
Chuangshanjia	穿山甲	Scale of scaly anteater
Chuanjiao	川椒	Pericarpium Zanthoxyli
Chuanlianzi	川楝子	Chinaberry fruit
Chuanxinlian	穿心莲	Common andrographis
Chuanxiong	川芎	Ligusticum wallichii
Chuipencao	垂盆草	Sedum
Cishi	磁石	Iodestone
Congbai	葱白	White stem of shallot
Dahuang	大黄	Rheum officinale
Daizheshi	代赭石	Ruddle
Daji	大戟	Euphorbia pekinensis
Danggui	当归	Angelica sinensis
Dangshen	党参	Codonopsis pilosula
Dannanxing	胆南星	Arisaema cum bile
Danpi	丹皮	The root bark of the peony tree
Danshen	丹参	The root of red-rooted salvia
Daqingye	大青叶	Green leaf hopper
Difuzi	地肤子	Fructus kochiae
Dilong	地龙	Dried earthworm
Diyu	地榆	Sanguisorba officinalis
Dongguaren	冬瓜仁	Winter melon kernel
Dongguazi	冬瓜子	Semen benincasae
Dongkuizi	冬葵子	Chingma abutilon seed
Douchi	豆豉	Fermented soya beans, salted or otherwise
Duhuo	独活	Levisticum
Duzhong	杜仲	The bark of eucommia
Eguanshi	鹅冠石	The root of kudzu vine
Ezhu	莪术	Curcuma zedoary
Fangfeng	防风	Saposhnikovia divaricata
Fangji	防己	The root of fangji (Stephania tetrandra)
Fanshi	矾石	Aluminite
Fengfang	蜂房	Apiary
Fengweicao	凤尾草	Phoenix-tail fern
Foshou	佛手	Bergamot

Fuling	茯苓	Poria cocos
Fuping	浮萍	Duckweed
Fushen	茯神	Indian bread hostwood
Fuxiaomai	浮小麦	Light wheat
Fuzi	附子	Aconitum carmichaeli
Gancao	甘草	(Mangnolia officinalis)
Gansong,	甘松	Coptis chinensis
Gansui	甘遂	Euphorbia kansui
Gaoben	藁本	Sakamoto
Gegen	葛根	The root of kudzu vine
Gehua	葛花	Flos puerariae
Gejie	蛤蚧	Gecko
Gouji	狗脊	Cibotium barometz
Gouqizi	枸杞子	Wolfberry fruit
Gouteng	钩藤	Radix Scutellariae
Guadi	瓜蒂	Muskmelon pedicle
Gualou	瓜蒌	Trichosanthes kirilowii Maxim
Guiban	龟板	Tortoise plastron
Guizhi	桂枝	Cinnamomi ramulus
Gusuibu	骨碎补	Drynaria rhizome
Haijinsha	海金沙	Lygodium japonicum
Haipiaoxiao	海螵蛸	Cuttle-bone
Haizao	海藻	Alga
Hanmolian	旱墨莲	Dry dark lotus
Hanshuishi	寒水石	Gypsum rubrum
Hehuanpi	合欢皮	Cortex albizziae
Heshouwu	何首乌	Polygonum multiflorum
Hezi	诃子	Chebule
Houpo	厚朴	Platycodon grandiflorum
Huajiao	花椒	Bunge pricklyash seed
Huangbo	黄柏	Golden cypress
Huangjing	黄精	Rhizoma polygonati
Huanglian	黄连	Tussilago
Huangqi	黄芪	Fossil fragments
Huangqin	黄芩	Scutellaria baicalensis
Huashi	滑石	Speckstone
Hubo	琥珀	Amber
Huoxiang	藿香	Agastache rugosus
Huzhang	虎杖	Polydatin
Jiangcan	僵蚕	Dried Silkworm
Jiaosanxian	焦三仙	Chared Shanzha, Maiya, Shenqu

Jiegen	桔梗	Platycodon grandiflorum
Jigucao	鸡骨草	Canton love-pea vine
Jineijin	鸡内金	Inner membrane of chicken stomach
Jingjiesui	荆芥穗	Schizonepeta spike
Jingli	荆沥	
Jinqiancao	金钱草	Desmodium
Jinqiaomai	金荞麦	Golden buckwheat
Jinyinhua	金银花	Honeysuckle
Jixingzi	急性子	Seed of garden balsam
Jixueteng	鸡血藤	Lignum millettiae
Juemingzi	决明子	Semen cassiae torae
Juhua	菊花	Chrysanthemum
Juluo	橘络	Tangerine pith
Jumai	瞿麦	Buckwheat
Kuandonghua	款冬花	Concha ostreae
Kufan	枯矾	Dried alum
Kuizi	葵子	Sunflower seed
Kuliangenpi	苦楝根皮	Melia azedarach root bark
Kunbu	昆布	Sea-tangle
Kushen	苦参	Radix sophorae flavescentis [flavescen]
Laifuzi	莱菔子	Semen raphani
Leigongteng	雷公藤	Tripterygium wilfordii
Lianqiao	连翘	Forsythia suspensa Vahl
Ligenbaipi	李根白皮	Peel of root of plum tree
Lilu	藜芦	Black false hellebore
Lingyangjiao	羚羊角	Cornu antelopis
Lizhihe	荔枝核	Semen litchi
Longdancao	龙胆草	Gentian
Longgu	龙骨	Fossil fragments
Loulu	漏芦	Globethistle Root
Lugen	芦根	Reed rhizome
Lujiaojiao	鹿角胶	Antler glue
Lujiaoshuang	鹿角霜	Ccornua cervi degelatinatum
Luoshiteng	络石藤	Trachelospermum jasminoides
Lurong	鹿茸	Pilose antler (of a young stag)
Luwei	芦苇	Ditch reed
Mabo	马勃	Bovista
Macixian	马齿苋	Herba portulacae
Mahuang	麻黄	Chinese ephedra
Maidong	麦冬	Lilyturf root
Maiya	麦芽	Malt

227

Mangchong	芒虫	Locust
Mangxiao	芒硝	Glauber salt
Manjingzi	蔓荆子	Fructus viticis
Maziren	麻子仁	Hempen kernel
Menshi	礞石	Chlorite schist
Miubangzi	牛蒡子	Fructus arctii
Moyao	没药	Myrrh
Mudanpi	牡丹皮	Bark of tree peony root
Mufangji	木防己	Cocculus trilobus
Mugua	木瓜	Fructus chaenomelis lagenariae
Muli	牡蛎	Oyster
Mutong	木通	Fiveleaf akebia root
Muxiang	木香	Radices saussureae
Muzeicao	木贼草	Equisetum hiemale Linne
Niuxi	牛膝	Maria glass, or plaster
Nuzhenzi	女贞子	Fructus ligustri lucidi
Oujie	藕节	Lutus root
Peilan	佩兰	Eupatorium
Pengsha	硼砂	Borax
Pianjianghuang	片姜黄	Piece of turmeric
Pugongying	蒲公英	Dandelion
Puhuang	蒲黄	Cattail pollen
Qiancao	茜草	Madder
Qianghuo	羌活	Notopterygium root
Qianhu	前胡	Angelica decursiva
Qianniuzi	牵牛子	Semen Pharbitidis
Qicao	蛴螬	Grub
Qingdai	青黛	Indigo naturalis
Qinghao	青蒿	Artemisia apiacea
Qingpi	青皮	Pericarpium citri reticulatae viride
Qingxiangzi	青葙子	Semen celosiae
Qinjiao	秦艽	Gentiana
Qinpi	秦皮	Fraxinus rhynchophylla Hance
Quanxie,	全蝎	Scorpio
Rendongteng	忍冬藤	Caulis lonicerae
Renshen	人参	Ginseng
Roucongrong	肉苁蓉	Herba cistanches
Roudoukou	肉豆蔻	Nutmeg
Ruxiang	乳香	Boswellia carterii
Sangbaipi	桑白皮	The root bark of white mulberry
Sangye	桑叶	Folium mori

Sangzhi	桑枝	Ramulus mori
Sanleng	三棱	Sparganium stoloni erum
Shancigu	山慈姑	Appendiculate cremastra flower
Shandougen	山豆根	Subprostrate sophora
Shanglugen	商陆根	Pokeweed root
Shangzha	山楂	Hawthorn
Shanyurou	山萸肉	Fructus Corni
Shaoyao	山药	Chinese yam
Sharen	砂仁	Fructus amomi
Shashen	沙参	The root of straight ladybell
Shechuangzi	蛇床子	Fructus cnidii
Shegan	射干	Blackberry lily
Shengdi	生地	Dried rehamnnia root
Shengma	升麻	Rattletop
Shenqieluo	生铁落	Iron flakes
Shenqu	神曲	Divine tune
Sheshecao	蛇舌草	Hedyotis diffusa
Shichangpu	石菖蒲	Acorus gramineus Soland
Shigao	石膏	Oulopholite
Shihu	石斛	Dendrobe
Shijunzi	使君子	The fruit of Rangoon creeper
Shinian	石楠	Moor besom
Shoufuzi	熟附子	Radix Aconiti Laterailis Prepareata
Shudi	熟地	Rehmannia glutinosa
Shuizhi	水蛭	Leech
Shujiao	蜀椒	Shu pepper
Shuti	蜀漆	Antifebrile dichroa branchlet and leaf
Shuyu	薯蓣	Yam
Suanzaoren	酸枣仁	Semen zizyphi spinosae
Sugen	苏梗	Perilla frutescens
Suye	苏叶	Beef-steak plant leaf
Suzi	苏子	Perillaseed
Taizishen	太子参	Pseudostellaria heterophylla
Tanxiang	檀香	White sandalwood
Tianhuafeng	天花粉	Radices trichosanthis
Tianma	天麻	Rhizoma gastrodiae
Tianmendong	天门冬	Radix asparagi
Tinglizi	葶苈子	Semen lepidii
Tongcao	通草	Ricepaper pith
Tubiechong	土鳖虫	Ground beetle
Tufuling	土茯苓	Tuckahoe

Tuguagen	土瓜根	Tucurbita root
Tusizi	菟丝子	The seed of Chinese dodder
Walengzi	瓦楞子	Concha arcae
Weilingxian	威灵仙	Radix clematidis
Weirui	葳蕤	Polygonatum odoratum
Wenhe	文蛤	Clam
whole Gualu	瓜蒌	Trichosanthes kirilowii Maxim
Wubeizi	五倍子	Chinese gall
Wugong	蜈蚣	Centipede
Wulingzi	五灵脂	Excrementum pteropi
Wumei	乌梅	Smoked plum
Wushaoshe	乌梢蛇	Zaocys dhumnade
Wutou	乌头	The rhizome of Chinese monkshood
Wuweizi	五味子	The fruit of Chinese magnoliavine
Wuyao	乌药	The root of three-nerved spicebush
Wuzeigu	乌贼骨	Cuttle-bone
Wuzhuyu	吴茱萸	Evodia rutaecarpa
Xiakucao	夏枯草	Selfheal
Xiangchi	香豉	Fermented soybean
Xiangfu	香附	Rhizoma cyperi
Xiangru	香薷	Herba elsholtziae
Xianhecao	仙鹤草	Hairyvein agrimony
Xianlingpi	仙灵脾	Elixir
Xiaohuixiang	小茴香	Fennel
Xiaoshi	硝石	Saltpetre
Xiebai	薤白	Longstamen onion bulb
Xinjiang	新绛(茜草)	Madder
Xinyi	辛夷	Magnoliae,flos
Xionghuang	雄黄	Realgar
Xixin	细辛	Asarum sieboldi Mig.
Xuanfuhua	旋覆花	Inula britannica chinensis
Xuanmai	玄麦	Xuan wheat
Xuanshen	玄参	Radix scrophulariae
Xuduan	续断	Teasel root
Yangqishi	阳起石	Chrysotilum
Yangzhi	羊脂石	Lambstone
Yanhua	芫花	Flos genkwa
Yejiaoteng	夜交腾	Polygonum multiflorum Thunb
Yimucao	益母草	Motherwort
Yinchenhao	茵陈蒿	Artemisia capillaris Thunb
Yinyanghuo	淫羊藿	Epimedium

Yitang	饴糖	Malt sugar
Yiyi kernel	薏苡仁	Semen Coicis
Yuanhu	元胡	Corydalis tuber
Yuanhua	芫花	Flos genkwa
Yuanminfeng	玄明粉	Refined mirabilite
Yuanshen	元参	Radix scrophulariae
Yuanzhi	远志	Polygala root
Yujin	郁金	Curcuma rcenyujin
Yunmu	云母	Mica
Yuxingcao	鱼腥草	Houttuynia cordata
Yuyuliang	禹余粮	Limonitum
Yuzhu	玉竹	Radix polygonati officinalis
Zaojia	皂荚	Chinese honey locust
Zaojiaoci	皂角刺	Spina gleditsiae
Zelan	泽兰	Eupatorium japonicum Thunb
Zeqi	泽漆	Euphorbia helioscopia
Zexie	泽泻	Rhizoma alismatis
Zhe Beimu	浙 贝母	Fritillaria thunnanensis
Zhechong	蛰虫	Dormant insect
Zhenzhumu	珍珠母	Mother of pearl
Zhigancao	炙甘草	Prepared radix glycyrrhizae
Zhike	枳壳	Fructus aurantii
Zhimu	知母	Unpeeled rhizoma anemarrhenae
Zhishi	枳实	Fructus aurantii immaturus
Zhizi	栀子	Cape jasmine
Zhufu	猪肤	Port skin
Zhuli	竹沥	Bamboo juice
Zhuling	猪苓	Grifola
Zhuru	竹茹	Bambusae caulis im taeniam
Zhusha	朱砂	Cinnabar
Zhuye	竹叶	Folia bambosae
Zicao	紫草	Radix lithospermi
Zigen	紫根	Root of Sinkiang Arnebia
Zihua Diding	紫花地丁	Tokyo violet herb
Zishen	紫参 (石见穿)	salvia chinensis
Zishiying	紫石英	Amethyst
Zisu	紫苏	Purple perilla
Zisuzi	紫苏子	Perillae,fructus
Ziwan	紫菀	Aster

Our other publications

- More Than Acupuncture
- Acupuncture for Emergencies
- Acupuncture Styles in Current Practice
- What We Can Learn from Acupuncture Research in Western Countries
- Does Nora Five-element Acupuncture Depend mostly on Psychological Effect?
- Current Opinion on Shanghan Lun
- Jingfang Today

Books are available in Amazon.com

References

[1] Liu Guantao. Jiang Jianguo talks about "thousand years "puzzling" of Jueyin diseases. 【刘观涛力荐姜建国谈 "千古疑案"厥阴病】 http://blog.sina.com.cn/s/blog_5f856c9a0101f6uq.html

[2] Hu Xishu. *Shanghan Lun* lecture 【胡希恕讲伤寒论】 http://www.tcm100.com/user/hxsjshl/zzbook2.htm

[3] Liu Duzhou. *Shanghan Lun* Lecture 【刘渡舟伤寒论讲稿】 http://www.tcm100.com/user/ldzshljg/index.htm

[4] Hao Wanshan. *Shanghan Lun* lecture 【郝万山讲伤寒论】 http://www.tcm100.com/user/hwsjshl/index.htm

[5] Ni Haixia. *Shanghan Lun* Lecture 【倪海厦人纪-伤寒论】 http://www.zyy123.com/zazhiall/74887.html

[6] Tan Jiezhong. Follow JT uncle to learn *Shanghan Lun*. 【JT 叔叔伤寒杂病论慢慢教】 老恕的博客 http://blog.sina.com.cn/s/blog_61b024da0102eo17.html

[7] Li Keshao, Zhang Guizhen, Zhang Hongcai, Li Jiapu. 【伤寒论语释】 Shandong Science and Technology Press. Shangdong, China. 1982

[8] Di Lengxian. My opinion about Shanghan disease and Warm disease. 【翟冷仙:伤寒杂病:我对伤寒与温病的 看法．】 http://blog.sina.com.cn/s/blog_4b3d991e0102v917.html

[9] Xu Chenghe. Several questions that must be made clear during lecture for *Shanghan Lun* 【徐成贺:伤寒论太阳 病"教学必须要搞清的几个问题．】 http://blog.sina.com.cn/s/blog_5e38503701015dlv.html

[10] Gui Liang. Experience and ideas of one of my students in study of *Shanghan Lun*. 【桂亮: 笔者某学生研究 《伤寒论》体会： 《伤寒论》第七条和第十一条释．】 http://blog.sina.com.cn/s/blog_6069fe530100yg43.html

[11] Cai Changfu. Several ways of thinking about *Shanghan Lun*. 【蔡长福老师对几种癌症的治疗思路】 http://blog.sina.com.cn/s/blog_69824c190102v73k.html

[12] Xiao Xiangru. The paragraph 326 is not the main outline for Jueyin disease. 【肖相如: 326 条不是厥阴病的提 纲】 http://www.gltcm.cn/?uid-15530-action-viewspace-itemid-26320

[13] Liao Houze. *Jingfang Lincheng Chuanxin Lu*. 【廖厚泽: 经方临证传心录】 Zhao Ningning Ed. People's Health Publishing House. China. 2011.

[14] Lao Zhuang. New explanation about *Shanghan Lun*. 【老庄:《伤寒论》全新破解】 https://wenku.baidu.com/view/572ee5a4d15abe23492f4d2f.html

[15] Huang Huang. *Shanghan Lun* lecture. 【黄煌讲伤寒论】 开心中医缘的博客 http://blog.sina.com.cn/s/blog_5f856c9a0101en2t.html

[16] Zhang Butao. Herbal table used by family Zhang. 【张步桃: 张氏汤方药物组成表】 http://www.baicao99.com/threads/6449/

[17] WHO International Standard technologies on traditional medicIne In the Western Pacific region (2007). http://www.wpro.who.int/publications/who_istrm_file.pdf

[18] Traditional Chinese Medicine/Chinese Medical Terms. Wikibooks. https://en.wikibooks.org/wiki/Traditional_Chinese_Medicine/Chinese_Medical_Terms.

[19] Nigel Wiseman.Translation of Chinese Medical Terms:

A Source-Oriented Approach (2000). http://www.paradigm-pubs.com/sites/www.paradigm-pubs.com/files/files/ex.pdf

[20] English-Chinese Chinese-English professional glossary 【专业英汉汉英词典】. https://zhuanye.911cha.com/

[21] Li Yuming. Herbal formula Gegen Tang is the main formula for the Taiyang stage of Shanghan disease. 【李宇铭.论葛根汤属太阳伤寒代表方】 Henan TCM. 2011;31(6): 569-571

[22] Dengdai Huakai. Discussion about the co-existing conditions in the *Shanghan Lun*. 【等待花开: 伤寒研究之合病解析】 http://blog.sina.com.cn/s/blog_5f856c9a0101dbpc.html)

[23] Wukong Daoke. Table of Getting-better in Six diseases. 【悟恐刀客: 六经病欲解时图】 http://www.360doc.com/content/10/1129/13/8186_73391042.shtml

[24] Hao Wanshan. The time rule of Taiyang disease development. 【郝万山: 讲太阳病病程的时间规律】 http://www.tcm100.com/user/hwsjshl/zzbook9.htm

[25] Chuancheng Zhongyi. The Getting-better and Getting-worse time zones of six diseases in *Shanghan Lun*. 【六经病的欲解时和欲作时】. Cited from Fuxing Zhongyi Website. http://aaaaaa2307a.lofter.com/post/1ccdcdd1_737d26a

[26] Hu Xishu. *Shanghan Lun* Lecture 【胡希恕讲伤寒论】 http://www.tcm100.com/user/hxsjshl/index.htm

[27] Zhang Zenkui blog. Jueyin disease- Wumeiwan. 【厥阴病 乌梅丸】. http://blog.sina.com.cn/s/blog_70db7a890102w088.html

[28] Lin Zhiman, Xiao Feng. Special and unique role of ancient TCM doctors. 【林之满, 萧枫:独领风骚的古代医家】 Liaohai Publishing House. China. 2008-02

[29] Xing Bin. Self-preface for book *Shanghan Lun* truth. 【邢斌: 伤寒论求真·自序】 http://blog.sina.com.cn/s/blog_aef2dc7e0101dr4q.html

[30] Cai Changfu. The reason and mechanism for Esophageal cancer, and its Six Jing diagnosis. 【蔡长福: 从食道癌的病因病机到六经辨证.】 http://blog.sina.com.cn/s/blog_500e196c0102emfh.html

[31] Feng Shilun. Different diagnosis systems used in *Shanghan Lun* and *Huangdi Nei Jing*. 【冯世纶:《伤寒论》与《内经》辨治方法不同】 http://www.haodf.com/zhuanjiaguandian/zhaodongqi_5257240398.htm

[32] Zhai Wanghao. The misunderstanding for *Shanghan Lun*. 【寨王潮: 对《伤寒论》的误解】 http://www.baijiahefu.com/article/explore/think/2013-03-28/469.html

[33] Fang Guoqiang. Medical sources of book *Shanghan Zabing Lun* by Dr. Zhang Zhongjing. 【方国强: 张机伤寒杂病论之医药学术源流】 http://blog.sina.com.cn/s/blog_70db7a890100r6p6.html

[34] Ma Wenhui. Discussion of time and space differentiation of three-yin and three-yang in Shanghan Lun. 【马文辉: 试论《伤寒论》的"六病"辨证及"三部"定位】 J Chin Integr Med, July 2005, 3 (4):257-259 · http://blog.sina.com.cn/s/blog_765a7af10100yee4.html

[35] Du Yumao. Explanation of questions about *Shanghan Lun* and clinic trying of the Classical formulas. 【杜雨茂: 伤寒论释疑与经方实验】 Chinese Medicine Science and Technology Press. 2001.

[36] Zhu Liangchun. Clinic application of *Shanghan Lun* theory. 【朱良春:《伤寒论》理论的临床应用】 医海一绝. http://blog.sina.com.cn/s/blog_66b5edc00102vxbd.html

37 Xu Jiadong. Review of therapeutic methods in *Shanghan Lun* – discussion about the diagnosis in Classical formula system. 【许家栋: 还原仲圣手段——经方辨证论治浅谈】 http://blog.sina.com.cn/s/blog_70db7a890102xioy.html

38 Liu Zhijie. The key theory of *Shanghan Lun* is the Six Gang diagnosis system. 【刘志杰: 伤寒论的理论核心是六纲辨证】 http://blog.sina.com.cn/s/blog_5e8a72a80100glsy.html

39 Ruan Jinping, Zhang Shaocai. The clinic experience and the characteristics of Dr. Kong Shaohua. 【阮劲平 张绍才: 孔少华先生临证经验及特点】 http://blog.sina.com.cn/s/blog_58d372a70102ee7t.html

40 Feng Xuegong. The treatment of stroke by Classical formulas, Can the marvelous results recur again? 【冯学功: 经方治疗中风病，奇效能否再现？】 Speech on a TCM conference. May 23, 2015. http://blog.sina.com.cn/s/blog_a3d866ea0102wh9j.html

41 Xiao Peng. Talks about TCM learning. 【肖鹏: 聊聊学习中医的话题】 http://blog.sina.com.cn/s/blog_616b76c70100qw7l.html

42 Gao Jianzhong. The smaller, the precise, the better. 【高建忠: 越小、越准、越好】 http://blog.sina.com.cn/s/blog_138ba8b160102vnza.html

43 Qiu Yu. Brief talk about Folk TCM and College TCM. 【邱岳: 浅谈民间中医与学院派中医】 http://www.360doc.com/content/17/1108/23/29842202_702210100.shtml

44 Xiong Jibai. Correction of some wrong concepts of TCM doctors. 【熊继柏: 纠正中医人的几个错误观念】 http://blog.sina.com.cn/s/blog_bf9957910102w262.html

45 Huang Huang. The sources and current situations of Classical formula TCM. 【黄煌: 经方医学的源流与现状分析】 http://blog.sina.com.cn/s/blog_70db7a890102xriw.html

46 Kaixin Zhongyi Yuan. My opinion about Shaoyang disease. 【少阳病之我见】 开心中医缘博客. http://blog.sina.com.cn/s/blog_5f856c9a0101bwns.html

47 Xing Bin. From the application of herbal formula Xuefu Zhuyu Tang to discuss TCM diagnosis. 【邢斌: 从血府逐瘀汤的运用谈中医的辨证思路】--转贴. http://blog.sina.com.cn/s/blog_66b5edc00102uzlm.html

www.ingramcontent.com/pod-product-compliance
Lightning Source LLC
Chambersburg PA
CBHW081556220526
45468CB00010B/2674